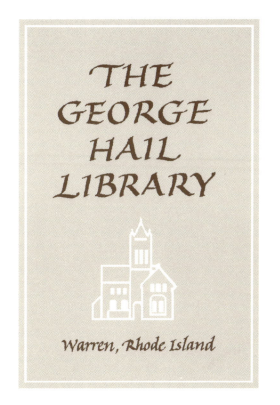

Vitamins and Minerals

Vitamins and Minerals

Zina Kroner, DO

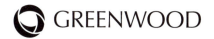

GREENWOOD

AN IMPRINT OF ABC-CLIO, LLC
Santa Barbara, California • Denver, Colorado • Oxford, England

Copyright 2011 by ABC-CLIO, LLC

Library of Congress Cataloging-in-Publication Data

Kroner, Zina.
   Vitamins and minerals / Zina Kroner.
     p. cm.
   Summary: "This insightful, objective, and evidence-based overview of the most commonly used supplements dispels misinformation and provides facts from a qualified physician's point of view"— Provided by publisher.
   Includes index.
   ISBN 978-0-313-38224-6 (hardback) — ISBN 978-0-313-38225-3 (ebook)
   1. Vitamins—Popular works.   2. Dietary supplements—Popular works.   3. Minerals in nutrition—Popular works.   I. Title.
   TX553.V5K76   2011
   613.2'86—dc22   2010051947

ISBN: 978-0-313-38224-6
EISBN: 978-0-313-38225-3

15 14 13 12 11   1 2 3 4 5

This book is also available on the World Wide Web as an eBook.
Visit www.abc-clio.com for details.

Greenwood
An Imprint of ABC-CLIO, LLC

ABC-CLIO, LLC
130 Cremona Drive, P.O. Box 1911
Santa Barbara, California 93116-1911

This book is printed on acid-free paper ∞

Manufactured in the United States of America

To my wonderful family...
thank you for everything.

Contents

Introduction

PROACTIVE VERSUS REACTIVE MEDICINE: PUTTING YOURSELF IN THE DRIVER'S SEAT

Half of all insured Americans are on prescription medications, according to a study done in 2007 by Medco Solutions Inc., a company that manages prescription medications for about one in five Americans. Specifically, approximately, two-thirds of women 20 years old and older, one-quarter of kids up to the age of 18, about one-half of adult men, and three-fourth of seniors are on at least one prescription medication. Among the seniors, 28 percent of women and nearly 22 percent of men take five or more medicines regularly. Do these statistics reflect worsening health of the American population, more aggressive prescription writing by physicians, lack of a systematic approach to get to the foundation of a problem, greater push by pharmaceutical companies to "get the word out" about certain drugs, or a potpourri of reasons?

Whatever the cause, this is a phenomenal statistic that needs to be actively and seriously addressed on multiple fronts. This statistic reflects a trend in American medicine that embraces a reactive rather than proactive approach to medicine. We are taught as physicians to focus on the presenting complaint and react to it once it has already peaked. We react to it by doing the appropriate tests, referring to specialists, and of course by prescribing medications. With this medical approach, the patient feels comforted that his or her medical care is in the hands of a well-wishing medical system. She or he tends to not question cause, rationale, or evidence supporting a particular plan of action and may unfortunately wind up taking a passive approach to the medical condition thereby relying solely on the medications given. This scenario is common but is not the rule.

I want to encourage serious discussions between you and your doctor on a number of fronts. First, there should be dialogue about the root cause(s) of your medical issue. You should not be satisfied with simply accepting a medical label, such

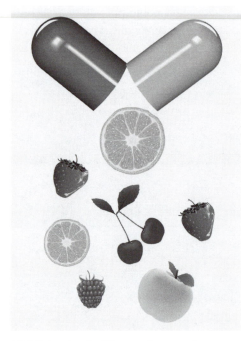

(© Mirjanabanjac/Dreamstime.com)

as chronic fatigue syndrome, or irritable bowel syndrome without delineating an appropriate cause and plan of action. Being told that you have heartburn or anxiety and treating it only with a medication is inappropriate.

Many patients and holistic practitioners take it upon themselves to take and prescribe, respectively, a unique concoction of supplements, disregarding all side effects and negative research. Their approach is such that supplements can do no harm and that medications are not a cure-all. This premise is of course skewed as well.

In this book, I will bring to light many of the common supplements, as they may play a significant role in helping to improve a variety of medical illnesses. I will discuss the supplements' mechanisms of action, the research behind them, and their evidence-based risks and benefits that you have to be aware of. Simply knowing this information allows you to be more involved with your own medical care. This book is not an endorsement of supplements, but a way for you to find out the fact versus the fiction behind the popularly used supplements.

It must be brought to your attention that every single study included in this book is from prominent medical journals that your physician is expected to read on a regular basis. The excuse that there is not enough evidence in the medical literature to actually recommend certain supplements on a regular basis is wrong and is a reflection of physicians not reading the journals that are put out by the very organizations that they belong to.

We should all expect a lot from our physicians. Physicians are there for you, not instead of you. My view of a physician is one who is sincere and has a close relationship with his or her patients; one who always practices a cause-oriented approach for every medical sign and symptom; one who is not quick to give a medication or neutraceutical to cover up a problem; one who discusses a variety of medical options, both medicinal and natural alike, addressing the risks and benefits of both; and one who always uses evidence-based medicine while staying abreast of the most current and pertinent medical literature.

Unfortunately, the state of medicine today makes the physician and patient feel rushed during an office visit. Most of the 10–15 minutes of time allotted to your physician to spend with you is spent on relatively urgent medical issues, checklist preventive medicine, and of course paperwork.

Please understand, the goal of this book is definitely not to put you on a slew of supplements. It is to show you the pros and the cons of many of the commonly prescribed neutraceuticals, so that you can be knowledgeable about the decision that you and your physician make. The physician should be your vehicle for recovery, but remember that you, and only you, are the driver.

1

5-Hydroxy-Tryptophan (5-HTP)

BRIEF OVERVIEW

Also known as 5-HTP, 5-hydroxytroptophan is a precursor to the neurotransmitter serotonin.

Serotonin is a major regulator of mood as well as having many other functions in the central nervous system. While there are many popular antidepressants that increase serotonin in the brain, 5-HTP is a natural substance that can be converted into serotonin.

Made from the amino acid L-tryptophan, which is essential to the human body, 5-HTP is in turn converted to serotonin by the enzyme tryptophan 5-monooxygenase. When 5-HTP is taken as a supplement, it will get into the body and pass through what is called the blood-brain barrier, a protective barrier that prevents the entry of many ingested chemicals and medicines into the brain. Then, 5-HTP will be converted to serotonin in the brain as well as other parts of the body.

THE HYPE

Since serotonin mediates so many different processes and states, anything that can raise serotonin levels will have a positive effect, from improving mood and sleep and decreasing pain to moderating cravings for food and drugs. Supplements of 5-HTP will be converted into serotonin, and thereby reduce depression, lessen insomnia, possibly decrease obesity and perception of pain, and potentially much more.[1] Furthermore, 5-HTP is safe to use, and may be free from some of the problems associated with selective serotonin reuptake inhibitors (SSRIs) like Prozac and Lexapro.

Safety: Eosinophilia-Myalgia Syndrome

(Symptoms of eosinophilia-myalgia syndrome can be found in "Potential Side Effects" below.)

The amino acid L-tryptophan is the precursor of 5-HTP and serotonin. Supplements of L-tryptophan were very popular in the 1980s. In 1989 and 1990, there was an outbreak of an illness named "eosinophilia-myalgia syndrome," which was linked to L-tryptophan supplements that were made by one manufacturer. At least 1,500 people were affected by the syndrome, although some have suggested there may have been many more cases. At least 38 people died. Sales of L-tryptophan were subsequently banned by the Food and Drug Administration (FDA).[2]

It is said that 5-HTP is free from the risk of the syndrome. It has been in use for more than 20 years and is being monitored by the FDA. As of 1998, there were 10 possible cases of eosinophilia-myalgia syndrome from 5-HTP and no deaths. Some researchers say that there has been only one actual case, in 1994.[3] However, there seems to be agreement that no new cases have been diagnosed since 1998.[2]

An analysis of the 5-HTP supplements related to possible cases in 1993 discovered a contaminant in the implicated supplements as well as in other, randomly chosen 5-HTP lots. It was named Peak X and subsequently identified as 4, 5-tryptophan-dione, a presumed neurotoxin. Peak X was found in all six of the random batches tested. This study raised concerns about the safety of 5-HTP.[4] Peak X was similar in structure to the contaminants in L-tryptophan.[2]

In 1994, one case of eosinophilia-myalgia syndrome occurred in a family taking 5-HTP. Two other family members developed only the high eosinophil count, which resolved. Analysis at the CDC found a possible contaminant.[5]

Subsequently, the methods of these analyses have been criticized, and the importance of Peak X has been cast into doubt.[3] Even so, to address the concerns about Peak X, some 5-HTP suppliers even test their products and label them as free of Peak X.[6]

The question remains, is 5-HTP safe in this regard? The answer at this point is, probably yes.

Safety: Serotonin Syndrome

(Symptoms of the serotonin syndrome can be found in "Potential Side Effects" below.)

The serotonin syndrome occurs when there is too much serotonin in the system. It has been observed in patients switching antidepressants of the SSRI class (selective serotonin reuptake inhibitors) or mixing antidepressants with other medicines that can raise serotonin. It occurred in one patient who took L-tryptophan along with fluoxetine, an SSRI. There have been no reports of the serotonin syndrome in patients taking just 5-HTP.[2]

Depression

The serotonin hypothesis of major depression states that a decreased amount of serotonin in the brain is related to the cause of depression. Very popular antidepressants are SSRIs, which means they stop serotonin from being taken up by cells and raise the amount of serotonin available at the nerve endings in the brain. SSRIs include Prozac and Lexapro, among others. Even older antidepressants inhibit serotonin reuptake to some degree.

5-HTP has been used for decades to treat depression. Since it can get into the central nervous system and undergo conversion to serotonin, it should be effective. Although there have been many studies demonstrating the effectiveness of 5-HTP, most were not done in a manner that would satisfy scientific requirements. If 5-HTP were a drug, the FDA would require two double-blind, placebo-controlled trials that would prove its safety and efficacy, with enough participants to make the results statistically significant. These studies have not been done. Many people working in the field want to see the appropriate trials done so the issue can be decided. Reviews of 5-HTP almost invariably end with a call for further studies.

The existing studies have not been long-term, or large-scale, or placebo-controlled, or in some other fashion are not completely definitive. A placebo control is especially important in studying a drug for depression. Responses to placebo can be as high as 60 percent in patients with depression. Trials need to be long term, because response to antidepressants often takes place over a matter of weeks to months.[7]

There have been many reviews of the available data. In 1998, an article in *Alternative Medicine Review* took the position of recommending 5-HTP as effective for depression.[8] However, a subsequent *Alternative Medicine Review* in 2000 was more in line with recent reviewers who are cautious about the supplement because of the quality of the research.[7]

A Cochrane Library analysis found the quality of most studies to be inadequate. A complete review in 2001, which was updated in 2004 and rechecked in 2008, looked at 111 trials and found only 2 trials involving 64 patients satisfactory for analysis. These reviewers included both tryptophan and 5-HTP together. The review states that both were probably better than placebo. However, due to the lack of good data as well as the risk of eosinophilia-myalgia syndrome, they could not recommend either substance.[9]

Other reviewers have used different approaches to look at the available information. In 2006, a review in *Pharmacology & Therapeutics* agreed that there were no definitive, large-scale studies to demonstrate safety and effectiveness of 5-HTP. However, the investigators did find 27 studies useful to review, which included 990 treated patients. They chose to analyze them in a descriptive manner.

Eleven studies were double-blind, meaning neither the patients nor the researchers knew what they were getting, and they were also placebo-controlled, meaning that 5-HTP was tested against a sugar pill. These studies were very different in terms of design and included very few people, but seven of them found 5-HTP superior to placebo. Other studies were open-label, which did not yield results that could be interpreted. There were studies comparing 5-HTP to other active drugs. A number of these found 5-HTP as effective as other antidepressants.

In summary, this review stated that there were three trials using 5-HTP alone that showed a benefit that was statistically significant, with very small numbers of patients. There was only one study that showed no benefit. They concluded that 5-HTP may have "at least limited efficacy" in treating depression.[2]

Anxiety Disorders Including Insomnia

It is possible that 5-HTP may be useful for treating insomnia.[10] Some small studies have found that it can increase REM sleep. However, there have been some reports of nightmares while taking 5-HTP.[8]

Many herbal supplements used for relaxation have components that contain 5-HTP. It is added to a number of other ingredients and sold as an anxiety-reducing dietary supplement or tea.[11]

Headache

Also, 5-HTP may be useful for treating various kinds of headache, including migraine and tension headaches. Migraine headaches can be related to a lack of serotonin.[8,10]

In one small, double-blind, randomized trial, 78 patients with chronic tension headaches were treated for eight weeks with 5-HTP or placebo, with a wash-out or follow-up period for three weeks afterward. There was no difference in frequency of headaches or headache intensity between the two groups. There was, however, a significantly decreased use of analgesic pain medicine in the 5-HTP group. In the three weeks after, there were fewer days with headache in the 5-HTP group. While the subjective impression of 5-HTP was good, there were more dropouts from the 5-HTP group and more who discontinued the 5-HTP due to adverse side effects. The numbers were very small. This is the kind of study that is hard to interpret.[12]

Fibromyalgia

Fibromyalgia is a rheumatologic disorder including multiple tender points, musculoskeletal pain, fatigue, and nonrestorative sleep. There is some evidence that fibromyalgia may be related to low serotonin levels.[13] A number of small studies have found 5-HTP effective in treating fibromyalgia. It may decrease tender points, pain, fatigue, stiffness, and improve sleep.[8,13]

Weight Control

There may be an association of low serotonin levels in obese patients with cravings and binge eating. Patients in a number of small studies given 5-HTP decreased their intake of food and were able to lose weight.[10]

To Counteract Effects of Ecstasy

There is little concrete information available, but according to some animal studies, 5-HTP may help prevent the negative effects of the drug Ecstasy. In animal studies it has been neuro-protective.[14] There is more information available on Internet forums discussing 5-HTP and Ecstasy (MDMA-3, 4-methylenedioxymethamphetamine) use.[15]

Hot Flashes

SSRIs have already been used as treatment for menopausal hot flashes. If they can be effective, 5-HTP might also be a possible treatment for hot flashes.[16] However, one recent, small, double-blind, placebo-controlled trial found no significant effect of 5-HTP on hot flashes.[17]

DEFICIENCY

As 5-HTP is not an essential nutrient, there is no deficiency state. It can be made in the body from L-tryptophan, which is an essential nutrient. Tryptophan occurs naturally in dietary protein from many sources.

FOOD SOURCES

5-HTP is not found in food in any significant quantity.

5-HTP supplements come from the seeds of an African plant called Griffonia simplifica.[1] The extract of the plant is also available, alone, or in conjunction with other herbal supplements.

MECHANISM OF ACTION: HOW DOES IT WORK?

5-HTP is part of the serotonin pathway. It can be made from the amino acid L-tryptophan and is converted to serotonin. Serotonin is a neurotransmitter required for normal brain activity and is also found in other parts of the body, specifically the gastrointestinal tract. 5-HTP works by being transformed to serotonin.

5-HTP is easily absorbed, and once in the bloodstream, crosses the blood-brain barrier where it can then be converted to serotonin. There is evidence that the levels of other active chemicals and neurotransmitters in the brain also increase after 5-HTP is taken. This includes dopamine, norepinephrine, melatonin, and beta-endorphin.[10]

In the brain, serotonin levels may impact mood, sleep, anxiety levels, aggression, appetite, sexual behavior, temperature, and the sensation of pain.

PRIMARY USES

Generally speaking, 5-HTP may be taken by people trying to stabilize mood and decrease pain and anxiety.

- 5-HTP is frequently used for depression by people who do not want to take medication, preferring a natural treatment. Some people even take it with prescription antidepressants, something that can be dangerous because of the serotonin syndrome. It is also taken together with other medicinal herbs that may combat depression, like St. John's wort.

- It is used by people as a relaxant, to combat insomnia, and to minimize anxiety.

- 5-HTP is taken by people with fibromyalgia. This is a difficult condition to treat, and patients frequently try alternative therapies.
- Similarly, it is taken by people with chronic headaches, both migraines and tension headaches.

Some of the other possible uses are less common, such as trying to lower cravings for food or drugs, and trying to reduce hot flashes.

More uses will become apparent as more research is done.

COMMON DOSAGES

5-HTP usually is available as 25 mg-, 50 mg-, or 100-mg capsules. It can also be found as the crude extract from the seeds of the plant G. simplifica. Because it is available in the United States under the Dietary Supplement Health and Education Act of 1994, it did not need prior FDA approval. No prescription is necessary.

For depression, 150 to 300 mg a day are usually used. Taking 5-HTP three times a day seems to work the best for depression. Treatment can start with 50 mg three times a day, and the dose can be increased if there is no response in two weeks. The usual maximum dose is 1,000 mg three times a day, although that much is rarely used. For insomnia, 100 to 300 mg should be taken before bedtime.[10]

For most indications except insomnia, 5-HTP should be taken three times a day.[18]

A medication called carbidopa, usually used in the case of Parkinson's disease, blocks the conversion of 5-HTP to serotonin in the body so that more gets into the brain, where it is then converted to serotonin. It can be used to increase the effect of 5-HTP.[2] Carbidopa requires a prescription.

5-HTP can also be found in preparations promoted as helpful for stress and anxiety, along with other natural ingredients. There are pills with multiple ingredients as well as teas and drinks.[11]

POTENTIAL SIDE EFFECTS

It is known that 5-HTP frequently causes gastrointestinal symptoms including heartburn and nausea, vomiting, and diarrhea. These symptoms may be from conversion of 5-HTP to serotonin in the intestinal tract. Other side effects have been reported, including headache, difficulty sleeping, and palpitations.[2] Starting with a low dose and slowly increasing it may decrease these side effects.[10]

If carbidopa is given with 5-HTP and serotonin is not made in the intestinal tract, these side effects may be minimized. This treatment is rarely recommended and quite controversial. A select few feel that the amount of 5-HTP required to treat depression without carbidopa is so high that it is very likely to cause intolerable side effects.[19]

The eosinophilia-myalgia syndrome is still a concern. Although 5-HTP probably does not cause the syndrome, it is a possibility. It needs to be recognized quickly and the use of the supplement stopped. The hallmarks of the syndrome are muscle pain (myalgia), spasm and later weakness, and an elevated number of eosinophils in the blood (eosinophilia). There are often skin lesions and swelling of the extremities and face. There can be lung and nerve problems. Many of the symptoms persist for years.

In order to avoid the serotonin syndrome, people who are taking SSRIs or have recently taken them may want to be careful when taking 5-HTP.[3] They should be mindful of the symptoms of serotonin syndrome, including high blood pressure, elevated temperature, flushing, sweating, dizziness, muscle jerks, and disorientation. These symptoms usually come on within hours of too high a serotonin elevation. The syndrome resolves in 24 hours in approximately 70 percent of cases. It is usually not serious, although there have been deaths. Now that the symptoms of this syndrome are known, it is easier to catch it early and prevent any complications.[2]

While SSRIs affect serotonin levels the most, other antidepressants can also raise serotonin levels, as can certain other medications including some used for migraine headaches. Anyone who is taking a prescription antidepressant or any other medication that raises serotonin should talk to his or her doctor before adding 5-HPT. If unsure about a particular medicine, it is safest to find out if it increases serotonin by asking a doctor or pharmacist.

Any supplement or medicine that can treat depression has the potential for triggering mania in bipolar patients, patients with both mania and depression. It is very difficult to treat bipolar illness; it should be done by or in conjunction with a physician who has experience treating patients with the disease.

FACT VERSUS FICTION

In general, 5-HTP is probably safe and effective for minor to moderate depression. It is not without risk, and it is not definitively effective. Bearing in mind the risk, it is reasonable for people to try it for depression. Even though it is a supplement, consulting a physician while taking the medication is still a good idea. A physician can make sure there are no other medicines being taken that might contribute to the serotonin syndrome.

There is less research available about other uses. 5-HTP is probably safe and somewhat effective for anxiety and chronic pain conditions including headaches and fibromyalgia.

It is reasonable for people with anxiety or pain to try 5-HTP, especially if standard medical treatment has not worked for them.

Most people who cannot tolerate 5-HTP discontinue it because of nausea or other gastrointestinal symptoms.

REFERENCES

1. Sarubin-Fragakis, A, Thomson, C. *The health professional's guide to popular dietary supplements*. 3rd edition. Chicago: American Dietetic Association, 2007.
2. Turner, EH, Loftis, JM, Blackwell, AD. Serotonin a la carte: Supplementation with the serotonin precursor 5-hydroxytryptophan. *Pharmacology & Therapeutics*. 2006;109(3):325–338.

3. Das, YT, Bagchi, M, Bagchi, D, Preuss, HG. Safety of 5-hydroxy-l-tryptophan. *Toxicol Lett*. 2004;150:111–122.

4. Klarskov, K, Johnson, KL, Benson, LM, Cragun, JD, et al. Structural characterization of a case-implicated contaminant, "Peak X," in commercial preparations of 5-hydroxytryptophan. *J Rheumatol*. 2003;30(1):89–95.

5. Michelson, D, Page, SW, Casey, R, et al. An eosinophilia-myalgia syndrome related disorder associated with exposure to L-5-hydroxytryptophan. *J Rheumatol*. 1994;21(12):2261–2265.

6. Turner, EH, Blackwell, AD. 5-hydroxytryptophan plus SSRIs for interferon-induced depression: Synergistic mechanisms for normalizing synaptic serotonin. *Medical Hypotheses*. 2005;65:138–144.

7. Meyers, S. Use of neurotransmitter precursors for treatment of depression. *Altern Med Rev*. 2000;5(1):64–71.

8. Birdsall, T. 5-hydroxytryptophan: A clinically-effective serotonin precursor. *Altern Med Rev*. 1998;3(4):271–280.

9. Shaw, K, Turner, J, Del Mar, C. Tryptophan and 5-hydroxytryptophan for depression. *Cochrane Database of Systematic Reviews*. 2002;1. Art. No.: CD003198. doi: 10.1002/14651858.CD003198.

10. Thorne Research, Inc. 5-hydroxytryptophan. *Altern Med Rev*. 1998;3(3):224–226.

11. Weeks, BS. Formulations of dietary supplements and herbal extracts for relaxation and anxiolytic action: Relarian™. *Med Sci Monit*. 2009;15(11):RA256–262.

12. Fontes Ribeiro, CA. l-5-hydroxytryptophan in the prophylaxis of chronic tension-type headache: A double-blind, randomized, placebo-controlled study. *Headache*. 2000;40:451–456.

13. Juhl, JH. Fibromyalgia and the serotonin pathway. *Altern Med Rev*. 1998;3(5):367–375.

14. Gudelsky, GA, Nash, JF. Carrier-mediated release of serotonin by 3,4-methylenedioxymethamphetamine: Implications for serotonin-dopamine interactions. *J Neurochem*. 1996;66:243–249.

15. DanceSafe.org. Ecstasy use and depression. http://www.dancesafe.org/documents/druginfo/depression.php#5htp. Accessed December 29, 2010.

16. Curcio, JJ, Kim, LS, Wollner, D, Pockaj, BA. The potential role of 5-hydroxytryptophan for hot flash reduction: A hypothesis. *Altern Med Review*. 2005;10(3):216–221.

17. Freedman, RR. Treatment of menopausal hot flashes with 5-hydroxytryptophan. *Maturitas*. 2010;65(4):383–385.

18. Health Canada. Monograph—5-HTP. December 17, 2007. http://www.hc-sc.gc.ca/dhp-mps/prodnatur/applications/licen-prod/monograph/mono_5-htp-eng.php. Accessed February 6, 2009.

19. Young, SN. Are SAMe and 5-HTP safe and effective treatments for depression? *J Psychiatry Neurosci*. 2003;28:471.

2

Alpha Lipoic Acid

One antioxidant getting a lot of attention on the free radical fighting scene is alpha lipoic acid. It is produced in the body as lipoic acid (LA), also sometimes called thioctic acid. It is absorbed from certain foods that we eat, but the body produces its own LA for metabolic use. LA plays a role in the Krebs cycle and cellular metabolism of carbohydrates and fats. In supplemental form, LA is known as alpha lipoic acid (ALA). ALA is not quite a vitamin and not quite a fatty acid, although it exhibits properties of each. Unlike other antioxidants, ALA is both water and fat soluble, enabling it to work throughout the body. As an antioxidant supplement, ALA neutralizes hydroxyl radicals and singlet oxygen and can also help regenerate oxidized vitamin C and vitamin E as well as glutathione and coenzyme Q_{10}.[1,2]

THE HYPE

There is a lot of hype around using ALA as a general antiaging supplement. It is probably one of the more popular antioxidant supplements around and is sold as a single supplement or as part of a complex (often together with vitamin C, vitamin E, and acetyl-L-carnitine). For 20 years, ALA supplements have been used to treat diabetes, cancer, neurological problems, vascular disease, cataracts and glaucoma.

DEFICIENCY

There are no reports of LA deficiency, suggesting that humans are able to synthesize enough for basic enzyme cofactor needs.[3]

LA is found in the mitochondrial cells, normally found in muscle cells. Due to this fact, vegetarians will take in less dietary LA than meat eaters. Vegetarians who don't eat green leafy vegetables (another source of LA) are theoretically at greater risk for deficiency.

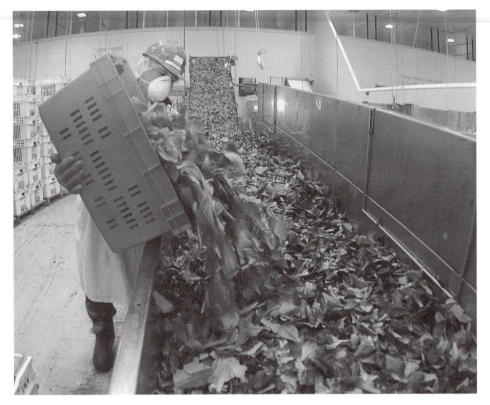

Harvested lettuce, spinach, and other vegetables are mixed together and sent down a conveyer belt to a wash and dry station at Earthbound Farms Plant in Yuma, Arizona. Leafy green vegetables are good food sources of lipoic acid. (AP Photo, Alfred J. Hernandez)

FOOD SOURCES

The richest sources of LA are animal proteins and green leafy vegetables. Liver, heart, and kidney are particularly high in LA, because of their high concentration of mitochondrial cells. Green vegetables that have a high concentration of chloroplasts are also rich in LA. Chloroplasts are key spots for energy production in plants, and they require LA for this activity. For this reason, broccoli, spinach, and other green leafy vegetables like collard greens, bok choy, or chard are good food sources of LA.[4]

MECHANISMS OF ACTION AND PRIMARY USES

ALA for Diabetes Management

The best-documented application for ALA in diabetes is its ability to help with symptoms of diabetic neuropathy.

ALA may have a more direct effect on diabetes too, by simply lowering blood sugar levels, through an increase in insulin sensitivity and a decrease in gluconeogenesis.

ALA works against insulin resistance by increasing the permeability of cell membranes, which is decreased by hyperglycemia. It also prevents the uptake of glucose. In human studies, oral supplementation with ALA has proven only marginally effective in helping to improve glycemic control, but intravenous infusions do help affect insulin-mediated glucose disposal and lower blood sugar.[5] A review study on the benefits of oral ALA in diabetes management supports the use of LA for glycemic control, and as a general antioxidant, but states that the major benefit of ALA supplementation is in patients with diabetic neuropathy.[6] ALA has been used in Germany for more than 30 years as a treatment for diabetic neuropathy. Many studies have been published in this regard and the beneficial effects have been reiterated time and again. Diabetic neuropathy is a painful and debilitating consequence of diabetes and is defined as deranged function and structure of peripheral motor, sensory, and autonomic neurons, involving either the entire neuron or selected levels.[7]

A large, randomized, placebo-controlled, multicenter, double-blind study involving 328 patients with type 2 diabetes revealed that intravenous Lipoic acid significantly improved symptoms of diabetic neuropathy, including sensations of burning, tingling, itching, and pain.[8] The same researchers later found that five weeks of oral supplementation with lipoic acid significantly improved the stabbing pain, burning pain, and numbness of the feet in patients suffering from diabetic neuropathy, with the dose-effectiveness range being 600–1,800 mg of lipoic acid dosed orally per day.[9] According to the authors, while some studies on orally administered ALA had suggested a reduction in neuropathic deficits associated with neuropathy, its effects on improving sensory symptoms is still in doubt.

ALA Prevents Cognitive Decline

ALA may play a role in the prevention of brain aging. Rat studies have pointed to an antioxidant protective effect of ALA on cortical neurons.[10] ALA protects against Alzheimer's by preventing the oxidative stress and energy depletion caused by deranged glucose metabolism and free radical production. In this study 600 mg of ALA was given daily to nine patients with Alzheimer's and related dementias for roughly a year and led to some stabilization of cognitive function.[11]

Studies using a combination of ALA and acetyl-L-carnitine show even more promise for prevention of age-related brain aging. A study showed that an antioxidant concoction including ALA and acetyl-L-carnitine reduced reactive oxygen species in normal mice by 57 percent and prevented the increase in reactive oxygen species normally observed in mice lacking murine ApoE (a gene that influences Alzheimer's disease).[12]

A review of studies on L-carnitine and ALA between 1966 and 2007 showed that L-carnitine and alpha lipoic acid are pleiotropic agents capable of offering neuroprotective and possibly cognitive-enhancing effects for neuropsychiatric disorders in which cognitive deficits are an integral feature.[13]

ALA for Cardiovascular Disease

Atherosclerosis (hardening of the arteries), caused by high LDL cholesterol levels and a variety of other factors, is America's biggest killer. ALA may play a role in the fight against cardiovascular disease by inhibiting monocyte adhesion and endothelial activation, which leads to oxidative stress and atherosclerosis due to oxidative stress.[14] In addition, ALA may help prevent hypertension, another risk factor for atherosclerosis and heart disease, through its ability to raise glutathione levels and suppress endothelin-1 (a substance produced in blood vessels that regulates their tone).[15,16] ALA has the potential to improve endothelial function and is part of one of the most powerful biological antioxidant systems; however, there is no consensus on dosage, dose frequency, form of administration, and/or preferred form of ALA.[17,18]

ALA and Cancer

The intracellular redox state plays an important role in controlling inflammation, a process that can lead to tumor progression. ALA has been hypothesized to be able to restore redox control and therefore inhibit inflammation and tumor progression.[19] One study showed that ALA is toxic to leukemia cells, inhibits proliferation of mitogen-stimulated human peripheral blood lymphocytes, and increases interleukin-2.[20] Another study showed that ALA is able to selectively inhibit the growth of tumorigenic as compared to nontumorigenic ovarian surface epithelial cells and may play a role in ovarian cancer prevention and management.[19] It has also been shown that ALA can effectively induce apoptosis (cell death) in human colon cancer cells by a mechanism that is initiated by an increased uptake of oxidizable substrates into mitochondria.[21]

ALA Offers Promise in Supporting Optimal Visual Health

Lipoic acid has been shown to offer protection against cataract formation in experimental animal models.[22,23] Scientists believe that lipoic acid may confer this benefit by increasing levels of essential endogenous antioxidant enzymes such as glutathione peroxidase.

Another cause of vision loss, common in diabetes, is glaucoma. A study in patients with open-angle glaucoma found that visual function and other measures of glaucoma were improved in a group that received either 75 mg of lipoic acid daily for two months or 150 mg of lipoic acid daily for one month, compared with a control group that received no lipoic acid.[24] A recent review of natural therapies for cataracts and glaucoma lists ALA as a potential therapy, but no conclusive evidence on effectiveness and recommended dosages can be given yet.[25]

ALA May Protect the Liver

ALA has various applications when it comes to liver function. In animal studies, lipoic acid has been shown to safeguard the liver against the effects of cadmium exposure (an environmental toxin that is also found in cigarette smoke).[26]

Fatty liver disease, a common symptom of metabolic diseases and diabetes, is associated with high levels of circulating fats, called triglycerides, in the blood. High triglycerides are also linked to an increased diabetes and heart disease risk. In animal studies ALA has been shown to improve hypertriglyceridemia by stimulating tria-cylglycerol clearance and down regulating liver triacylglycerol secretion.[27]

Another mechanism of action by which ALA lowers triglyceride levels and de-creases hepatic lipogenesis (fat production by the liver) is through its influence on adenosine monophosphate (AMP)-activated protein kinase (AMPK), a major regulator of energy metabolism. This effect on AMPK also results in an increase in insulin sensitivity.[28]

ALA for Healthy Skin

ALA may improve the health of the skin and is a commonly used ingredient in topical skin care products. A study of 33 women with an average age of 54 years found that twice-daily application of a cream containing 5 percent lipoic acid for three months reduced the roughness of the skin and decreased the appearance of photoaging, compared with a control cream.[29]

COMMON DOSAGES

The intravenous dose that seems to be effective for treating diabetic neuropa-thy is 600 mg per day. Oral dosages of anywhere between 300 mg and 600 mg have been used for reducing neuropathy symptoms. Most supplements of ALA are available in doses of 25–100 mg, with the higher doses being reserved for a specific condition such as diabetes.

TOXICITY

Intravenous administration of ALA at doses of 600 mg/day for three weeks did not result in serious adverse effects when used to treat diabetic peripheral neuropathy.[8] Adverse effects at high dosages include skin conditions, possible hypoglycemia in diabetic patients, and thiamine deficiency.[1] Intravenous ALA is often put into a dextrose solution so that a precipitous drop in blood glucose will not occur.

FACT VERSUS FICTION

ALA seems to live up to its reputation as a superior antiaging antioxidant. Its most promising role is the one it plays in diabetes management and in lessening the symptoms of diabetic neuropathy and glaucoma in particular. Its role in prevent-ing age-related cognitive decline also seems promising, but more human studies are needed in this regard. The role of ALA in the prevention and management of cardiovascular disease and cancer looks positive so far, but more studies are needed in this regard.

REFERENCES

1. Nichols, TW, Jr. Alpha-Lipoic acid: Biological effects and clinical implica-tions. *Alter Med Rev.* 1997;2(3):177–183.

 2. Packer, L, Witt, EH, Tritschler, HJ, et al. Antioxidant properties and clinical implications of alpha-lipoic acid. Chapter 22 in: Packer, L, Cadenas, E. (Eds). *Biothiols in health and disease.* New York: Marcel Dekker, 1995, 479–516.

 3. Biewenga, GP, Haenen, GR, Bast, A. The pharmacology of the antioxidant lipoic acid. *Gen Pharmacol.* 1997;29(3):315–331.

 4. Lodge, JK, Youn, HD, Handelman, GJ, et al. Natural sources of lipoic acid: Determination of lipoyllysine released from protease-digested tissues by high performance liquid chromatography incorporating electrochemical detection. *J Appl Nutr.* 1997;49(1 & 2):3–11.

 5. Evans, JL, Goldfine, ID. Alpha-lipoic acid: A multifunctional antioxidant that improves insulin sensitivity in patients with type 2 diabetes. *Diabetes Thechnol Ther.* 2000 Autumn;2(3):401–413.

 6. Singh, U, Jialal, I. Alpha-lipoic acid supplementation and diabetes. *Nutr Rev.* 2008 Nov; 66(11):645–657.

 7. Dyck, PJ. Current concepts in neurology: The causes, classification, and treatment of peripheral neuropathy. *N Engl J Med.* 1982;307(5):283–286.

 8. Ziegler, D, Hanefeld, M, Ruhnau, KJ, et al. Treatment of symptomatic diabetic peripheral neuropathy with the anti-oxidant alpha-lipoic acid. A 3-week multicentre randomized controlled trial (ALADIN Study). *Diabetologia.* 1995 Dec;38(12):1425–1433.

 9. Ziegler, D, Ametov, A, Barinov, A, et al. Oral treatment with alpha-lipoic acid improves symptomatic diabetic polyneuropathy: The SYDNEY 2 Trial. *Diabetes Care.* 2006 Nov;29(11):2365–2370.

10. Zhang, L, et al. Alpha-lipoic acid protects rat cortical neurons against cell death induced by amyloid and hydrogen peroxide through the Akt signalling pathway. *Neurosci Lett.* 2001 Oct 26;312(3):125–128.

11. Hager, K, et al. Alpha-lipoic acid as a new treatment option for Alzheimer type dementia. *Arch Gerontol Geriatr.* 2001 Jun;32(3):275–282.

12. Suchy, J, Chan, A, Shea, TB. Dietary supplementation with a combination of alpha-lipoic acid, acetyl-L-carnitine, glycerophosphocoline, docosahexaenoic acid, and phosphatidylserine reduces oxidative damage to murine brain and improves cognitive performance. *Nutr Res.* 2009 Jan;29(1):70–74.

13. Soczynska, JK, Kennedy, SH, Chow, CS, Woldeyohannes, HO, Konarski, JZ, McIntyre, RS. Acetyl-L-carnitine and alpha-lipoic acid: Possible neurotherapeutic agents for mood disorders? *Expert Opin Investig Drugs.* 2008 Jun; 17(6):827–843.

14. Zhang, WJ, Frei, B. Alpha-lipoic acid inhibits TNF-alpha-induced NF-kappaB activation and adhesion molecule expression in human aortic endothelial cells. *FASEB J.* 2001 Nov;15(13):2423–2432.

15. Decker, EA, et al. Inhibition of low-density lipoprotein oxidation by carnosine histidine. *J Agric Food Chem.* 2001 Jan;49(1):511–516.

16. El Midaoui, A, de Champlain, J. Prevention of hypertension, insulin resistance, and oxidative stress by alpha-lipoic acid. *Hypertension.* 2002 Feb; 39(2):303–307.

17. Ghibu, S, Richard, C, Delemasure, S, Vergely, C, Mogosan, C, Muresan, A. An endogenous dithiol with antioxidant properties: Alpha-lipoic acid, potential uses in cardiovascular diseases (article in French). *Ann Cardiol Angeiol* (Paris). 2008 Jun;57(3):161–165. Epub 2008 Jun 4. http://www.ncbi.nlm.nih. gov/pubmed/18571145. Accessed December 29, 2010.

18. Wollin, SD, Jones, PJ. Alpha-lipoic acid and cardiovascular disease. *J Nutr.* 2003 Nov;133(11):3327–3330.

19. Vig-Varga, E, Benson, EA, Limbil, TL, Allison, BM, Goebl, MG, Harrington, MA. Alpha-lipoic acid modulates ovarian surface epithelial cell growth. *Gynecol Oncol.* 2006 Oct;103(1):45–52.

20. Pack, RA, et al. Differential effects of the antioxidant alpha-lipoic acid on the proliferation of mitogen-stimulated peripheral blood lymphocytes and leukaemic T cells. *Mol Immunol.* 2002 Feb;38(10):733–745.

21. Wenzel, U, Nickel, A, Daniel, H. Alpha-Lipoic acid induces apoptosis in human colon cancer cells by increasing mitochondrial respiration with a concomitant O2 generation. *Apoptosis.* 2005 Mar;10(2):359–368.

22. Kojima, M, Sun, L, Hata, I, Sakamoto, Y, Sasaki, H, Sasaki, K. Efficacy of alpha-lipoic acid against diabetic cataract in rats. *Jpn J Opthalmol.* 2007 Jan–Feb;51(1):10–13.

23. Sun, L, Zhang, JS. Effects of DL-alpha-lipoic acid on the experimentally induced diabetic cataract in rats. *Zhonfhua Yan Ke Za Zhi.* 2004 March; 40(3):193–196.

24. Filina, AA, Davydova, NG, Endrikhovskii, SN, Shamshinova, AM. Lipoic acid as a means of metabolic therapy of open-angle glaucoma. *Vestn Oftalmol.* 1995 Oct–Dec;111(4):6–8.

25. Head, KA. Natural therapies for ocular disorders, part two: Cataracts and glaucoma. *Altern Med Rev.* 2001 Apr;6(2):141–166.

26. Muller, L, Menzel, H. Studies on the efficacy of lipoate and dihydrolipoate in the alteration of cadmium2+ toxicity in isolated hepatocytes. *Biochim Biophys Acta.* 1990 May 22;1052(3):386–391.

27. Butler, JA, Hagen, TM, Moreau, R. Lipoic acid improves hypertriglyceridemia by stimulating triacylglycerol clearance and downregulating liver triacylglycerol secretion. *Arch Biochem Biophys.* 2009 May 1;484(1):63–71.

28. Park, KG, Min, AK, Koh, EH, Kim, HS, Kim, MO, Park, HS, Kim, YD, Yoon, TS, Jang, BK, Hwang, JS, Kim, JB, Choi, HS, Park, JY, Lee, IK, Lee, KU. Alpha-lipoic acid decreases hepatic lipogenesis through adenosine monophosphate-activated protein kinase (AMPK)-dependent and AMPK-independent pathways. *Hepatology.* 2008 Nov;48(5):1477–1486.

29. Beitner, H. Randomized, placebo-controlled, double blind study on the clinical efficacy of a cream containing 5% alpha-lipoic acid related to photoageing of facial skin. *Br J Dermatol.* 2003 Oct;149(4):841–849.

3

Beta-Sitosterol

BRIEF OVERVIEW

Although the term beta-sito*sterol* may seem unfamiliar, it is similar to another word everyone has heard, chole*sterol*. The sterol, which is a ringed compound, is in fact how the two are similar. Sterols are present in the cell membranes of both animals and plants. Although too much cholesterol, or the wrong kind, is unhealthy, cholesterol itself is absolutely necessary to maintain cell membranes in humans. Beta-sitosterol is the most abundant phytosterol (plant sterol), which performs the same function in plants that cholesterol performs in humans. Phytosterols include sterols and stanols, similar types of molecules that can also be called plant fats.

Even though cholesterol can be bad for blood vessels and the heart, it turns out that consumption of beta-sitosterol can actually lower cholesterol in humans. In order to do the most good, beta-sitosterol (along with other phytosterols) must be consumed in the right amount. If this is done, LDL (low-density lipoprotein) cholesterol can be lowered.

Beta-sitosterol has also been shown to decrease the symptoms of prostatic hyperplasia. It is usually taken as a supplement for this purpose. Beta-sitosterol may have other uses, but they are not yet clearly defined.

THE HYPE

Effects on Cholesterol

In the human body, cholesterol is both absorbed from food sources as well as made by the body. There is a balance between synthesis and absorption. Beta-sitosterol and other plant sterols and stanols can decrease total cholesterol and LDL cholesterol. When added to the diet in the range of 1 to 2 g a day, they will lower LDL cholesterol approximately 10 percent. They therefore can be expected to decrease the risk of coronary artery disease significantly. They are safe to take.

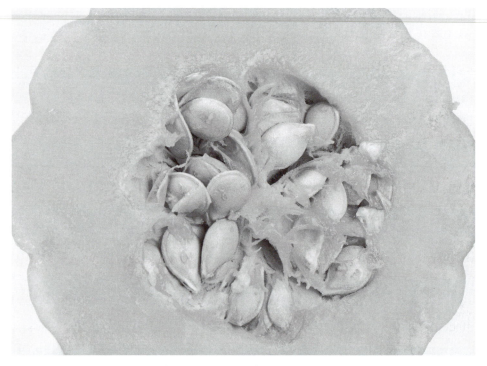

Pumpkin seeds are a source of beta-sitosterol. (© Sergei Rodionov/Dreamstime.com)

Beta-sitosterol, alone, or with other phytosterols, reduces cholesterol probably by blocking cholesterol absorption from the gastrointestinal tract. Although it is only absorbed in very small amounts, some beta-sitosterol will eventually be transported by lipoproteins and incorporated into cell membranes.

Phytosterols have been shown to lower total cholesterol and LDL cholesterol without affecting HDL cholesterol. They have been effective when used with dietary modifications like a National Cholesterol Education Step 1 diet for people trying to lower cholesterol.[1] They also lower cholesterol when added to a normal diet. For this purpose, phytosterols can be made into a fat-containing spread or ingredient for salad dressing by a process called esterification. It is not known definitively if the process of esterification changes the properties of the sterols.[2]

In general, consumption of approximately 2 to 3 g a day of phytosterol will lower LDL cholesterol by approximately 10 percent. This occurs whether a normal or low-fat diet is eaten.[2] The supplement can be taken with meals.

Phytosterols have been tested the most in vegetable spreads. Other studies have shown that sterols in low-fat milk can still lower LDL.[3] Phytosterols can even been added to low-fat ground beef with success.[4]

Some studies have suggested that stanols work better at lowering cholesterol, but other studies have favored sterols like beta-sitosterol.[5] There have been varying results comparing sterols to stanols, liquid to solid forms (spreads), and once a day versus multiple doses a day, among other variables. A recent review found a slight advantage of multiple daily doses as well as solid forms of sterols or stanols in terms of lowering LDL cholesterol.[6]

Esterified sterols are more stable in food products and are the most frequently used form of sterols in food. Esterification does not diminish their effectiveness in lowering LDL cholesterol.[7]

Phytosterols including beta-sitosterol are absorbed at a very low rate, approximately 4 to 5 percent. They can be measured in the blood. If enough (or too much) is ingested, beta-sitosterol can be incorporated into atheromas, the plaques of fat and cholesterol that cause vascular disease. Most mouse models show that phytosterols use decreases the formation of atheromas, but whether or not they can promote atherosclerosis is not completely clear.[2]

Phytosterols together with an exercise regimen can lower LDL and raise HDL.[8]

Phytosterols work along with statin medications to lower cholesterol further. This has been shown in various populations, including postmenopausal women who have had heart attacks and need to lower their cholesterol. Use of sitostanol ester margarine has also made it possible to lower statin doses.[9] For some people, the phytosterols by themselves might be enough to lower LDL without the side effects associated with statins. For others with higher LDL cholesterol, statins and sterols together may be of great benefit.[7]

Some investigators have tried to show the public health benefits of getting various populations to consume phytosterols. One such calculation shows that if 25 million Europeans used plant sterols, there would be 117,000 less cases of coronary heart disease during the following 10 years. This would save approximately $25 billion in healthcare costs.[2]

In 2001, the National Cholesterol Education Program (NCEP) recommended adding 2 g of plant sterols a day to the diet, aimed at lowering cardiovascular risk in the United States. Other groups that recommend including plant sterols in the diet are the International Atherosclerosis Society, which did so in 2003, and the National Foundation of Australia, in 2001.

The data so far confirms that phytosterols and stanols can decrease LDL cholesterol by around 10 percent. It is inferred by some experts that this would lower risk of cardiovascular disease by about 25 percent. Lowered cholesterol by other means has been documented to lower the risk of cardiovascular disease. There is not yet direct proof linking dietary sterols and stanols to lowered cardiovascular risk.[10] However, it is logical to assume that they will reduce risk like other cholesterol-lowering methods. Some experts expect a 20 percent reduced risk over a person's lifetime.[11]

Prostate Enlargement (Hyperplasia/Hypertrophy)

Beta-sitosterol has been used in Europe to lessen the symptoms of enlarged prostate glands for decades. It is a low-cost choice for a problem that affects many older men.

A review of existing data performed by the Cochrane Prostatic Diseases and Urologic Cancers Group, published in 1998 and verified up to date in 2008, summarized a number of high-quality trials. The group concluded that beta-sitosterol improves symptoms of prostatic hypertrophy including improved urinary flow and decreased residual urine after voiding, meaning the bladder is more completely emptied. Beta-sitosterol did not decrease prostate size. Long-term effects and safety were not assessed in these studies.[12] Some other reviewers have come to similar conclusions.[13]

Men are continuing to use beta-sitosterol for this reason, with few side effects. They also take saw palmetto, which contains phytosterols and fatty acids. There are urologists (doctors specializing in the urinary tract) that consider this therapy a reasonable alternative with some evidence beginning to accumulate.[14] Somewhere between 2 and 4 percent of men actually take saw palmetto, depending on their age, among other factors.[15]

In one study, saw palmetto clearly improved symptoms but not measurable results in terms of urinary flow or retention.[16] The investigators stated, "Saw palmetto led to a statistically significant improvement in urinary symptoms in men with lower urinary tract symptoms compared with placebo. Saw palmetto had no measurable effect on the urinary flow rates. The mechanism by which saw palmetto improves urinary symptoms remains unknown."

Other

Beta-sitosterol and other phytosterols have been said to possess immune-modifying properties. They are said to balance the immune system and have been suggested as useful in lowering fevers, controlling blood sugar, reducing inflammation in rheumatoid arthritis, helping tuberculosis as well as cancer cases. Most of the data on these uses are from animal studies or epidemiologic observations and not human trials.[17]

SAMPLE STUDIES USING BETA-SITOSTEROL

Cancer

Beta-sitosterol is used the most frequently in testing. It has been shown to inhibit tumor growth in vitro (in a lab). In mice it has slowed tumor metastases. Since beta-sitosterol is incorporated into cell membranes, changes there could affect the growth or death of cancerous cells.[18]

One in vitro study looked at beta-sitosterol along with tamoxifen to see its effect on breast cancer cells in a laboratory setting. Tamoxifen is an antiestrogen drug used to treat breast cancer. Looking at cells treated with both indicated that beta-sitosterol might increase the effectiveness of tamoxifen.[19]

Not every investigation has found a correlation between plant sterols and lowered risk of cancer. One study in the Netherlands found no relationship between a high intake of phytosterols and colon or rectal cancers.[20]

Multiple Sclerosis

In one study, beta-sitosterol modulated the release of inflammatory chemicals from blood cells of a patient with multiple sclerosis in a laboratory setting.[21]

There are many ongoing trials of phytosterols in laboratory settings, using animals and cell cultures. There are epidemiologic studies looking at associations between phytosterols and various diseases. Most of the research involving clinical testing is in the cholesterol-lowering area, trying to define the best doses and vehicles for phytosterols. There is also research on benign prostatic hyperplasia.

DEFICIENCY

There is no deficiency state of beta-sitosterol or any other phytosterols.

FOOD SOURCES

Beta-sitosterol is found in many plants. It is found in black cumin seed, nigella sativa, pecans, saw palmetto, avocados, curcurbita pepo (pumpkin seeds), pygeum africanum, cashew fruit, rice bran, wheat germ, corn oils, soybeans, sea-buckthorn wolfberries, and Wrightia tinctoria.

More generally, plant sterols are found in vegetable oils, nuts, seeds, and grains.

Phytosterols include beta-sitosterol, campesterol, and stigmasterol. These can be found in plants in their free form, esterified, or as glycosides. Stanols are closely related compounds—they are hydrogenated (or saturated) phytosterols (no double bonds in ring structure). These include sitostanol and campestanol.[5]

Normally, the proportions of sterols in plants are 65 percent beta-sitosterol, 30 percent campesterol, and 5 percent stigmasterol.

MECHANISM OF ACTION: HOW DOES IT WORK?

Beta-sitosterol and other phytosterols (as well as phytostanols) are believed to reduce cholesterol by decreasing absorption in the intestine. The phytosterols as well as stanols have similar effects, although some trials have favored one over the other. The effect of adding phytosterols to the diet is a lowering of total cholesterol, in particular the LDL or bad cholesterol.[5]

Phytosterols are believed to decrease the intestinal absorption of cholesterol as well as increasing its excretion in bile and feces.[22]

In the intestine, there are little packages of fats called micelles that are surrounded by bile from the gall bladder. This is how fats are absorbed. It is believed that phytosterols and stanols replace cholesterol in the micelles, so that less cholesterol is absorbed and more is excreted.[11]

Phytosterols are incorporated into the cell membrane of enterocytes, the cells lining the intestinal tract. This may inhibit the entrance of more cholesterol into the cells. It has also been suggested that phytosterols may prevent the esterification of cholesterol, which can decrease absorption.[4]

Since beta-sitosterol is incorporated into cell membranes, that may be part of the mechanism by which it affects cancer cells and immune cells.

PRIMARY USES

- Beta-sitosterol is used to lower LDL cholesterol and total cholesterol. It is used by healthy individuals who want to improve their cholesterol profile.

- Phytosterols can also lower LDL cholesterol in diabetics, children with familial hypercholesterolemia, and people who already have heart disease.

- Beta-sitosterol and other phytosterols are used on a population level to lower LDL cholesterol. Having products such as foods enriched with phytosterols available in stores can have an impact on the health of people across the board, without a visit to a doctor. These products are recommended in the United States, many places in Europe, Australia, and other countries.

- Bet-sitosterol and related products are taken by men to improve the symptoms of benign prostatic hyperplasia.

COMMON DOSAGES

In order to be incorporated into food, phytosterols and phytostanols must be esterified. The recommended dose of phytosterols is 1 to 2 g per day. This is often consumed as part of a margarine-like spread, so the dose is not exact. Amounts above 3 g do not show any further benefit but can lower vitamin levels in the bloodstream due to its effect on absorption.

Many trials have given the sterol or stanol three times a day. However, the same LDL cholesterol-lowering effects have been seen using one daily dose, putting the sterol or stanol in milk or meat, and adding it to a normal or low-fat diet. Most of the data indicate that LDL cholesterol will be lowered in any of these ways.[11]

Capsules of 300 mg are sold, often containing a mixture of all the sterols.

POTENTIAL SIDE EFFECTS

There has been no long-term toxicity of phytosterols and stanols discovered as yet, in animal trials or in humans. There have been no very long-term studies in humans.

Because phytosterols get into the micelles in the intestine that are transporting fats as well as cholesterol, there is a concern that their consumption can lower the levels of fat-soluble vitamins such as vitamin A, vitamin E, and carotenes. This seems to be the case at high levels of phytosterol ingestion, around 6.6 g a day. There is no reason to take this much. Beyond 3 g a day, there is no significant further lowering of LDL cholesterol. At that level, there may be a slight decrease in some vitamins, which can be offset by increasing the amount of green, leafy vegetables in the diet.[7]

It is possible that esterified sterols interfere with vitamin absorption more than free sterols.[23]

Many studies have confirmed that at doses of 1 to 2 or 2.5 g a day, phytosterols do not affect vitamin A and E concentrations but can lower beta-carotene.[24] Beta-carotene can be lowered by 8 to 19 percent. Lowering of vitamin D has not been observed.[10] Studies have also confirmed that eating high-carotenoid foods along with the plant-sterol–enriched spreads maintains normal carotenoids levels. One serving of high-carotenoid fruit or vegetable a day is enough. Examples would be carrots, apricots, and tomatoes.[25] There is no evidence of long-term problems associated with these possibly lowered carotene levels at the current time. Long-term follow-up will be needed to tell if the lowered levels of carotenes have any adverse effects on health.[11]

For individuals taking phytosterols, it might be a good idea to increase fruit and vegetable consumption or take a multivitamin until there is more information.[26] More research needs to be done to define the best way to prevent low levels of carotenoids and to make sure that no other vitamin deficiencies appear in the long term.

As sterols, phytosterols could be atherogenic like cholesterol. That means that they could contribute to the development of fatty plaques in arteries that cause coronary and other arterial disease. However, so little phytosterol is absorbed that this has not proven to be a problem.

About 5 percent of ingested beta-sitosterol is absorbed, as opposed to the 45 to 50 percent of cholesterol that is normally absorbed.[10] There have been studies indicating that plant sterols do not contribute to plaque formation, as well as studies that conclude that they might. This question has not been answered definitively.[7,11]

There is an extremely rare condition called phytosterolemia, also called sitosterolemia, in which sitosterol absorption is much higher than normal. People with this disease absorb 15 to 25 percent of phytosterols, whereas normal individuals absorb up to 5 percent. This is an inherited disease that is recessive, meaning that a person has to get the gene from both parents. Approximately 1 in 5 million people are homozygous for this gene, which means they have the two abnormal copies. They are more likely to have coronary heart disease and early atherosclerosis. Heterozygous people (1 abnormal gene) may have slightly elevated or normal absorption of phytosterols.[11] This rare condition should not change the public health aspects of trying to lower cholesterol on a population level. However, people who have early atherosclerosis in their family may wish to discuss supplementation with their doctors.

It has been found that 1 to 2 percent of men taking beta-sitosterol for benign prostatic hyperplasia have experienced slight gastrointestinal upset. Less than 1 percent complained of impotence in one study.[13]

FACT VERSUS FICTION

The FDA considers the following proved:

- "Scientific evidence demonstrates that diets that include plant sterol/stanol esters may reduce the risk of CHD."
- "The scientific evidence establishes that including plant sterol/stanol esters in the diet helps to lower blood total and LDL cholesterol levels."

- "Nature of the substance . . . . Plant sterol esters prepared by esterifying a mixture of plant sterols from edible oils with food-grade fatty acids. The plant sterol mixture shall contain at least 80 percent beta-sitosterol, campesterol, and stigmasterol (combined weight)."

The FDA allows these statements to be placed on the appropriate foods, along with other required language.[27] These products have the GRAS label—Generally Regarded As Safe.

Phytosterols in general, and beta-sitosterol in particular, can be included in the diet to lower LDL cholesterol. Personal preference and availability may dictate the way in which these supplements are taken or consumed. They can be added to medication taken to lower LDL cholesterol. If under a doctor's care, a person who takes these supplements should continue to get recommended blood tests.

Men with benign prostatic hyperplasia often feel better taking beta-sitosterol, mixed phytosterols, or saw palmetto. Since these supplements are safe, it is reasonable to try them for relief of symptoms only.

REFERENCES

1. Maki, KC, Davidson, MH, Umporowicz, DM, et al. Lipid responses to plant-sterol-enriched reduced-fat spreads incorporated into a National Cholesterol Education Program Step I diet. *Am J Clin Nutr.* 2001;74:33–43.
2. Clifton, P. Lowering cholesterol: A review on the role of plant sterols. *Australian Family Physician.* 2009;38(4):218–221.
3. Hansel, B, Nicolle, C, Lalanne, F, et al. Effect of low-fat, fermented milk enriched with plant sterols on serum lipid profile and oxidative stress in moderate hypercholesterolemia. *Am J Clin Nutr.* 2007;86:790–796.
4. Matvienko, OA, Lewis, DS, Swanson, M, et al. A single daily dose of soybean phytosterols in ground beef decreases serum total cholesterol and LDL cholesterol in young, mildly hypercholesterolemic men. *Am J Clin Nutr.* 2002;76:57–64.
5. Jones, PJ, Raeini-Sarjaz, M, Ntanios, FY, et al. Modulation of plasma lipid levels and cholesterol kinetics by phytosterol versus phytostanol esters. *J Lipid Res.* 2000;41:697–705.
6. Demonty, I, Ras, RT, van der Knaap, HCM, et al. Continuous dose-response relationship of the LDL-cholesterol-lowering effect of phytosterol intake. *J Nutr.* 2009;139:271–284.
7. Patch, CS, Tapsell, LC, Williams, PG, Gordon, M. Plant sterols as dietary adjuvants in the reduction of cardiovascular risk: Theory and evidence. *Vascular Health and Risk Management.* 2006;2(2):157–162.
8. Varady, KA, Ebine, N, Vanstone, CA, et al. Plant sterols and endurance training combine to favorably alter plasma lipid profiles in previously sedentary hypercholesterolemic adults after 8 wk. *Am J Clin Nutr.* 2004;80:1159–1166.
9. Gylling, H, Radhakrishnan, R, Miettinen, TA. Reduction of serum cholesterol in postmenopausal women with previous myocardial infarction and cholesterol

malabsorption induced by dietary sitostanol ester margarine. *Circulation.* 1997;96:4226–4231.

10. Law, M. Plant sterol and stanol margarines and health. *BMJ.* 2000; 320:861–864.

11. Katan, MB, Grundy, SM, Jones, P. Efficacy and safety of plant stanols and sterols in the management of blood cholesterol levels. *Mayo Clin Proc.* 2003;78:965–978.

12. Wilt, T, Ishani, A, MacDonald, R, Stark, G, Mulrow, CD, Lau, J. Beta-sitosterols for benign prostatic hyperplasia. *Cochrane Database of Systematic Reviews.* 1999;3. Art. No.: CD001043. doi: 10.1002/14651858. CD001043.

13. Barry, MJ, Roehrborn, CG. Benign prostatic hyperplasia. *BMJ.* 2001; 323(7320):1042–1046.

14. Gerber, GS. Phytotherapy for benign prostatic hyperplasia. *Curr Urol Rep.* 2002;3(4):285–291.

15. Kelly, JP, Kaufman, DW, Kelly, K, et al. Recent trends in use of herbal and other natural products. *Arch Intern Med.* 2005;165(3):281–286.

16. Gerber, GS, Kuznetsov, D, Johnson, BC, Burstein, JD. Randomized, double-blind, placebo-controlled trial of saw palmetto in men with lower urinary tract symptoms. *Urology.* 2001;58(6):960–964.

17. Alternative Medicine Review. Plant sterols and sterolins. *Altern Med Rev.* 2001;6(2):203–206.

18. Awad, AB, Fink, CS. Phytosterols as anticancer dietary components: Evidence and mechanism of action. *J Nutr.* 2000;130:2127–2130.

19. Awad, AB, Barta, SL, Fink, CS, Bradford, PG. Beta-Sitosterol enhances tamoxifen effectiveness on breast cancer cells by affecting ceramide metabolism. *Mol Nutr Food Res.* 2008;52(4):419–426.

20. Normén, AL, Brants, HAM, Voorrips, LE, et al. Plant sterol intakes and colorectal cancer risk in the Netherlands Cohort Study on Diet and Cancer. *Am J Clin Nutr.* 2001;74:141–148.

21. Desai, F, Ramanathan, M, Fink, CS, et al. Comparison of the immunomodulatory effects of the plant sterol β-sitosterol to simvastatin in peripheral blood cells from multiple sclerosis patients. *International Immunopharmacology.* 2009;9(1):153–157.

22. Racette, SB, Lin, X, Lefevre, M, et al. Dose effects of dietary phytosterols on cholesterol metabolism: A controlled feeding study. *Am J Clin Nutr.* 2010;91:32–38.

23. Richelle, M, Enslen, M, Hager, C, et al. Both free and esterified plant sterols reduce cholesterol absorption and the bioavailability of beta-carotene and beta-tocopherol in normocholesterolemic humans. *Am J Clin Nutr.* 2004; 80:171–177.

24. Ntanios, FY, Homma, Y, Ushiro, S. A spread enriched with plant sterol-esters lowers blood cholesterol and lipoproteins without affecting vitamins A and E in normal and hypercholesterolemic Japanese men and women. *J Nutr.* 2002;132:3650–3655.

25. Noakes, M, Clifton, P, Ntanios, F, et al. An increase in dietary carotenoids when consuming plant sterols or stanols is effective in maintaining plasma carotenoids concentrations. *Am J Clin Nutr.* 2002;75:79–86.
26. EBSCO CAM Review Board. iHerb.com. Herbs and supplements. Stanols/Sterols. Last review and update February 1, 2010. http://healthlibrary.epnet.com. Accessed February 1, 2011.
27. Code of Federal Regulations. Title 21, Volume 2. Revised as of April 1, 2009. 21CFR101. *Sec. 101.83 Health claims: Plant sterol/stanol esters and risk of coronary heart disease (CHD).* http://www.accessdata.fda.gov/scripts/cdrh/cfdocs/cfcfr/CFRSearch.cfm?CFRPart=101&showFR=1. Accessed February 13, 2010.

4

Biotin

BRIEF OVERVIEW

Biotin is an essential, water-soluble vitamin. It is known to be involved in a whole host of biochemical reactions in humans and other animals. It is a coenzyme for five carboxylases, all of which are catalysts involving the metabolism of many nutrients. It can also modify material that can change the expression of genes.

Biotin deficiency appears to be rare in humans. This is because biotin is ubiquitous in nature, found in plant-based food sources and even made by the bacteria that live in the human intestine.

While biotin was discovered in 1927, it took close to 40 years for it to be designated a vitamin. After being overlooked for decades, it has become the focus of much research because it is involved in so many different steps in the life of a cell or an organism.

Animals deficient in biotin can produce offspring that have birth defects. One question is, does that happen in humans? This is one of the many active areas of research involving biotin.

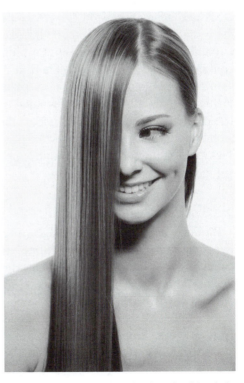

Biotin supplements can lead to healthy hair. (© Valua Vitaly/Dreamstime.com)

THE HYPE

There are some claims about biotin deficiency and biotin treatment that may prove to be true. There are other claims that were made in the 1980s that were not further evaluated, probably because of inadequate evidence. Research continues in many areas.

Borderline Deficiency during Pregnancy

There is increasing evidence of borderline biotin deficiency during many pregnancies. This has been hard to prove due to the difficulty of finding the best test to demonstrate biotin deficiency (see "Deficiency" below). There have been studies showing that greater than 50 percent of pregnant women have higher-than-normal amounts of a specific acid (3-hydroxyisovaleric acid) in their urine, which usually indicates biotin deficiency. However, this could also be due to changes in kidney function during pregnancy.

Investigators have found the activity of one of the carboxylases (propionyl-CoA or PCC) decreased in white blood cells of pregnant women, which is also an indicator of biotin deficiency. Even though the levels of the deficiencies in pregnant women are marginal, the same level of deficiency in animals is teratogenic. The low levels cause genetic damage to the offspring of many animals, including fetal malformations, for example, in rats, chickens, and turkeys. The babies can be born with cleft lip, cleft palate, and/or shortened long bones. In humans, orofacial clefts (cleft palate and lip) occur in approximately 1 out of 1,000 births.[1]

Enough evidence has accumulated to reach a consensus among researchers in the area that there is reason for concern. The understanding that biotin can affect DNA and gene expression (see "Mechanism of Action" below) even shows that there is a direct way for biotin deficiency to cause fetal damage.[2]

While there is an agreement that biotin deficiency is a concern, there is not a consensus about what to do, aside from further research.[3]

In one small study, investigators used white blood cell PCC levels and found them to be low in 10 out of 12 women during early pregnancy, and 8 out of 10 in late pregnancy. The same investigators then gave supplemental biotin to 4 pregnant women with low PCC levels. After two weeks, the PCC levels rose 95 percent. This small study showed that biotin supplementation in pregnant women does lead to higher levels of biotin activity.[1]

Diabetes

Biotin is involved in many stages of glucose metabolism. It has activity in the liver, pancreas, and muscle that affect the handling of glucose. Biotin deficiency could be expected to worsen diabetes. People with deficiency of the carboxylases that need biotin as a coenzyme (see "Mechanism of Action" below) can appear to have severe diabetes.[4]

Research has revealed a number of ways in which biotin may affect blood sugar. At high doses, biotin can increase the activity of an intermediate (guanylate cyclase) that helps control sensitivity to insulin as well as the glucose output from the liver. It has been suggested that these properties mean that biotin could aid in the treatment of diabetes.[5]

In laboratory studies, biotin has been shown to increase the activity of glucokinase from the pancreas, as well as increase insulin secretion. Biotin's actions in glucose metabolism may be due to its activity as a coenzyme or as a gene modifier.[6]

In the past, small studies have indicated some improvement in diabetics given biotin.[7] A recent study of biotin's effects on blood sugar as well as lipids did not show an effect on glucose in diabetics. In this study, 18 diabetic and 15 nondiabetic subjects were randomized into two groups. One group got a placebo, the other got biotin. After 28 days, there was no effect of biotin on blood sugar, insulin levels, or cholesterol. There was an improvement in VLDL (very low density lipoproteins) and triacylglycerol (therefore triglycerides).[8]

Biotin's role in the treatment of diabetes is not clear. The evidence of improvement of triacylglycerol and VLDL in the above study shows a possible use as a treatment for elevated triglycerides.

Biotin for Elevated Lipids

As noted above, biotin may lower triglycerides.[8] Triacylglycerol is another name for triglycerides, which can be measured in the blood and also contained in VLDL. Other small studies have found lipid-lowering effects of biotin.[7]

Biotin for Treatment of Peripheral Neuropathy

Biotin has been used to treat peripheral neuropathy (damaged nerves) because of kidney failure. It is possible that biotin absorption decreases along with decreasing kidney function. In one small study, nine patients on dialysis with neuropathy were treated with 10 mg of biotin a day for between one and four years. Within three months, all of the patients reported improvement in symptoms. The improved symptoms included paresthesias, difficulty walking, and restless legs.[9]

After this very small study the same researchers tried biotin for paresthesias in diabetic patients. They gave 3 patients 10 mg of injected biotin daily for six weeks, then three times a week for six weeks, then orally at 5 mg a day. All 3 patients reported some relief of symptoms.

These two studies included a total of 12 patients and were all open, nonblinded, without controls. It is very hard to make conclusions from this kind of data.[9]

Low Biotin can Cause SIDS

In 1980, a couple of articles appeared making a case for a connection between SIDS (sudden infant death syndrome) and low biotin. Apparently, young broiler chickens that die when stressed have low levels of biotin in their livers. Autopsies were performed on 204 human infants, and those who died from SIDS had lower levels of biotin in their livers than those who died of other causes.[10] As noted in the *Handbook of Vitamins* in 2001, significantly more data would be needed to consider this theory, but there has been no apparent further study to confirm or refute this hypothesis since the early 1980s.[11]

Infant Seborrhea and Other Skin Problems

Biotin deficiency does affect the skin, but if the deficiency is severe enough to cause skin problems, there will be other symptoms of biotin deficiency. Although it has been said to correct Leiner's disease, which is a very severe form of a skin disease called seborrheic dermatitis in infancy, as well as other forms of seborrhea, studies have not proven biotin effective.[7,11] In at least two double-blind trials, biotin did not improve seborrhea any more than placebo.[12,13]

Brittle Nails

The hooves of pigs and horses can have problems that are treated with biotin. Because of this, there were some trials done to see if biotin could improve brittle human nails. A few small studies did indicate that biotin might improve brittle nails, but there has been little other work in this area.[7,14]

DEFICIENCY

One of the problems in understanding biotin deficiency has been trying to find the best way to detect it. One way is measuring the amount of biotin in the urine. Another is measuring a specific acid (3-hydroxyisovaleric acid) in urine that increases if there is a lack of biotin. The combination of decreased urinary biotin along with increased urinary concentration of 3-hydroxyisovaleric acid has been found in biotin-deficient individuals. A third way is measuring the activity of one of the carboxylases (propionyl-CoA) for which biotin is a cofactor (see "Mechanism of Action" below) in white blood cells.[15] This may be the most accurate test.[16,17]

Some of the research necessary to discover how to measure biotin has come from studies in which biotin deficiency was induced by feeding raw egg whites to healthy individuals.[18] Raw eggs contain a substance called avidin that binds biotin so that it cannot be absorbed. People who regularly eat raw eggs can develop biotin deficiency.[17] Avidin binds biotin so strongly that the bond is used for other purposes, including helping administer radiation therapy to cancer patients.[19]

Symptomatic biotin deficiency is very rare. Information about it has been drawn from a number of small studies or observations. These include cases of both adults and infants given total intravenous nutrition without biotin; these would be cases of malabsorption in which the intestinal tract could not be used, and biotin was omitted because there was no knowledge of the deficiency syndrome.

Children with severe protein/energy malnutrition can show symptoms of biotin deficiency. This may be a problem in many developing countries.

In adults, biotin deficiency affects the skin and nervous system. The symptoms include thinning hair, often accompanied by a loss of hair color, and a red, scaly rash that is most prominent on the face. Adults often suffer depression and fatigue, as well as hallucinations and symptoms of nerve irritation in the arms and legs. These symptoms take months or years to develop.[17]

Infants who are not getting any biotin start to show symptoms in three to six months. A rash like the one seen in adults becomes very prominent around the eyes, mouth, and nose. There is also a change in where the fat is under the babies' skin. All the facial features are called "biotin deficiency facies" because they are specific to biotin deficiency. The rash can also be seen around the ears and in the diaper area. The diaper area rash looks like a yeast infection, and also somewhat like the rash seen in zinc deficiency.[17] The rash can also resemble seborrhea.

In infants, after six to nine months of total parenteral nutrition without biotin, hair loss may be seen, including eyelashes and eyebrows. The babies' development will be delayed. They are hypotonic (which means floppy), not very alert, with an unusual type of behavior that may be the infant equivalent of depression.[17]

Levels of biotin in the blood do not reflect accurately biotin levels in the body. However, the activity of the enzyme in white blood cells mentioned above is a very good way to diagnose deficiency. Even in the best laboratories, getting accurate numbers from these various reactions and chemicals has proved difficult. Results tend to be different from one laboratory to another.[17]

When biotin deficiency exists, the cells in the intestine absorb more of any available biotin. If a patient with clinical biotin deficiency is treated with biotin, the symptoms will resolve fairly quickly, and there will be increased urinary biotin and decreased 3-hydroxyisovaleric acid. The rash will resolve and healthy hair will start to grow in as few as one to two weeks. Infants will resume normal development,[20] unless they have been deficient for a very long time.

In addition to raw egg consumption, excessive alcohol intake can cause biotin deficiency. Smoking causes a faster breakdown of existing biotin.[16] Patients on anticonvulsant medications, including carbamazepine, phenytoin, and phenobarbital can become biotin deficient.[21] The medicines may interfere with absorption of biotin, or they may cause it to be metabolized more quickly.[20] Supplementing patients with biotin does not interfere with their medical treatment.

Biotinidase deficiency is a congenital lack of the enzyme that is critical for normal use and metabolism of biotin. People with biotinidase deficiency also show symptoms of biotin deficiency.[20] There is another disorder, deficiency of holocarboxylase synthetase, which causes similar problems to biotinidase deficiency and biotin deficiency. Biotin deficiency, biotinidase deficiency, and holocarboxylase synthetase deficiency have similar but not identical symptoms.

Another rare, congenital disorder of part of the brain called the basal ganglia can be treated with biotin. It appears to be a defect in transporting biotin into the brain, so there is biotin deficiency in the brain. Affected individuals have multiple symptoms, including encephalopathy (widespread brain dysfunction), seizures, and disorders of movement.[7,22]

FOOD SOURCES

Mammals do not make biotin. They ingest it. It is made by bacteria, fungi, yeasts, molds, and some other plants. Biotin winds up in much human food, but amounts vary.[20] People eating a normal diet who have no genetic problem handling biotin, no specific medical condition, or any specific medication that interferes with biotin absorption or utilization will get enough biotin.

There are national surveys done to assess adequacy of many parameters of the diet, and none of them report biotin values. Calculations based on food intake in the United States in the past estimated that young women are probably getting approximately 40 μg of biotin a day in the diet. Average intakes calculated for the United Kingdom are between 33 and 35 μg a day. Canadians may be taking in around 62 μg a day.[17] The Swiss take in about 70 μg a day.[20]

MECHANISM OF ACTION: HOW DOES IT WORK?

Biotin is a coenzyme for five different carboxylases. That means it is necessary for these carboxylases to function. They catalyze reactions that include fatty acid synthesis, glucose production, and regulation of certain genes. The carboxylases exist in the cytoplasm of cells as well as mitochondria (powerhouses of the cell). All in all, biotin is critically involved in macronutrient metabolism, including lipid formation, insulin release, amino acid and cholesterol metabolism. Biotin must be present for the body to function normally. It is especially important for the heart and brain.[16]

Biotin itself is made into biocytin or other short compounds with biotin-linked residues. Biotinidase breaks these down into biotin so it can be reused. This is another reason there is not a lot of biotin deficiency. The body recycles it.

Biotinidase also helps break biotin from ingested protein so it can be absorbed in the intestine. If biotinidase is absent or nonfunctioning, the body cannot use biotin efficiently. It cannot absorb it normally or reuse it.[17]

Biotin is transported into the cells of the upper intestine and also the lower intestine. Some biotin may be derived from the bacteria in the intestine. Once absorbed, it is partly free and partly bound to proteins in the blood.

Biotin does cross the placenta and get to the fetus.[17] It is not clear, however, how much biotin gets to the fetus, especially if the mother has marginal amounts of biotin in her system.[16] It is also found in breast milk.

While the classic understanding of how biotin works is as a coenzyme for the 5 carboxylases, it has been discovered that biotin is also able to modify histones, which are part of chromatin. This gives biotin the ability to modify genetic material and gene expression. The ability of biotin to modify histones might give biotin the ability to repair DNA or trigger cell death via DNA.[23] Through its effects on histones, biotin can affect gene regulation and stability. This is a very active area of research.[24]

PRIMARY USES

Inborn Errors of Metabolism That Prevent Normal Biotin Absorption or Use

- Biotin is used to treat biotinidase deficiency. Patients with this disease need large, pharmacologic doses of biotin. The earlier in life that biotinidase deficiency is treated, the more likely a child is to develop normally.

- Biotin is also used to treat holocarboxylase synthetase deficiency. It can be harder to treat and take higher doses of biotin.
- Biotin-responsive basal ganglia disease must also be treated with biotin.

Biotin Deficiency Must Be Prevented

- Infant formula must contain biotin.
- Anyone receiving all his or her nutrition by vein must have biotin in the mixture he or she is given.
- People on medicine for epilepsy need to take more biotin.
- People who have serious intestinal problems that might prevent normal absorption need biotin.
- People with kidney failure need more biotin.
- Those with other chronic diseases should be evaluated, depending on the illness and treatment.
- Alcoholics may need more biotin.

Other Uses

- Serious consideration should be given to supplementing pregnant women.
- Other uses may become more clear, such as treating peripheral neuropathy with biotin or treating people with high triglycerides.

NEW USE: MULTISTEP IMMUNE TARGETING FOR RADIOIMMUNOTHERAPY

This is not a use for biotin as a supplement. It is interesting to note that research about biotin as a nutrient has led to other uses.

It is hard to reach solid tumors with radiation without damaging adjacent tissue. The avidin-biotin bond is so strong that it is being used in new ways to deliver radiotherapy.[19] An avidin compound bound to antibodies against the tumor cells is given to patients by vein. A biotin-containing compound (a clearing agent) is given to collect all the free avidin that is not attached to tumor cells. Then a radioactive biotin compound is given, which is taken up only by tumor cells with avidin. A larger dose of radioactivity can get directly to the tumor cells, and the excess is quickly excreted. This is called multistep immune targeting, and there are many different compounds used that have the biotin-avidin bond as a central point.[25,26]

COMMON DOSAGES

In 1986, approximately 17 percent of American adults were taking biotin in supplements.

As a vitamin, the Adequate Intake (AI) for adults has been set at 30 μg a day. However, there is no definitive data on what amount adults actually need.

The AI values from infants zero to six months of age are based on the amount of biotin in human milk given to babies who show no symptoms of deficiency. This value is then used to calculate an adequate intake for children and adults by the Institute of Medicine (IOM). The AI for infants is 5 µg a day. This progresses upward to 12 µg a day for ages 4 to 8, 20 µg a day for ages 9 to 13, 25 µg a day ages 14 to 18, and finally 30 µg a day for adults of all ages, except for breast-feeding women, who need 35 µg a day.[17]

In the past, biotin requirements have not been thought to increase during pregnancy. However, as noted above, more recent studies have detected evidence of borderline biotin deficiency during pregnancy.[17,20]

People taking medicine for epilepsy often need more biotin. So do people with kidney failure on dialysis. People with intestinal malabsorption may need more, as may alcoholics. The suggested dose to lower triglycerides is 15 mg a day. As noted above in "The Hype," the connection between low biotin levels and other conditions, such as SIDS, brittle nails, and infant seborrhea, has not been proven.[20]

People with biotinidase deficiency usually need 10 mg of biotin a day. For patients with holocarboxylase synthetase deficiency, treatment is more difficult. Affected individuals may need to take up to 100 mg of biotin a day, sometimes with only a partial response. Patients with basal ganglia disease may need thiamine in addition to biotin.[7]

POTENTIAL SIDE EFFECTS

There has been no biotin toxicity reported in people or animals.[17] There have been laboratory experiments where large doses have been given. There have also been patients treated with large doses with no ill effects. Therefore the IOM has not established an upper limit or a risk characterization.

Up to 200 mg by mouth and 20 mg given by vein have been used when treating biotin deficiencies from various causes, and there have been no reports of toxicity.[20]

FACT VERSUS FICTION

Biotin is a vitamin that is critical to the human body. While it is hard to become biotin deficient, it is not impossible. People who are deficient need to be treated, and deficiency should be prevented whenever possible. People with congenital deficiencies in biotin metabolism can usually be treated successfully with high doses of biotin.

Many claims for biotin will probably never be substantiated. There is no reason to think biotin deficiency causes SIDS or that it will cure infants with seborrhea.

However, it does seem possible that borderline deficiency of biotin may be dangerous to a growing fetus and that pregnant women should be taking biotin supplements in the same way they take folic acid supplements.

It also may turn out to be useful in ways that have not been discovered or proven. Since it is nontoxic, taking it as a supplement is safe.

REFERENCES

1. Mock, DM. Marginal biotin deficiency is common in normal human pregnancy and is highly teratogenic in mice. *J Nutr.* 2009;139:154–157.

2. Mock, DM, Said, H. Introduction to: Advances in understanding of the biological role of biotin at the clinical, biochemical, and molecular level. *J Nutr.* 2009;139:152–153.

3. Said, HM. Biotin: The forgotten vitamin. *Am J Clin Nutr.* 2002;75:179–180.

4. Hou, JW. Biotin responsive multiple carboxylase deficiency presenting as diabetic ketoacidosis. *Chang Gung Med J.* 2004;27:129–133.

5. McCarty, MF. cGMP may have trophic effects on beta cell function comparable to those of cAMP, implying a role for high-dose biotin in prevention/treatment of diabetes. *Med Hypotheses.* 2006;66:323–328.

6. Romero-Navarro, G, Cabrera-Valladares, G, German, MS, et al. Biotin regulation of pancreatic glucokinase and insulin in primary cultured rat islets and in biotin-deficient rats. *Endocrin.* 1999;140:4595–4600.

7. Biotin. *Altern Med Rev.* 2007;12(1):73–78.

8. Revilla-Monsalve, C, Zendejas-Ruiz, I, Islas-Andrade, S, et al. Biotin supplementation reduces plasma triacylglycerol and VLDL in type 2 diabetic patients, and in nondiabetic subjects with hypertriglyceridemia. *Biomed Pharmacother.* 2006;60:182–185.

9. Head, KA. Peripheral neuropathy: Pathogenic mechanisms and alternative therapies. *Altern Med Rev.* 2006;11(4):294–329.

10. Johnson, AR, Hood, RL, Emery, JL. Biotin and the sudden infant death syndrome. *Nature.* 1980;285:159–160.

11. Mock, DM. Biotin. Chapter 11 in: Rucker RB (Ed). *Handbook of vitamins.* New York: Marcel Decker, 2001, 397–426.

12. Keipert, JA. Oral use of biotin in seborrhoeic dermatitis of infancy: A controlled trial. *Med J Aust.* 1976;1(16):584–585.

13. Erlichman, M, Goldstein, R, Levi, E, et al. Infantile flexural seborrhoeic dermatitis. *Arch Dis Child.* 1981;56:560–562.

14. Colombo, VE, Gerber, F, Bronhofer, F, Floersheim, GL. Treatment of brittle fingernails and onychoschizia with biotin: Scanning electron microscopy. *J Am Acad Dermatol.* 1990;6(1):1127–1132.

15. Stratton, SL, Bogusiewicz, A, Mock, M. Lymphocyte propionyl-CoA carboxylase and its activation by biotin are sensitive indicators of marginal biotin deficiency in humans. *Am J Clin Nutr.* 2006;84(2):384–388.

16. Zempleni, J, Hassan, YI, Wijeratne, SSK. Biotin and biotinidase deficiency. *Expert Rev Endocrinol Metab.* 2008;3(6):715–724.

17. Institute of Medicine. Biotin. *Dietary reference intakes for thiamin, riboflavin, niacin, vitamin B6, folate, vitamin B12, pantothenic acid, biotin, and choline.* 1998:374–389.

18. Mock, DM, Henrich, CL, Carnell, N, Mock, NI. Indicators of marginal biotin deficiency and repletion in humans: Validation of 3-hydroxyisovaleric acid excretion and a leucine challenge. *Am J Clin Nutr.* 2002;76:1061–1068.

19. Breitz, HB, Weiden, PL, Beaumier, PL, et al. Clinical optimization of pre-targeted radioimmunotherapy with antibody-streptavidin conjugate and 90Y-DOTA-biotin. *J Nucl Med.* 2000;41:131–140.

20. Mock, DM. Biotin. Chapter II in: *Modern nutrition in health and disease.* Philadelphia, PA: Lippincott Williams & Wilkins, 2006, 497–507.

21. Gaby, A. Natural approaches to epilepsy. *Altern Med Rev.* 2007;12(1):9–24.

22. Debs, R, Depienne, C, Rastetter, A, et al. Biotin-responsive basal ganglia disease in ethnic Europeans with novel *SLC19A3* mutations. *Arch Neurol.* 2010;67(1):126–130.

23. Hassan, YI, Zempleni, J. Epigenetic regulation of chromatin structure and gene function by biotin. *J Nutr.* 2006;136:1763–1765.

24. Zempleni, J, Chew, YC, Hassan, UI, Wijeratne, SSK. Epigenetic regulation of chromatin structure and gene function by biotin: Are biotin requirements being met? *Nutr Rev.* 2008;66(Suppl 1):S46–S48.

25. Boerman, OC, van Schaijk, FG, Oyen, WJ, et al. Pretargeted radioimmuno-therapy of cancer: Progress step by step. *J Nucl Med.* 2003;44:400–411.

26. Forster, GJ, Santos, EB, Smith-Jones, P, et al. Pretargeted radioimmuno-therapy with a single-chain antibody/streptavidin construct and radiolabeled DOTA-biotin: Strategies for reduction of the renal dose. *J Nucl Med.* 2006;47(1):140–149.

5

Calcium

BRIEF OVERVIEW

Calcium is a naturally occurring mineral that is an essential component of the human body. It is absolutely necessary in order for all the systems of the body to function properly.

Most of the calcium in the human body is found in bones and teeth. There is a complicated regulatory process that keeps the blood level of calcium stable when a person is in good health. This involves the absorption of calcium from food, the storage of calcium in bone, the elimination of excess calcium in the urine, and the resorption of calcium into the blood from the bone if levels get low. A number of hormones and vitamins help regulate this process. The main hormone is called parathyroid hormone, and it is necessary for the body to maintain a normal calcium level. Vitamin D is also essential for the body to absorb and use calcium.[1]

For most people, the level of calcium in the blood stays normal and never causes a problem. However, many people develop a deficiency of calcium in the bones as they age. They have not been ingesting enough calcium in their diet for years, and the body has used the calcium from bones to keep the levels up. Eventually, people low on calcium will have lower bone mass, as well as a deterioration of bone tissue. This is called osteoporosis. People can feel fine and be completely unaware of this problem until they break a bone or a doctor screens them for osteoporosis.[2]

THE HYPE

Calcium can Treat/Prevent Osteoporosis

Calcium can help to both prevent and treat osteoporosis. Most people do not get enough calcium in their diet. The questions are, when should people take supplemental calcium, how much should they take, and how long should they take it? All of these questions are being tested in clinical trials.

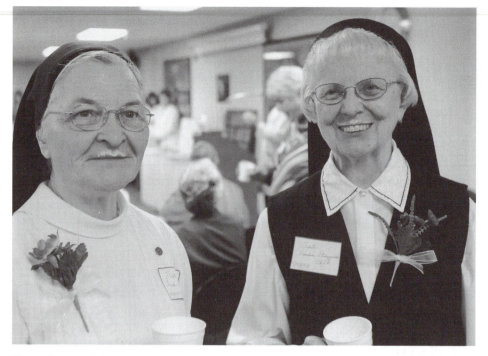

Sister Cecelia, left, and Sister Charlene Stuczynski sport milk mustaches at a reunion in Omaha, Nebraska, 2007. Forty years before, in 1967, nearly 200 nuns from the Omaha area enrolled in the study run by Creighton University researcher Dr. Robert Heaney. Results gathered over 25 years of in-hospital studies, and later from biyearly checkups, serve as the basis for calcium intake recommendations for adult women. (AP Photo/Nati Harnik)

It is accepted that adequate calcium intake is necessary for healthy bones, but it is a complicated process, not just related to how much calcium a person ingests.[2,3]

Calcium Ingestion can Help Weight Loss

There have been studies that showed that people who ingest a lot of calcium-containing dairy products while they diet, or take supplemental calcium, may lose more weight than people who do not. This may only be true for calcium in dairy products and not in supplements. Or it may not be true at all.

Data gathered while a group of people was taking calcium for treatment of osteoporosis indicated that those taking more calcium tended to weigh less.[4] However, a review of nine studies containing data on weight and calcium ingestion was conducted, and there was little evidence that dairy products or calcium supplements had an effect on weight or fat mass.[5] Studies need to be done to specifically address this question.

Coral Calcium Is Better

Calcium is found in combination with other substances. These compounds, which can also be called calcium salts, include, among others, calcium carbonate and calcium citrate. Calcium salts differ in how much actual elemental calcium they contain (see "Common Dosages" below). They also differ in how well they are absorbed, and how many side effects (mainly digestive) people get from taking them. Calcium citrate is often easiest to digest in terms of side effects, while calcium carbonate has more elemental calcium in it, so less pills are needed.

"Coral calcium" comes from ocean coral. It contains calcium carbonate, and this is the same chemical no matter where it comes from. There are a number of problems with coral calcium, which have been investigated over the last 5 to 10 years.[6]

Calcium Supplementation Leads to Increase in CV Events and Mortality

Some studies following the progress of groups of people over time noted an increased risk of cardiovascular disease possibly associated with calcium intake. These were incidental findings, at first, which led to more close scrutiny and trials specifically looking at calcium supplements and cardiovascular disease, such as strokes and heart attacks. A randomized trial in Australia showed a trend toward more cardiovascular events in postmenopausal women given calcium.[7] This study included just under 1,500 women and used just calcium, not calcium plus vitamin D. Many studies are ongoing to confirm these findings.

Calcium Supplementation Leads to an Increase in Prostate Cancer

Some studies have shown an increased risk of prostate cancer in men associated with higher levels of dairy products and/or calcium intake. However, different studies have conflicting results.[8]

Calcium Supplements Decrease the Risk of Colon Cancer and Possibly Other Cancers

Early studies looking at the association of colon cancer and calcium intake in the 1990s were inconclusive. The Calcium Polyp Prevention Study found a decrease in colorectal adenomas with supplemental calcium. Since some polyps can progress to cancer, this was evidence that calcium supplementation might prevent some colon cancer.[9]

DEFICIENCY

The human body does everything it can to keep the amount of calcium in the blood within a normal range. If enough calcium is not ingested in food or supplements, the body will start pulling calcium out of the bones. It will also allow less calcium to leave the body in urine. If all the hormones in the body are working properly, including a high enough level of vitamin D, the level of calcium in the blood will be normal.

One cause of hypocalcemia, which means low calcium in the blood, is hypoparathyroidism. This means the parathyroid glands are not working properly. The parathyroid glands are in the neck, on either side of the thyroid gland, around the level of the Adam's apple. The parathyroid glands can be removed accidentally during thyroid surgery. They can be infiltrated by cancer. There are genetic (inherited) conditions that can cause low parathyroid hormone.

There are other problems that affect calcium metabolism. Inadequate levels of vitamin D or abnormal levels of magnesium can contribute to low calcium levels. The kidneys also play a role in keeping the amount of calcium in the blood constant.[1] Research has shown that there are many more factors regulating calcium level than were previously identified, in terms of other minerals, cofactors, and vitamins.[10]

The most common problem associated with actual calcium deficiency is osteoporosis. A person will feel fine and not suspect anything is wrong, until she fractures a bone.

Any condition in which the level of calcium in the blood is low (hypocalcemia) can be very dangerous. If the calcium level gets very low, multiple body systems will start to malfunction, from the nerves and muscles to the heart and brain.[11] Many symptoms occur because of malfunction of nerves and/or muscles, called neuromuscular irritability. These include:

- Muscle cramps
- Muscle twitches
- Muscle spasms
- Numbness
- Abnormal sensations
- Seizures
- Spasm of the larynx (voicebox), leading to trouble breathing
- Spasm of the bronchial tubes, also leading to trouble breathing
- Tetany, which is a lot of these symptoms together with muscle spasm and aching

A person with hypocalcemia can have a change in brain function. Low calcium can cause the heart muscle to fail. It can also cause arrhythmias—abnormalities in the way the heart beats. A person with very low calcium can have depression, dementia, and even psychosis. If this goes on long enough, there can be swelling in the brain, cataracts in the eye, and permanent heart damage. Very low calcium levels can be fatal.[1]

FOOD SOURCES

Calcium in food comes from dairy products, which means milk and milk products. There are smaller amounts of calcium in some green leafy vegetables and other foods including soy, certain kinds of fish, sesame seeds, and some dried fruit.

For people who cannot digest lactose, there are lactose-free dairy products. They can also take pills containing the enzyme lactase with milk products. Rice milk and almond milk are now fortified with calcium and readily available.

Packaged foods are labeled with their calcium content. The labels reflect a recommended total of 1,000 mg of calcium a day. So if a label says 20 percent DV it has 200 mg of calcium. Foods fortified with calcium include breads, breakfast cereals, orange juice, soy milk, and bottled water, among other products.

Some foods can decrease the absorption of calcium, including large amounts of protein and caffeine.[12] Therefore, heavy coffee drinkers are warned by their physicians to be careful about its effects on their bones.

MECHANISM OF ACTION: HOW DOES IT WORK?

Calcium is necessary for many critical body functions and cell functions.

Of the body's calcium, 99 percent is in bone; 1 percent is not in bone, but it is present in blood, other body fluids, inside cells, and inside certain parts of cells.

The amount of calcium in cells is tightly regulated. Calcium goes in and out of the cells through cell membranes and parts of the cells (called organelles), including the mitochondria, the so-called workhouses of the cell. Calcium acts as a messenger. It is involved in cell-to-cell signaling. It is a part of neural transmission—the signals from nerve to nerve. It is necessary for normal muscle function, including heart muscle. Part of the blood coagulation system, it is a cofactor for many enzymatic reactions and the activation of other messengers. It is involved in secretion of many chemicals, including hormones. It is critical in the mineralization of bone.[11]

Calcium's mechanisms of action are multiple and complicated. It is mainly important to know that calcium has to be present in the correct amount for the nerves and muscles to talk to each other and work as they should. This includes everything from thinking to moving. Research on the actions of calcium, vitamin D, and other cofactors and hormones is constantly in progress.

Calcium needs to be present in enough quantities to give strength to bone. As children grow, bone is growing with them and needs enough calcium to be strong. Bone is constantly being "remodeled," meaning damaged bone is cleaned up and new bone is deposited in its place. A lack of calcium at any time can cause weakened bone. Up until around age 30, more bone is made by cells called osteoblasts than removed by cells called osteoclasts. The body eventually shifts to removing more bone than forming new bone.

Calcium in the body is also related to the amount of phosphate, magnesium, and other chemicals. It is tightly regulated by a number of hormones (including testosterone and female hormones), vitamins, factors, cotransporters and receptors, all of which interact to keep the blood calcium level normal, and ideally, to get enough calcium to the bones.[1,13,14]

PRIMARY USES

Treating Hypocalcemia (Low Levels of Calcium in the Blood)

- This can come on gradually or be a medical emergency. It is not from a lack of dietary calcium, but from malfunctions of the complicated systems that control the level of calcium in the blood, usually because of low parathyroid hormone. It can also be from a severe lack of vitamin D. If all the systems controlling calcium in the blood are working, calcium will be pulled out of bone to keep the blood level normal.

- Someone with hypoparathyroidism will be low on calcium and supplementation will be necessary for life.[1] In this situation, low amounts of calcium in the blood can be fatal if not treated.

Preventing Osteoporosis

- Calcium (along with vitamin D, exercise, and other factors) can help prevent osteoporosis in older men and women. Since many people do not get the recommended amounts of calcium as teenagers and young adults, does that make them more likely to develop osteoporosis later in life? Studies have shown that bone mineral content and size can be increased in boys 16 to 18 by giving them supplementary calcium.[15] Similar studies show increases in bone mineral content but without increasing size in 16- to18-year-old girls.[16]

- Many studies have confirmed that bone mineral density increases in children who get more calcium in their diet or have supplements. However, this effect disappears when the supplements are stopped.[17]

- It will be some time before anyone can say with certainty that starting supplemental calcium at a young age will increase bone strength going into middle age and give more of a cushion before development of osteoporosis. It seems reasonable to think this might be the case; it also seems unlikely that most people will take supplemental calcium all of their lives.

To Treat Osteoporosis

- People with osteoporosis need treatment with calcium, vitamin D, and often medication in order to prevent fractures. Fractures in people with osteoporosis can often occur with minimal or no trauma. They can also be serious enough to cause the serious decline of an older person. As many as 25 percent of people who sustain a hip fracture wind up needing long-term care in a nursing home.[2] Of patients over age 50 who have a hip fracture, about 24 percent of them die during the year after their fracture.[18]

- Osteoporosis usually becomes evident in women after menopause and in men more slowly as they age, because testosterone as well as estrogen affects the amount of calcium in the bone. More bone is resorbed by osteoclasts and less is replaced by osteoblasts, especially if there is not enough calcium and vitamin D around.

- There is not complete agreement as to when to screen for osteoporosis, who to screen, or who to treat.

- Usually, women are assessed perimenopausally for osteoporosis. The U.S. Preventive Services Task Force recommends that women be screened at age 65 or age 60 to 64 if they are at higher risk for osteoporosis. The National Osteoporosis Foundation recommends screening women age 65 and older, men at age 70, and others based on risk factors or history of fracture.[2]

- Risk factors in women include low body weight, low level of physical activity, excessive alcohol intake (more than two drinks per day), caffeine and tobacco use, low calcium and vitamin D intake, no hormone therapy for menopause, increasing age, history of falls, family history of osteoporotic fracture, personal history of fracture, and white or Asian background.

- Some of the same risk factors apply to men.

- There are also many illnesses and medications that can cause osteoporosis in men and women. Illnesses include but are not limited to autoimmune diseases like rheumatoid arthritis, lupus and ankylosing spondylitis, inflammatory bowel disease, and kidney failure. Endocrine abnormalities can cause osteoporosis, including diabetes, hyperparathyroidism, hyperthyroidism, and hypogonadism, among others. Glucocorticoids (like prednisone), immunosuppressants, and medicines that suppress sex hormones are some of the more common medications that can cause osteoporosis.[2]

- The way to check for osteoporosis is with a special x-ray test, a DEXA scan, which means dual energy x-ray absorptiometry, usually checked at the hip and spine. Bone density is compared to the bone density of healthy young women (or men when screening men). If a test is significantly lower, osteoporosis is present. The results are expressed as how far a test differs from the reference (healthy) value. This number is called a T score. What patients need to know is that a T score of -1 to just under -2.5 means the bones are thin, called osteopenia. When the T score is equal to or below -2.5, it means osteoporosis.

- There are calculations that can be made to get an idea of the risk of fracture based on a person's DEXA score and other factors. Treatment decisions are usually made on the basis of DEXA scores, history of hip or vertebral fracture, and risk of fracture based on a number of criteria.

- The World Health Organization, for example, recommends treatment based on a low DEXA score, less than or equal to -2.5 at the hip or spine, or if the person has sustained a hip or vertebral fracture, or if the DEXA scan is not as low but there are lots of risk factors, for patients in the United States.[19]

- Treatment of osteoporosis involves many things. This chapter is about calcium, which is part of the treatment of osteoporosis, along with vitamin D, and a number of medicines that can help strengthen bone.[2,3]

COMMON DOSAGES

There are differences of opinion as to exactly how much calcium should be taken for optimal health.

Calcium intake as suggested by the NIH (National Institutes of Health)

	(Calcium in mg/day)
Infants to 6 months	210
Infants 6 to 12 months	270
Children 1 to 3 years	500
Children 4 to 8 years	800
9 to 18 years	1,300
Adult 19 to 50 years	1,000
Adults 50 years and older	1,200
Pregnant and lactating women	
18 years or younger	1,300
19 to 50 years	1,000

The National Osteoporosis Foundation also advises adults 50 and over to take 1,200 mg of calcium a day.[21] Their guidelines differ only slightly from the NIH suggestions.

Calcium supplements should be split up during the day and not taken all at once if possible.

Osteoporosis Treatment

Adults with osteoporosis need to ingest at least 1,200 mg of calcium plus vitamin D.[2]

It is important to remember that each person needs to take that much elemental calcium. Calcium carbonate is 40 percent elemental calcium. Calcium citrate is 21 percent elemental calcium. These are the two most commonly used supplements. Calcium carbonate is not well absorbed and must be taken with meals. Stomach acid must be present to absorb it. Calcium citrate does not need to be taken with meals and is more completely absorbed.

Calcium can decrease the absorption of many other medications, including some medicines for high blood pressure, some antibiotics, and some of the medications used to treat osteoporosis.

POTENTIAL SIDE EFFECTS

Most forms of calcium can cause gastrointestinal side effects, including gas, cramps, bloating, and constipation. Calcium citrate causes these symptoms somewhat less often than calcium carbonate.

When starting supplementation, sometimes beginning with a low amount and increasing it slowly may reduce some of these symptoms. If the gas and constipation are problems while taking calcium carbonate, a switch to citrate may help. Sometimes just taking a different brand of calcium supplement helps.[21]

Hypercalcemia, or too much calcium in the blood, is caused by disorders in the body and not overdoses of calcium.[22]

FACT VERSUS FICTION

Prevention and Treatment of Osteoporosis

This has been covered above under primary usages, because it is fact.

Weight Loss

A one-year study of young healthy women did not detect any difference in weight when the women were given the same number of daily calories but in calcium-rich dairy products.[23]

In another study, calcium supplements or placebo were given to premenopausal and postmenopausal women on calorie-restricted diets for 25 weeks, and there was no difference in weight loss or fat mass decrease between the groups.[24]

A recent study designed to see if calcium supplements would prevent overweight women from gaining weight showed absolutely no benefit to the supplements.[25]

This is still being investigated. There seems to be more evidence that calcium and dairy products do not help people lose weight than the other way around.

Coral Calcium Is Better

Coral calcium, from ocean coral, contains calcium carbonate just like Tums or other chewable antacids, but at a premium price. It does contain other biologically active ingredients, magnesium, for example, and also contaminants like lead some of the time.

Both the FDA (Food and Drug Administration) and the FTC (Federal Trade Commission) investigated companies selling coral calcium. They were making health claims that could not be substantiated. Companies were forced to stop their infomercials and some of their ads.[26]

The NIH warned consumers as follows: "Consumers should be aware that claims that coral calcium can treat or cure cancer, multiple sclerosis, lupus, heart disease, or high blood pressure are not supported by existing scientific evidence. These claims go far beyond the existing scientific evidence regarding the recognized health benefits of calcium."[27]

Researchers also looked at exactly what was in a number of coral calcium supplements. Some of the coral calcium bottles did not have the amount of calcium stated, some of it was in a form that was hard to digest, and some had elevated lead levels. In addition to the high price and contamination, coral calcium promoters continue to make false claims about their product curing cancer and many other illnesses.

The National Osteoporosis Foundation, as well as other agencies, recommends that people buy calcium and other supplements from well-known companies and that the calcium should be pure. Look for either a well-known brand, or the USP symbol (United States Pharmacopeia), which indicates that the product has been found to meet standards of quality and purity.[28]

Calcium Supplementation Leads to Increase in CV Events and Mortality

In a large study, more than 36,000 postmenopausal women were randomly assigned to receive calcium and vitamin D or placebo and were followed for seven years. There was no difference in coronary or cerebrovascular adverse events.[29] These findings predated the Australian study mentioned above.

An observational study looking at results of trials of women ages 60 to 89 given calcium and vitamin D found that they did not have any higher risk of cardiovascular events or deaths than women not given supplements.[30]

Since research has been yielding contradictory results, it is not possible to state with certainty either way. It seems that perhaps calcium with vitamin D may be safe. Women in these age groups who are at risk for both osteoporosis and heart disease need to discuss choices with their physicians.

Prostate Cancer

Does increased calcium increase the risk of prostate cancer? This question has not been answered. Some investigators have found a higher risk of prostate cancer; some have found a very slightly increased risk.[31] Investigations are ongoing. Men with osteoporosis need to discuss this with their own physicians.

Lung, Colorectal, and Other Cancers

The decreased incidence of colon polyps associated with increased calcium intake has been shown to last at least five years.[32] One recent study found evidence of decreased distal colon cancer with increased calcium intake, enough to encourage further research.[33] Others studies have found similar results.[34]

Some studies have shown a reduced risk of all cancers, but especially the intestinal tract.[35]

Another study of postmenopausal women given calcium, calcium plus vitamin D, or placebo found that calcium plus vitamin D reduced the risk of all cancers over four years. The effect was most apparent in the women given both calcium and vitamin D.[36] This is an area of ongoing research.

There are countless areas to explore as all the functions of calcium, especially in conjunction with vitamin D, are investigated. It seems likely that calcium and vitamin D, probably together, exert their effects on many more body systems than was originally believed.

REFERENCES

1. Shoback, D. Hypoparathyroidism. *N Engl J Med.* 2008;359:391–403.
2. Sweet, MG, Sweet, JM, Jeremiah, MP, Galazka, SS. Diagnosis and treatment of osteoporosis. *Am Fam Physician.* 2009;79(3):193–200, 201–202.
3. Nieves, JW. Osteoporosis: The role of micronutrients. *Am J Clin Nutr.* 2005;81(Suppl):1232S–1239S.
4. Davies, KM, Heaney, RP, Recker, RR, et al. Calcium intake and body weight. *J Clin Endocrinol Metab.* 2000;85:4635–4638.
5. Barr, SI. Increased dairy product or calcium intake: Is body weight or composition affected in humans? *J Nutr.* 2003;133:245S–248S.

6. Osteoporosis Foundation. FAQ on calcium. http://www.nof.org/osteoporosis/faq.htm. Accessed October 7, 2009.

7. Bolland, MJ, Barber, PA, Doughty, RN, et al. Vascular events in healthy older women receiving calcium supplementation: Randomised controlled trial. *BMJ.* 2008;336(7638):262–266.

8. Giovannucci, E, Liu, Y, Stampfer, MJ, Willett, WC. A prospective study of calcium intake and incident and fatal prostate cancer. *Cancer Epidemiology, Biomarkers & Prevention.* 2006;15:203.

9. Baron, JA, Beach, M, Mandel, JS, van Stolk, et al. Calcium supplements for the prevention of colorectal adenomas. Calcium Polyp Prevention Study Group. *N Engl J Med.* 1999;340:101–107.

10. Taylor, JG, Bushinsky, DA. Calcium and phosphorus homeostasis. *Blood Purif.* 2009;27(4):387–394.

11. Lewis, JL (reviewer). Endocrine and metabolic disorders: Disorders of calcium concentration. *Merck medicus online.* 2009. http://www.merck.com/mmpe/sec12/ch156/ch156g.html. Accessed October 6, 2009.

12. National Osteoporosis Foundation. What you should know about calcium. http://www.nof.org/prevention/calcium2.htm. Accessed October 7, 2009.

13. Rizzoli, R, Bonjour, JP. Calciotropic hormones and integrated regulation of calcemia and calcium balance. *Rev Prat.* 1998;48(11):1178–1184.

14. Deftos, LJ. Calcium and phosphate homoestasis. Chapter 2 in: Singer, F (Ed). Diseases of bone and mineral metabolism. *Endotext.org.* http://www.endotext.org/parathyroid/index.htm. Accessed October 6, 2009.

15. Prentice, A, Ginty, F, Stear, S, Jones, S, et al. Calcium supplementation increases stature and bone mineral mass of 16- to 18-year-old boys. *The Journal of Clinical Endocrinology & Metabolism.* 2005;90(6):3153–3161.

16. Stear, SJ, Prentice, A, Jones, SC, Cole, TJ. Effect of a calcium and exercise intervention on the bone mineral status of 16–18-y-old adolescent girls. *Am J Clin Nutr.* 2003;77:985–992.

17. Lee, W, Leung, S, Leung, D, Chen, J. A follow-up study on the effects of calcium-supplement withdrawal and puberty on bone acquisition of children. *Am J Clin Nutr.* 1996;64:71–77.

18. National Osteoporosis Foundation. Fast facts on osteoporosis. http://www.nof.org/osteoporosis/diseasefacts.htm. Accessed October 8, 2009.

19. World Health Organization Collaborating Centre for Metabolic Bone Diseases, University of Sheffield, UK. http://www.shef.ac.uk/FRAX/tool.jsp?locationValue=9. Accessed October 9, 2009.

20. Nutrition and Bone Health. reviewed January 2009. http://www.niams.nih.gov/Health_Info/Bone/Bone_Health/Nutrition/default.asp. Accessed October 8, 2009.

21. National Osteoporosis Foundation. What you should know about calcium. http://www.nof.org/prevention/calcium2.htm. Accessed October 8, 2009.

22. Hypercalcemia. http://www.cancer.gov/cancertopics/pdq/supportivecare/hypercalcemia/patient/allpages. Accessed October 8, 2009.

23. Gunther, CW, Legowski, PA, Lyle, RM, McCabe, GP, et al. Dairy products do not lead to alterations in body weight or fat mass in young women in a 1-y intervention. *American Journal of Clinical Nutrition.* 2005;81(4):751–756.

24. Shapses, SA, Heshka, S, Heymsfield, SB. Effect of calcium supplementation on weight and fat loss in women. *J Clin Endocrinol Metab.* 2004;89:632–637.

25. Yanovski, JA, Parikh, SJ, Yanoff, LB, Denkinger, BI, et al. Effects of calcium supplementation on body weight and adiposity in overweight and obese adults: A randomized trial. *Ann Intern Med.* 2009;150(12):821–829.

26. Federal Trade Commission. FTC charges marketers of Coral Calcium Supreme dietary supplement and a pain-relief product with making false and unsubstantiated claims. Press release June 10, 2003. http://www.ftc.gov/opa/2003/06/trudeau.shtm. Accessed October 9, 2009.

27. National Institutes of Health. Coral calcium. Press release June 10, 2003. http://nccam.nih.gov/news/alerts/coral/coral.htm. Accessed October 9, 2009.

28. National Osteoporosis Foundation. FAQ on calcium. http://www.nof.org/osteoporosis/faq.htm. Accessed October 9, 2009.

29. Hsia, J, Heiss, G, Ren, H, et al. Calcium/vitamin D supplementation and cardiovascular events. *Circulation.* 2007;115:846–854.

30. Shah, SM, Carey, IM, Harris, T, Dewilde, S, Cook, DG, et al. Calcium supplementation, cardiovascular disease and mortality in older women. *Pharmacoepidemiology and Drug Safety.* September 15, 2009. http://www.ncbi.nlm.nih.gov/pubmed/19757413. Accessed February 1, 2011.

31. Gao, X, LaValley, MP, Tucker, KL. Prospective studies of dairy product and calcium intakes and prostate cancer risk: A meta-analysis. *J Natl Cancer Inst.* 2005;97:1768–1777.

32. Grau, MV, Baron, JA, Sandler, RS, Wallace, K, et al. Prolonged effect of calcium supplementation on risk of colorectal adenomas in a randomized trial. *J Natl Cancer Inst.* 2007;99:129–136.

33. Wu, K, Willett, WC, Fuchs, CS, Colditz, GA, et al. Calcium intake and risk of colon cancer in women and men. *J Natl Cancer Inst.* 2002;94(6):437–446.

34. Cho, E, Smith-Warner, SA, Spiegelman, D, et al. Dairy foods, calcium, and colorectal cancer: A pooled analysis of 10 cohort studies. *J Natl Cancer Inst.* 2004;96:1015–1022.

35. Park, Y, Leitzmann, MF, Subar, AF, Hollenbeck, A, Schatzkin, A. Dairy food, calcium, and risk of cancer in the NIH-AARP Diet and Health Study. *Arch Intern Med.* 2009;169(4):391–401.

36. Lappe, JM, Travers-Gustafson, D, Davies, KM, et al. Vitamin D and calcium supplementation reduces cancer risk: Results of a randomized trial. *Am J Clin Nutr.* 2007;85:1586–1591.

6

Chromium

Chromium is a mineral, tiny amounts of which are needed by human beings. In the 1950s, investigators discovered that a substance in brewer's yeast could prevent diabetes in lab animals. It was determined that this substance was in fact trivalent chromium.[1]

Chromium is known to enhance the activity of insulin when tested in a lab (in vitro), and evidence is accumulating that it does the same in the body. There is no known natural deficiency state at the current time or clear evidence about how much chromium might cause toxicity. The FNB (Food and Nutrition Board) has only been able to establish a suggested adequate intake level.[2]

THE HYPE

Supplemental Chromium can Help People Lose Weight and Supplemental Chromium can Help Control Diabetes

It is important to note that many people are already taking chromium in multivitamins or other supplements, and this may or may not be noted in studies. It is common practice among diabetics.[3]

There are three general areas related to weight and glucose control that may be affected by chromium. One is obesity. Another is any type of diabetes. The third is the metabolic syndrome, which includes impaired fasting blood sugar or type 2 diabetes, high blood pressure, central obesity, elevated triglycerides, and decreased HDL ("good cholesterol").

Chromium picolinate (CrPic) is said to help people lose weight, reduce body fat while building muscle, lower triglycerides and cholesterol, and improve insulin function.[3] If this proves to be true, it should help people with the metabolic syndrome as well as those with just diabetes and/or obesity. While low chromium levels impair insulin function, there is no definitive proof that extra chromium will help treat diabetes, improve lipid levels, or affect body composition.

In one placebo-controlled, double-blind study of patients with impaired glucose metabolism, half were given 400 µg of chromium picolinate twice a day. No difference in any parameter of metabolism was changed after three months. BMI (body mass index), glucose tolerance, cholesterol, and lipids, for example, were no different in the supplemented group than in the group that did not receive supplements.[4]

In another double-blind, placebo-controlled trial, nonobese patients with the metabolic syndrome were given chromium picolinate or placebo. After 16 weeks, there were essentially no differences in glucose metabolism or measures of inflammation and stress between the two groups.[5]

A large analysis of existing trials found that, overall, patients using chromium picolinate lost approximately 1.1 kg more weight than dieters not using the supplement. Many of these studies did not provide sufficient information about side effects or enough about the participants to see if specific subgroups were more likely to lose weight than others.[6]

In 2004, an article in the *American Family Physician* summarized the evidence and said that patients should be cautioned about using chromium for weight loss, because there is not enough data to prove that it will help them, and the toxic amount is unclear.[7]

On the other hand, a large analysis of studies done by different investigators two years later determined that almost all of the trials show that chromium picolinate is beneficial for diabetics. Diabetics taking chromium picolinate may have reduced glucose levels, reduced cholesterol and triglycerides, reduced need for insulin and other medication. These researchers suggested that chromium picolinate is more bioavailable than other forms of chromium, and studies using chromium picolinate should have better outcomes than studies using different chromium compounds.[8] Other researchers have suggested that the amount of chromium used be significantly more than 200 µg a day, and that chromium picolinate is the preferred form. There is evidence that chromium picolinate supplementation reduces glucose levels in type 1 and type 2 diabetes and also gestational (pregnancy-induced) and steroid-induced diabetes.[1]

Other Diseases

There have been a number of studies that show an inverse relationship between toenail levels of chromium and cardiovascular disease. However, taken altogether, the evidence for the use of chromium to prevent cardiovascular disease is not yet robust enough to make definitive decisions.[1]

Some have studied supplementary chromium as a substance that might decrease carbohydrate craving in atypical depression. One small study indicated that chromium could be useful for this disorder.[9]

DEFICIENCY

In 1977, a number of patients on Total Parenteral Nutrition (TPN) developed what looked like diabetes, but it could not be controlled by insulin. Their blood sugars where high, they lost weight, and they had damage to peripheral nerves. Once chromium was added to their TPN formula, their symptoms improved significantly and they did not need insulin.[1]

Apart from the specific situation of patients receiving TPN without chromium for prolonged periods, there is no recognized disease associated with low levels of chromium[2,3] occurring in people outside of a hospital setting.

There is not even complete consensus on how to measure chromium in the body. It has been measured in blood, hair, and sweat, as well as urine, but these values may not indicate the amount of chromium in the body.[3]

Some people may need more chromium than others. It is possible that older people need more chromium.

Normal plasma levels may be in the range of 0.05 to 0.5 µg/l.[3] That is a 100-fold difference and means it is difficult to know if someone has too much or too little chromium.

Absolute deficiency of chromium does seem to cause impaired glucose tolerance, and chromium may be of benefit in treating type 2 diabetes.[10] It is possible that some diabetics are deficient in chromium, and that is why supplementation helps them.

FOOD SOURCES

Chromium is found throughout the earth's crust and oceans. It is contained in many foods. However, there is no good way to determine how much. The very methods used to measure chromium can contaminate the food sample with chromium. Even in specific foods, different harvests or different lots vary in their chromium content.

Processing food and drink increases its chromium content. Wine and beer both may have significant amounts of chromium. Chromium in small amounts can be found in meats including liver, whole grains, nuts, some spices (molasses), some vegetables (carrots and broccoli), and some fruit. If a food is high in simple sugars like fructose, it will be low in chromium.[3,10]

The only definite cases of deficiency have been in patients on total parenteral hyperalimentation that did not contain chromium. Otherwise, people get enough of it sprinkled throughout their diet.

If a person's diet contains an excessive amount of simple sugars, so that more than 35 percent of the calories come from the sugars, more chromium will leave the body in the urine. Chromium can also be lost from the body during stress, such as infection, trauma, heavy exercise, and pregnancy.[10]

When chromium is paired with picolinate, more chromium is absorbed by the body. Picolinate is a byproduct of tryptophan.

MECHANISM OF ACTION: HOW DOES IT WORK?

Chromium is found naturally in a number of forms. What is called chromium III (or trivalent chromium) is the most stable and thought to be what is found in food. Chromium VI (or hexavalent chromium) is a byproduct of countless manufacturing processes. If inhaled, it is carcinogenic. On the skin, it causes irritation. Workplace exposures can lead to lung cancer and perforation of the septum of the nose.[2,3]

Substances in food will convert chromium VI to III. Chromium concentrates in the liver, spleen, soft tissue, and bone.

Its principal mechanism of action is not absolutely clear,[10] but it does promote glucose tolerance.[3,5] It is known to be able to enhance the action of insulin. It seems to be involved in activation of the insulin receptor tyrosine kinase.[2] Through a number of steps, chromium gets into insulin-dependent cells and binds to a substance that then binds to the insulin receptor, which activates tyrosine kinase.

At the current time, the sequence of events is thought to be this: chromium is ingested. When it gets into the blood, it is bound to transferrin. Insulin activates insulin receptors, which trigger the movement of chromium into cells. There, it is then bound to a substance called chromomodulin. Insulin also mediates this reaction. The chromomodulin with chromium attached binds to the insulin receptor and activates tryosine kinase. Tyrosine kinase potentiates insulin activity.[11]

Chromium's ability to potentiate insulin has attracted the most attention. Chromium also is involved in the metabolism of carbohydrates, fats, and proteins. Its other actions are not clear. It is not known if more chromium will enhance metabolism and help treat diabetes in all people. It is not known if some people are actually deficient and benefit from taking it.[10] It is not known if it will help those that are not deficient. It is not even clear how to decide who is deficient.

With increased aerobic exercise, more chromium may be ingested and excreted.[2] Chromium may also interact with iron. It competes for one of the binding sites on transferrin, which transports iron. People with the disease hemochromatosis have too much iron, and they are often diabetic. The excess iron may affect the transport of chromium, which may, in turn, be part of the reason for the diabetes seen in this condition.[2]

PRIMARY USES

- Chromium is added to total parenteral nutrition (TPN) formulas because it is believed that some chromium is necessary for the normal functioning of the human body.

- Many people, especially diabetics, take chromium supplements.

COMMON DOSAGES

It is very difficult to tell how much chromium healthy people have ingested from dietary sources. For this reason, there has not been an RDA (Recommended Dietary Allowance) determined.[2,10]

The Institute of Medicine, Food and Nutrition Board has set an Adequate Intake (AI) level of chromium at 35 µg per day for young men, and 25 µg per day for young women.[1] The "estimated safe and adequate daily dietary intake" range for chromium has been set at 50 to 200 µg for adults and adolescents.[1,5] Generally similar levels have been set in other areas, such as the United Kingdom, which also states the difficulties in setting these standards.[12] There is a clear need for more study about safe and effective levels of chromium.

Adult men and women should meet their AIs with normal diets. Many multivitamin and mineral supplements include chromium at the 35-µg level. Separate supplements are available with much higher dosages.

POTENTIAL SIDE EFFECTS

As stated above, some forms of chromium may be carcinogenic and damage DNA. Some may cause irritation and ulcers in the gastrointestinal tract. Chromium supplements reduce iron absorption.[3]

Chromium picolinate taken for weight control can cause renal failure and other toxicities if ingested in excess.[2,13] Supplements need to be checked for their total chromium content. Chromium supplements have caused both acute tubular necrosis (death of tubules in the kidney) and interstitial nephritis (diffuse kidney disease), both of which can cause renal failure.[14] There have been reports of liver problems.[2] Rhabdomyolysis, which is damage to muscle that releases cell contents into the blood, has also been reported, but this may have been due to other factors such as weight lifting.[2]

Overall, chromium is probably quite safe to take.[1] However, some of the potentially very dangerous side effects have occurred at levels used in many supplements.

It is not known how much chromium should be added to TPN even now. Recently there have been reports of temporary decreases in kidney function with chromium added to TPN, and it has been suggested that the amount added to TPN routinely is too high. More research is needed.[15]

FACT VERSUS FICTION

There is no question that much research needs to be done in order to understand the functions of chromium in the body. A normal level of chromium in the body has to be established. It is also important to be able to measure the amount of chromium in food more accurately.

Chromium is an essential micronutrient. People receiving total parenteral nutrition must have some chromium in their formulas. Diabetics of all types will probably benefit from chromium supplements, but how much is not clear. It is not clear if chromium supplements are helping people who are low in chromium but do not know it, or if adding more chromium helps all diabetics.

There is not enough evidence yet to say whether or not chromium can significantly help with weight loss or help reverse the metabolic syndrome.

The small amount of chromium in most multivitamin/multimineral supplements is safe, as is significantly more. But the absolute upper limits of safety are not yet known.

REFERENCES

1. Cefalu, WT, Hu, FB. Role of chromium in human health and in diabetes. *Diabetes Care.* 2004;27(11):2741–2751.
2. Institute of Medicine. Food and Nutrition Board. *Dietary reference intakes for vitamin A, vitamin K, arsenic, boron, chromium, copper, iodine, iron, manganese, molybdenum, nickel, silicon, vanadium, and zinc.* Washington, DC: National Academies Press, 2001.
3. The Merck Manuals Online Medical Library for Healthcare Professionals. Chromium. Last full review/revision May 2009 by Ara DerMarderosian, PhD. Content last modified May 2009. http://www.merck.com/mmpe/sec22/ch331/ch331e.html#sec22-ch331-ch331e-244 http://www.merck.com/mmpe/sec01/ch005/ch005a.html#BABHDJDB http://www.merck.com/media/mmpe/pdf/Table_005–1.pdf. Accessed November 18, 2009.
4. Gunton, JE, Cheung, NW, Hitchman, R, et al. Chromium supplementation does not improve glucose tolerance, insulin sensitivity, or lipid profile. *Diabetes Care.* 2005;28(3):712–713.
5. Igbal, N, Cardillo, S, Volger, S, et al. Chromium picolinate does not improve key features of metabolic syndrome in obese nondiabetic adults. *Metabolic Syndrome Related Disorders.* 2009;7(2):143–150.
6. Pittler, MH, Stevinson, C, Ernst, E. Chromium picolinate for reducing body weight: Meta-analysis of randomized trials. *International Journal of Obesity.* 2003;27:522–529.
7. Saper, RB, Eisenberg, DM, Phillips, RS. Common dietary supplements for weight loss. *American Family Physician.* 2004;70(9):1731–1738.
8. Broadhurst, CL, Domenico, P. Clinical studies on chromium picolinate supplementation in diabetes mellitus: A review. *Diabetes Technology & Therapeutics.* 2006;8(6):677–687.
9. Docherty, JP, Sack, DA, Roffman, M, et al. A double-blind, placebo-controlled, exploratory trial of chromium picolinate in atypical depression: Effect on carbohydrate craving. *J Psychiatr Pract.* 2005;11(5):302–314.
10. Office of Dietary Supplements, NIH Clinical Center, National Institutes of Health. Dietary supplement fact sheet: Chromium. http://ods.od.nih.gov/factsheets/chromium.asp. Accessed November 18, 2009.
11. Vincent, JB. The biochemistry of chromium. *Journal of Nutrition.* 2000;130:715–718.
12. Expert Group on Vitamins and Minerals. Review of chromium. 2002. www.foodstandards.gov.uk/multimedia/pdfs/reviewofchrome.pdf. Accessed November 22, 2009.
13. Cerulli, J, Grabe, DW, Gauthieer, I, et al. Chromium picolinate toxicity. *The Annals of Pharmacotherapy.* 1998;32(4):428–431.
14. Gabardi, S, Munz, K, Ulbricht, C. A review of dietary supplement–induced renal dysfunction. *Clin J Am Soc Nephrol.* 2007;2:757–765.
15. Moukarzel, A. Chromium in parenteral nutrition: Too little or too much? *Gastroenterology.* 2009;137:S18–S28.

7

Coenzyme Q$_{10}$ (CoQ$_{10}$)

BRIEF OVERVIEW

Coenzyme Q$_{10}$ is a molecule used by the human body during aerobic cellular respiration. CoQ$_{10}$ does much of its work in the mitochondria, parts of the cell where energy is produced. It is a critical link in the mitochondrial respiratory chain. CoQ$_{10}$ is also an antioxidant, and like other antioxidants, can help protect the body from damage caused by free radicals and other reactive chemicals. CoQ$_{10}$ is the most fat-soluble antioxidant, so that it protects areas with fats (like the linings of blood vessels) against oxidative damage.

There is CoQ$_{10}$ everywhere in the body. The highest amounts are in the kidneys, liver, pancreas, and heart, whereas the lungs have much less. Levels of CoQ$_{10}$ in the blood can be decreased during oxidative stress; low levels are often found in people with cancer, as well as people with chronic neurologic diseases.

Mitochondrial dysfunction is present in many chronic diseases. Because CoQ$_{10}$ helps mitochondria produce energy, it has potential as a treatment for many diseases, including cardiovascular disease and disorders of the immune system. As an antioxidant as well as an immune system stimulant, it may be able to help with cancer treatments.

Most CoQ$_{10}$ is made by the body, but some comes from the diet. It is not a vitamin because its class of molecule can be made by all animals including humans. These are called ubiquinones because they are present everywhere; CoQ$_{10}$ is also known as ubiquinone.

THE HYPE

Because CoQ$_{10}$ is needed for essentially all cellular processes dependent on energy, low CoQ$_{10}$ is often associated with disease states; supplemental CoQ$_{10}$ may help treat many diseases.

There is evidence of mitochondrial dysfunction in many degenerative diseases; CoQ$_{10}$ might be able to help treat these. Similarly, oxidative stress is thought to cause many disease states and CoQ$_{10}$ would be expected to help treat these as well.

There is a lot of evidence from laboratory work on cells in culture and on animals demonstrating the activity of CoQ_{10}. There are also preliminary human studies, many of which have been small and not properly designed. Even some of the best trials have yielded different outcomes, evaluating CoQ_{10} treatment of the same conditions. For most diseases, there have not yet been enough well-designed human studies to consistently determine benefit.[1] Researchers continue to call for clinical trials to try and answer some of the questions posed by earlier work, and there are ongoing trials.

Cancer

Decreased levels of CoQ_{10} have been found in patients with many kinds of cancer, including breast, lung, prostate, kidney, colon, pancreas, head and neck, myeloma, and lymphoma. Both increased and decreased levels have been found in actual cancerous tissue.[1]

Laboratory and animal testing has been done with CoQ_{10} since the 1960s. All of CoQ_{10}'s properties may be important to prevent or treat cancer. It stimulates the immune system in animals and humans, including increasing antibody levels, and affects helper T cells (immune cells). The antioxidant activities of CoQ_{10} have also been studied as they relate to cancer. There is some evidence that analogs (chemicals with similar properties) of CoQ_{10} may stop cancer cells from growing.

There have actually been limited studies in humans. CoQ_{10} does limit the toxicity to the heart caused by certain agents used to treat cancer, called anthracyclines. A study showed this benefit in regard to doxorubicin, a chemotherapeutic agent. Monitoring heart function in patients on doxorubicin is standard. Perhaps its depletion of CoQ_{10} is to blame.

There have been uncontrolled tests with incomplete data indicating a benefit to using CoQ_{10} in treating breast cancer patients with metastases. There are other anecdotal reports and case reports but not well-designed clinical trials.[1,3]

An analysis of the reports and studies completed in 2003 found that there was no evidence that CoQ_{10} can treat or prevent cancer.[2]

Heart Disease

CoQ_{10} has been considered for prevention and treatment of cardiovascular disease related to atherosclerosis, hypertension, diabetes, and other common risk factors. LDL ("bad cholesterol") in the walls of arteries can be oxidatively damaged and that may be an initiating event leading to atherosclerosis. In these cases, the antioxidant function of CoQ_{10} might be beneficial. There are other properties of CoQ_{10} that are of interest, such as its ability to decrease the amount of a specific substance on the surface of cells that can collect on the blood vessel walls.[2]

An analysis of available research in 2003 found conflicting results. Some improvement in cardiac function was observed in some studies but not confirmed in others.[4]

CoQ_{10} is considered as a possible treatment for cardiomyopathy, which is an abnormality or disease of the cardiac muscle. Improvements in cardiac output have been found in some small studies. It has also been shown to help congestive heart failure as the result of coronary heart disease in other small studies. Again, there is a need for more large-scale clinical trials.[2,5]

Levels of CoQ_{10} have been considered as an independent predictor for outcome in patients with chronic heart failure. Those with lower levels have a higher risk of death. In one recent study, the correlation was strong enough for investigators to call for more interventional studies using CoQ_{10} to treat heart failure.[6]

This same pattern repeats for almost all types of cardiovascular disease and treatment. From the treatment of angina (lack of blood supply to the heart muscle), to high blood pressure and damage of the lining of the blood vessels, there is limited evidence of benefit from CoQ_{10} and a need for more studies.[2]

Diabetes Mellitus

Multiple small trials have shown no effect of CoQ_{10} on diabetes. It does not improve glucose control or lower insulin needs in type 1 diabetes; it does not improve glucose control or lipid profiles in type 2 diabetics.[2]

CoQ_{10} has been tested to see if it can improve endothelial function in diabetics. A number of small studies have reported success. For example, a double-blind, crossover study of 23 statin-treated type 2 diabetics found that 200 mg a day of CoQ_{10} did improve measures of endothelial function in 12 weeks. Not surprisingly, the authors of this study concluded by suggesting a clinical endpoint trial.[7]

CoQ_{10} has not been shown to improve heart function in diabetics, at least in small trials like one testing 74 type 2 diabetics with dysfunction of the left side of the heart.[8]

Neurodegenerative Diseases

Evidence of both mitochondrial dysfunction and oxidative damage is found in neurodegenerative diseases including Parkinson's disease, Huntington's disease, and Alzheimer's disease. CoQ_{10} levels in the brain decrease with aging. The substantia nigra, which is the area affected in Parkinson's disease, has the lowest CoQ_{10} amounts in the brain.

While supplemental CoQ_{10} raises blood levels in humans, only animal studies have shown that it crosses the blood-brain barrier. As of 2009, no testing has been done on humans to see if it crosses the human blood-brain barrier.[9]

Many tests in the lab show the protective effect of CoQ_{10} in stressed cells in vitro. Oral administration of CoQ_{10} increases CoQ_{10} levels in the brain of older lab animals but not young ones. There are many models of neurodegenerative disorders in animals that are meant to mimic those in humans, and tests have shown that CoQ_{10} can help prevent or ameliorate the symptoms of these diseases.

The results in animal studies have been favorable enough to encourage human clinical studies. Trials of CoQ_{10} for Parkinson's disease have yielded mixed results. There does appear to be some benefit in patients' movement abilities, particularly activities of daily living and also motor control, cognition, behavior, and mood.[10] However, CoQ_{10} has not reduced the time to when dopamine is needed to treat disability. A large, randomized, Phase III trial is said to be currently underway.

One multicenter, randomized, double-blind, placebo-controlled, strati-fied, parallel-group, single-dose trial involving 131 patients with Parkinson's who were stabilized on treatment used nanoparticular CoQ_{10} at 300 mg a day (comparable to 1,200 mg regular CoQ_{10}) for three months. While the supple-ments were well tolerated and increased CoQ_{10} plasma (blood) levels, there was no statistically significant change in any measurable outcome from the supplementation.[11]

Trials using CoQ_{10} to treat Huntington's disease have also yielded unclear re-sults; a Phase III trial is underway for Huntington's disease and CoQ_{10}. Tests using CoQ_{10} for amyotrophic lateral sclerosis have showed little enough benefit that stage II testing is as far as the testing will go. CoQ_{10} has not been tested for Alzheimer's disease, although a number of studies have looked at the analogue idebenone. Results have been mixed.[9] Researchers in this field stress the need for more definitive, large-scale testing.

(See "Deficiency.")

Statin Administration

CoQ_{10} and cholesterol share part of the same biochemical pathway, and statin drugs lower cholesterol by blocking one of the steps. Patients on statins have low blood levels of CoQ_{10}. They can also have muscle pain, myopathy, and even break-down of muscle tissue with myoglobin in the urine. It has been hypothesized, but not proven, that the myopathy associated with statin use occurs because of a CoQ_{10} deficiency. Tests have not shown definitely low levels of CoQ_{10} in affected muscle. There are those who believe that people on statins should take supplemental CoQ_{10} based on the incomplete current information.[12]

There have also been studies that do not show relief of myopathic symptoms by giving CoQ_{10} to patients with myopathy on statins. Some have postulated that there may be a subgroup of people with genetic subtypes that are more likely to need CoQ_{10} supplementation and benefit from it.[13]

Others suggest that since CoQ_{10} is so safe, there is no reason not to give it to individuals with statin myopathy, even though it has not been proved effective. At the same time, more testing is suggested, both of the effectiveness of CoQ_{10} for this purpose, as well as to determine genetic subtypes that may benefit.[14]

(See "Deficiency.")

Miscellaneous Other Uses

CoQ_{10} has been used to treat migraine headaches as well as cyclic vomiting syndrome, a related condition. It may be better tolerated and at least as effective as amitriptyline for these conditions.[15]

CoQ_{10} improves exercise tolerance in patients with genetic deficiencies; perhaps supplements can improve exercise performance in other people. The controlled studies to date do not support this idea. CoQ_{10} has not been found to improve exer-cise tolerance in normal individuals.[2]

DEFICIENCY

There is no deficiency syndrome related to insufficient CoQ_{10}. Enough is made by the body and ingested to meet the needs of healthy people. Approximately 25 percent of CoQ_{10} may come from dietary sources. However, no regulatory agency has suggested a recommendation for amounts of intake.

There are genetic disorders leading to a decrease in production of CoQ_{10} but these are very rare.[16]

Genetic CoQ_{10} deficiencies are autosomal-recessive conditions. They involve, in varying degrees, myopathy (muscle abnormalities), encephalopathy (problems with the brain), encephalopathy and myopathy together, atrophy of the cerebellum (balance center) with ataxia (difficulty keeping balance), and an infantile variant involving multiple organs including the kidneys. This can appear as growth retardation, with deafness, seizures, and cognitive impairment.[9,17]

The genetic defects are just beginning to be understood. Early identification of patients and their siblings may allow prompt treatment with CoQ_{10}. All patients improve with CoQ_{10} administration, but they need high doses and long-term administration. The muscular and peripheral symptoms improve more than the central nervous system abnormalities; CoQ_{10} may not get through the blood-brain barrier, or the damage may be irreversible. There are other genetic mutations in other areas that can interfere with CoQ_{10} synthesis and cause the same types of symptoms.

Since deficiency of CoQ_{10} decreases antioxidant capacity and causes mitochondrial dysfunction (see "Mechanism of Action"), other diseases with these defects in the central nervous system may respond to CoQ_{10}. This could include Parkinson's disease, Alzheimer's disease, Friedreich's ataxia, and others.[17] Most are being studied.

There are many other mitochondrial diseases. A CoQ_{10} synthesis defect is one of the few treatable mitochondrial diseases. As the genetic defects are isolated, earlier treatment will be possible.[18]

Deficiency of CoQ_{10} has been reported with many types of cancer, as well as other diseases including diabetes, congestive heart failure, and progressive neurological disorders as noted. CoQ_{10} levels also decrease with age.[2] The significance of all of this is not completely understood as yet.

FOOD SOURCES

The best sources of CoQ_{10} are fish, poultry, and meat. Nuts, soybean, and canola oils also contain a relatively large amount of CoQ_{10}. Other foods, including fruits, vegetables, dairy products, and eggs contain some CoQ_{10}.

Most people probably consume less than 10 mg a day of CoQ_{10}. As examples, 3 ounces of fried chicken has 1.4 mg of CoQ_{10}, while one orange has 0.3 mg.[2]

MECHANISM OF ACTION: HOW DOES IT WORK?

CoQ_{10} is required for energy production in every cell. Most of its work is in the mitochondria, the powerhouse of the cell, to synthesize ATP, which is a kind of fuel. CoQ_{10} accepts and then transfers electrons as needed. CoQ_{10} also transfers protons. With these processes, energy in the form of ATP is generated.[2]

CoQ_{10}, as stated, is an electron carrier during mitochondrial respiration. It also transports electrons elsewhere in cells. It regulates permeability of a number of membranes, including the mitochondrial pores. It can affect the amount of certain substances carried by a type of blood cell called a monocyte. It has an effect on the lining of blood vessels called the endothelium. CoQ_{10} is able to cause alterations in yeast and bacteria. Many of these actions have been understood because of what is found in people with genetic deficiencies of CoQ_{10}.[17]

CoQ_{10} exists in a reduced form and an oxidized form. CoQ_{10} is an antioxidant in its reduced form. Since it is fat-soluble, it works in cell membranes and lipoproteins, preventing damage to them. Lipoproteins are the packages that carry cholesterol. CoQ_{10} can also prevent oxidative damage to the mitochondria.[2]

CoQ_{10} is synthesized in three steps. Part of its structure comes from an amino acid. A second part is mevalonate. The two parts are joined; this is regulated by hydroxymethylglutaryl (HMG)-CoA reductase. This enzyme is necessary for cholesterol synthesis and is the target of statin therapy. One of the effects of statin therapy to reduce cholesterol is a reduction in CoQ_{10}.[2]

As people with genetic deficiencies of CoQ_{10} have been identified, it has been estimated that there are five general groups of symptoms, which are related to different errors in the biosynthesis of CoQ_{10}.[17] More genetic defects are still being found and analyzed.

PRIMARY USES

- CoQ_{10} must be given to anyone with a genetic condition causing the inability to manufacture it. These are rare problems, and not all are treatable with CoQ_{10}. However, if the genetic abnormality can be identified early in patients or siblings and CoQ_{10} is administered, it can improve many symptoms, especially those outside the central nervous system.

- It can be used for migraine headaches and cyclical vomiting.

- CoQ_{10} has not been proved beneficial for most of the conditions for which people take it. Individuals may choose to take it to try and improve their cardiovascular health or exercise tolerance, to gain better control of their diabetes or lipids, to prevent cancer or Alzheimer's disease. Patients on statins can take CoQ_{10} to try and avoid muscle problems. It can be used for any of the diseases discussed above.

- People who choose to take CoQ_{10} for any serious medical condition should discuss it with their doctor. They should not stop any prescribed medication.

COMMON DOSAGES

As a supplement, CoQ_{10} doses are usually between 30 to 100 mg a day. Softgel capsules range in price from $20 to $60 for 60 to 120 100-mg capsules, or for 30 400-mg capsules.[9]

As treatment for various conditions, doses of 100 mg to 300 mg may be used. Doses above 100 mg should be split up. CoQ_{10} is absorbed best when taken with a meal that contains fats.

Doses as high as 3,000 mg a day have been used to treat Parkinson's disease.[2]

While it is fairly certain that supplements of CoQ_{10} increase blood levels and also lipoprotein levels of CoQ_{10}, it is not certain that supplements increase tissue concentrations in normal individuals. There has not been enough research in this area.[2]

CoQ_{10} is available in many different forms. It is dissolvable in lipids or fats, not water. It can be found as a powder, suspension, oil solution, and solubilized form. Creams, wafers, tablets, capsules with both hard and soft shells are all available. There are newer forms that aim to increase the amount of CoQ_{10} available to the body, such as nanoparticular CoQ_{10}. There is also an analog of CoQ_{10} that has been made, called idebenone. This substance may be able to more easily dissolve in water.[9]

Administration of CoQ_{10} does raise its blood levels. Using a lipid (fat) formulation or taking it with foods containing fat improves its absorption.

POTENTIAL SIDE EFFECTS

CoQ_{10} is well tolerated. Insomnia has occurred at doses of 100 mg or higher. At doses of 300 mg a day for long periods of time, there have been elevations of liver enzymes but no actual liver damage. CoQ_{10} can cause nausea and stomach pain, heartburn, rash, dizziness, fatigue, irritability, and the sensitivity of the eyes to light, called photophobia.[1]

The doses used in trials of CoQ_{10} as treatment for neurodegenerative diseases, as high as 3,000 mg a day, have been well tolerated. Patients have had headaches, gastrointestinal symptoms, upper respiratory infections, all in similar numbers to patients taking placebo. In one study evaluating tolerability of CoQ_{10} up to 3,000 mg a day, participants complained of headache, rash, urinary tract infections, edema (swelling), gastrointestinal symptoms, and joint pain. It is believed that mild gastrointestinal symptoms are the most likely side effects from CoQ_{10}.[9]

Some studies have pointed out that there are essentially no differences between placebo and CoQ_{10} in terms of side effects.[11]

FACT VERSUS FICTION

Right now it is early in the story of CoQ_{10}. It may live up to all its potential, or it may not. There is no way to know what well-designed trials will discover about this supplement. In the future, researchers may be able to say authoritatively what CoQ_{10} can and cannot do. For now, none of this is proved. On the other hand, most of it has not been disproved.

In the meantime, it can be taken by people with cardiovascular risk factors or diabetes. Patients on statins can take it to try and avoid muscle problems. Patients with cancer can try it. People with neurodegenerative diseases can also take it. Because it seems to be very safe and can be obtained inexpensively, there are not many objections to trying it. However, it has not been proved useful for these conditions.

REFERENCES

1. National Cancer Institute. Coenzyme Q_{10} (PDQ®). Revised December 18, 2007. http://www.cancer.gov/cancertopics/pdq/cam/coenzymeQ10/healthpro fessional/allpages#Reference4.2. Accessed May 27, 2010.

2. Higdon, J. Coenzyme Q_{10}. Micronutrient Information Center. Linus Pauling Institute. February 2003; updated February 2007. http://lpi.oregonstate.edu/ infocenter/othernuts/coq10/#deficiency. Accessed May 27, 2010.

3. Coulter, I, Hardy, M, Shekelle, P, et al. *Effect of the supplemental use of antioxidants vitamin C, vitamin E, and the coenzyme Q_{10} for the prevention and treatment of cancer.* Summary, Evidence Report/Technology Assessment: Number 75. AHRQ Publication Number 04-E002, October 2003. Agency for Healthcare Research and Quality, Rockville, MD. http://www.ahrq.gov/clinic/ epcsums/aoxcansum.htm. Accessed June 2, 1010.

4. Shekelle, P, Morton, S, Hardy, M. *Effect of supplemental antioxidants vitamin C, vitamin E, and coenzyme Q_{10} for the prevention and treatment of cardiovascular disease.* Summary, Evidence Report/Technology Assessment: Number 83. AHRQ Publication Number 03-E042, June 2003. Agency for Healthcare Research and Quality, Rockville, MD. http://www.ahrq.gov/clinic/epcsums/ antioxsum.htm. Accessed June 2, 2010.

5. Dallner, G, Stocker, R. Coenzyme Q_{10}. In: Coates, PM. (Ed). *Encyclopedia of dietary supplements.* New York: Marcel Dekker, 2005, 529–538.

6. Molyneux, SL, Florkowski, CM, George, PM, et al. Coenzyme Q_{10}: An independent predictor of mortality in chronic heart failure. *J Am Coll Cardiol.* 2008;52:1435–1441.

7. Hamilton, SJ, Chew, GT, Watts, GF. Coenzyme Q_{10} improves endothelial dysfunction in statin-treated type 2 diabetic patients. *Diabetes Care.* 2009;32:810–812.

8. Chew, TG, Watts, GF, Davis, TME, et al. Hemodynamic effects of fenofibrate and coenzyme Q_{10} in type 2 diabetic subjects with left ventricular diastolic dysfunction. *Diabetes Care.* 2008;31:1502–1509.

9. Spindler, M, Beal, MF, Henchcliffe, C. Coenzyme Q_{10} effects in neurodegenerative disease. *Neuro Dis and Treat.* 2009;5:597–610.

10. Kidd, PM. Neurodegeneration from mitochondrial insufficiency: Nutrients, stem cells, growth factors, and prospects for brain rebuilding using integrative management. *Altern Med Rev.* 2005;10(4):268–293.

11. Storch, A, Jost, WH, Vieregge, P, et al. Randomized, double-blind, placebo-controlled trial on symptomatic effects of coenzyme Q_{10} in Parkinson's disease. *Arch Neurol.* 2007;64(7):938–944.

12. Lamperti, C, Naini, AB, Lucchini, V, et al. Muscle coenzyme Q_{10} level in statin-related myopathy. *Arch Neurol.* 2005;62:1709–1712.

13. Molyneux, SL, Young, JM, Florkowski, CM, et al. Coenzyme Q_{10}: Is there a clinical role and a case for measurement? *Clin Biochem Rev.* 2008;29:71–82.

14. Marcoff, L, Thompson, PD. The role of coenzyme Q_{10} in statin-associated myopathy: A systematic review. *J Am Coll Cardiol.* 2007;49:2231–2237.

15. Boles, RG, Lovett-Barr, MR, Preston, B, et al. Treatment of cyclic vomiting syndrome with coenzyme Q$_{10}$ and amitriptyline: A retrospective study. *BMC Neurology*. 2010;10:10.

16. Natural Standard Research Collaboration. Medline Plus. Coenzyme Q$_{10}$. http://www.nlm.nih.gov/medlineplus/druginfo/natural/patient-coenzymeq10. html. Accessed May 27, 2010.

17. Quinzii, CM, DiMauro, S, Hirano, M. Human coenzyme Q$_{10}$ deficiency. *Neurochem Res*. 2007;32:723–727.

18. Duncan, AJ, Bitner-Glindzicz, M, Meunier, B, et al. A nonsense mutation in CoQ$_9$ causes autosomal-recessive neonatal-onset primary coenzyme Q$_{10}$ deficiency: A potentially treatable form of mitochondrial disease. *Am J of Human Gen*. 2009;84:558–566.

8

Copper

BRIEF OVERVIEW

Copper is a naturally occurring mineral. It is present in the soil and water in most areas of the world. Like many other metals, it is an essential micronutrient. Copper is a critical part of multiple enzymes with many functions throughout the human body.

Although obvious dietary copper deficiency is rare, it does occur in some situations. There may also be a marginal state of deficiency that is not yet well understood.

People can consume copper from a variety of different plant and animal sources. There is usually copper in drinking water. The Environmental Protection Agency (EPA) regulates the amount of copper in water so there is not too much.

Too much copper can definitely cause toxicity. It is seen clearly in Wilson's disease, a genetic disorder that prevents the body from eliminating copper. The excess copper damages the liver, the brain, and other organs including the kidneys. Paradoxically, there is also a genetic disorder called Menkes' disease that causes the symptoms of deficiency because the body cannot absorb copper normally.

Researchers continue to search for the best balance—not too much and not too little copper.

One researcher looks at copper this way, "Copper: two sides of the same coin."[1]

THE HYPE

Copper administration is said to improve many conditions. Some of the time, the people taking the copper may have been copper deficient, and the copper reversed the deficiency. For these conditions, copper may not be a general treatment, but a treatment for the condition that occurs as a result of copper deficiency.

Examples of this include certain kinds of anemia that can be caused by low copper levels and reversed by copper administration. The same is true of certain

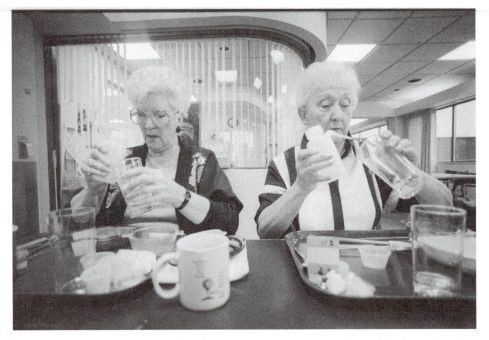

Bonnie Ferguson, left, and Pat McCarty rinse every last morsel of their breakfast into glasses at the U.S. Department of Agriculture Human Nutrition Research Center in Grand Forks, North Dakota. The women, paid volunteers, were among the subjects of a 1993 study to determine whether a lack of copper in the diet affects postmenopausal women. (AP Photo/Eric Hylden)

rare nervous system disorders caused by low copper. Osteoporosis in children due to low copper can be improved when copper is given. Some of these will be described briefly under "Deficiency."

Copper deficiency can be difficult to diagnose, as will be described later. Although rare, it does occur. Because there is not uniform agreement about how to measure copper in humans, it is hard to compare studies.

Elevated copper levels are also said to cause a number of problems.

It is important to note that some illnesses are caused by genetic defects in enzymes or proteins that use or transport copper. Some may be improved by increasing or decreasing copper intake depending on the problem, but not cured, because the underlying problem is not the copper.

The Copper Tracking Theory

All organisms need copper, but it can be toxic in many forms. Organisms from yeast to humans have developed copper "chaperones," compounds inside cells that protect the rest of the cell from copper and move copper to where it needs to be. This movement inside the cell is called copper tracking.[2,3]

A whole new field of study has developed to attempt to measure copper and other metals in biologic systems. During these kinds of studies, high levels of copper have been found in association with certain diseases, and low levels have also been found. Sometimes the ratio of copper to other metals like zinc and iron may be out of balance. For example, some studies have found that there is an imbalance of copper with other metals in patients with coronary heart disease.[4]

This new understanding may explain why investigators have found both high and low levels of copper in certain disease states.

Degenerative Neurologic Disorders

In some patients with Alzheimer's disease, there is a high level of copper in the fluid surrounding the brain and spinal column, but a normal copper level in the blood (plasma). There are certain characteristic findings in Alzheimer's—plaques and tangles in the brain made of a substance called amyloid; copper can interact with amyloid precursors. It is possible that elevated copper in the brain may cause or worsen Alzheimer's disease but this is far from certain.[5]

Studies have found both high and low copper levels in patients with Alzheimer's disease.[6] In one recent clinical trial, patients with Alzheimer's disease were given 8 mg a day of copper for 12 months. There was no effect on the patients' disease, neither improvement nor worsening. There was also no change in serum copper levels even after 12 months of supplementation. The researchers were looking for substances that can indicate the amount of copper in the brain and found one such substance that decreased less in patients treated with copper than placebo over the 12 months.[7]

Huntington's disease is an inherited condition in which there is an abnormal protein that damages the brain, causing a severe movement disorder and eventually death. There are also elevated levels of copper in the brains of patients with this disease, which may cause some of the damage.[5]

It has been suggested that copper may play a role in the development of Parkinson's disease.

Patients with Wilson's disease have some of the same type of movement disorders as patients with Parkinson's.[5]

New research is showing ways that copper might cause damage to the brain in all of these diseases. There are cellular proteins that are "misfolded" in neurodegenerative disorders, and these may cause some of the damage to cells in the nervous system. The ubiquitin-protease system is supposed to eliminate these potentially damaging clumps of protein. Copper binds strongly to ubiquitin and can compromise the ability of this system to protect cells in the central nervous system.[8]

Copper also binds to a protein that accumulates in the nerve cells of patients with Parkinson's disease.[9]

It is possible that copper binding to proteins is part of the problem in many or all of these neurodegenerative disorders.

Cholesterol

Copper status may have an effect on cholesterol. Elevated cholesterol has been reported with both low and high levels of copper intake.[6,10]

Diabetes

Disturbed copper regulation or elevated levels of copper have been found in diabetics. Copper chelators, which attach to excess copper so it can be eliminated, have been proposed as treatment for diabetes and diabetic complications.[11]

One trial of a copper chelator in diabetics with heart muscle abnormalities showed some positive effect.[12]

Immune System

Studies have shown that both low and high copper intakes may cause changes in markers of immune function over periods of many months.[13]

Copper has been proposed as helpful in treating rheumatoid arthritis and other arthritis, as well as systemic lupus erythematosus, but with no clear proof.[6] Wearing copper bracelets is a type of alternative therapy that is still used by some patients with arthritis.[14]

Elevated copper levels have also been found in patients with rheumatoid arthritis.[15] Other investigators have found that copper chelators, which remove copper from the system, may improve some of these conditions, at least in animal trials.[16]

Cancer

Copper chelating agents have also been tried as agents to suppress tumor growth, both in animals and in limited human trials. Chelating agents may lower angiogenic factors, which are factors that make blood vessels grow. Angiogenic factors can control the blood supply and thereby growth of tumors.[6]

In one Phase II trial, patients with metastatic kidney cancer were given a copper chelator. It did lower copper levels but did not make any clinically detectable change in cancers of the 15 patients.[17]

DEFICIENCY

Copper deficiency can lead to decreased function of copper-containing enzymes (see "Mechanism of Action" below). Some deficiency states have been observed in animals; others have also been documented in humans. Theoretically, there can be connective tissue problems that damage skeletal or blood vessel structures. There can be problems in the central nervous system. There may also be defects in immune function and heart function. There is a lot of research going on at the current time trying to delineate how copper is normally used in the body, how much copper is ideal, and what happens under conditions of copper deficiency or copper excess in normal people.[10]

Copper deficiency is rare in people without genetic disorders of copper metabolism. It only occurs in unusual circumstances. Malnourished infants given cow's milk can become copper deficient. Premature babies given milk formulas can also become copper deficient, as can patients receiving all their nutrition by vein. People with intestinal diseases that interfere with its ability to absorb nutrients can become copper deficient.[6,10] People can become deficient after gastric bypass surgery, which is increasingly more common.[18]

Patients with dietary deficiency of copper usually have low blood cell counts, both red and white. Babies and children who are copper deficient can have osteoporosis (thin bones). Copper stores are rapidly replenished once copper is administered, and blood counts return to normal.[6,10]

There are other symptoms that can be prominent in a person with serious copper deficiency, in which the neurologic are the most obvious. The damage to the nervous system and peripheral nerves can be severe. One specific group of problems is called "copper deficiency myelopathy" or "human swayback." These patients will have low blood counts as well, which can be corrected quickly with copper. Copper does not necessarily significantly improve the neurologic damage, although further damage can be prevented. A group of 25 cases of human swayback was described in 2006, in which the low copper levels were explained in 16 cases. Causes included high zinc and iron ingestion, stomach surgery for peptic ulcers or weight control, and general malabsorption. No cause was determined in nine patients.[19]

In animals, low copper levels can cause heart damage. However, the type of damage is not related to human coronary artery disease. There are questions about the effect of low copper levels on the heart rhythm as well as the heart muscle. Other areas of study involve copper's effect on blood sugar, blood pressure, immune function, certain blood-clotting chemicals, and bone metabolism. These are areas in which results have not been consistent.

Copper deficiency is not always easy to diagnose. Copper status can be followed by measuring copper in blood as well as ceruloplasmin. Generally speaking, ceruloplasmin and copper levels are only low in moderate to severe copper deficiency. Copper deficiency can also be diagnosed by finding a low level of other enzymes that need copper. Investigators are still trying to find the best way to diagnose early copper deficiency, as well as early excess, reviewing existing tests and finding new ones.[20]

One way that the amount of copper in the body is kept at the correct level is by increasing or decreasing the amount absorbed from the intestine. Stomach acid helps separate copper from compounds in the diet. The percentage of copper absorbed depends on the amount available. With low copper intake, as much as 75 percent may be absorbed. If the intestine is presented with a lot of copper, absorption can decrease to less than 12.5 percent. Absorbed copper goes to the liver. Most copper is bound to ceruloplasmin and released to the circulation. In the liver, before binding to ceruloplasmin or being excreted in bile, there are other necessary ATPases that transport copper. When there is a lot of copper available, more is excreted, which also helps keep the copper level normal. A defect in the genes involved in transporting copper (an ATPase) in the liver causes Wilson's disease, which involves an abnormal accumulation of copper.

A defect in the gene coding for a copper-transporting ATPase that regulates copper absorption in the intestine as well as passage across the placenta causes Menkes' disease, a disease with reduced available copper.[10] In Menkes' disease, copper cannot leave the intestinal cells. Because this causes the dysfunction of many critical enzymes, patients have severe neurologic dysfunction as well as connective tissue problems.[1] With Menkes' disease, copper cannot cross the blood-brain barrier and get into the central nervous system. Children with Menkes' disease usually do not live past three years of age.[5] There are apparently a number of different genetic mutations that cause Menkes' disease. Some cause only a dysfunction of the ATPase as opposed to a complete absence of it. These can be treated with a form of injectable copper if it is started soon after birth.[21]

Inherited Diseases Involving Copper-Containing Enzymes or Copper Metabolism

There are problems involving copper-containing enzymes that are not caused by high or low copper intake but by genetic defects. These defects can cause a lack of useable copper, as noted above in Menkes' disease, or too much copper accumulation, as noted above in Wilson's disease.

A congenital defect in another enzyme called ceruloplasmin, which is involved in iron transport, can lead to an abnormal accumulation of iron.[10]

There is also an inherited condition (autosomal-recessive) in which no ceruloplasmin is made, called aceruloplasminemia. There seems to be some doubt about what damages the nervous system in this case, copper or iron accumulation. It is also unclear if there is always liver damage, although there does seem to be copper accumulation in the liver.[5,22]

A defect in the gene for copper/zinc superoxide dismutase causes Lou Gehrig's disease, otherwise known as amyotrophic lateral sclerosis. Copper itself may cause the neurologic damage in this disease.[5]

FOOD SOURCES

Most drinking water contains copper, although the levels are regulated. Copper can be found in plant-derived foods, including vegetables, legumes, fruits, nuts, whole grains, avocado, and cocoa. It can also be found in shellfish and other seafood and beef organs such as liver.[6,10] A lot of dietary copper in the United States comes from foods with low levels of copper that are consumed a lot, such as milk, potatoes, chicken, and tea.[10]

The amount of copper absorbed from the diet has very little to do with the type of food. It is influenced more by how much copper is in the diet. A higher percentage is absorbed when there is less total copper in the diet; however, with increasing available amounts, even with a smaller percentage absorbed, more copper is ingested.[10]

Surveys indicate that the average dietary copper intake for women in the United States is about 1 to 1.1 mg a day. Men ingest between 1.2 to 2.6 mg a day. These amounts meet the RDAs for copper.

Large amounts of zinc and also iron can interfere with copper absorption, but this is usually not from the amounts of zinc or iron found in food.

MECHANISM OF ACTION: HOW DOES IT WORK?

Copper is part of many metalloenzymes that act as oxidases. In these reactions, molecular oxygen (O_2) accepts an electron and is converted to either water (H_2O) or hydrogen peroxide (H_2O_2). These reactions are critical to life.

There are many known copper metalloenzymes in humans.[10] Some of the enzymes include:

- Amine oxidases. Diamine oxidase inactivates histamine, a key component in allergic reactions. Monoaminoxidase is part of the breaking down of serotonin as well as the metabolism of other central nervous system chemicals such as norepinephrine and dopamine. Lysyl oxidase uses components in collagen and elastin to make some of the links holding tissues together in bone and lung.

- Ferroxidases are found in plasma (in the blood), and are copper-containing enzymes involved in the oxidation of iron. Iron must be oxidized in order for it to bind to transferrin, the protein that carries it around the body. There are a number of these. As previously noted, a genetic defect in one called ceruloplasmin can lead to an abnormal accumulation of iron.

- Cytochrome c oxidase catalyzes the reaction that turns O_2 into H_2O on a cellular level. It allows ATP to be made, which can transport energy around the cell. This is especially important in the brain, the heart, and the liver.

- Dopamine ß tyrosinase helps make dopamine into norepinephrine. These are both neurotransmitters in the brain.

- There are two different forms of an enzyme called superoxide dismutase. One uses copper and zinc and is a big part of the defense of damage to cells from oxygen radicals. This enzyme is called copper/zinc superoxide dismutase. Mutations in the gene that codes for this enzyme cause Lou Gehrig's disease, otherwise known as amyotrophic lateral sclerosis.[10]

PRIMARY USES

- The primary use of copper is to treat copper deficiency, which can occur in any case of malabsorption.

- Copper must be included in infant formulas or nutrition given by vein to infants. Low lactose diets, as well as cow-milk formulas, are low in copper. Infants with severe diarrhea, malnutrition, or with an inability to absorb nutrients normally from the intestine, and infants with cystic fibrosis may need copper as well as other trace nutrients. There is no infant supplement available. Physicians must add copper to intravenous nutrition or formula.[6]

• Copper can be given in high doses intravenously to some patients with Menkes' disease. In certain cases, if started within days of birth, copper may prevent the devastating and fatal neurologic damage that occurs in the disease.

COMMON DOSAGES

Recommended supplement dosages are based on how much copper is needed; 900 µg of copper a day will meet the RDA for adults (see below). In 1989 about 15 percent of adults took a dietary supplement containing copper.

In order to reach recommendations for copper intake, the Institute of Medicine used copper concentration in the blood, ceruloplasmin concentrations, as well as the activity of a number of the copper-containing dismutases in red blood cells to try and determine adequate amounts of copper intake.

Low serum copper concentrations usually reflect copper deficiency. So do low ceruloplasmin levels. Both of these go up when copper supplementation is given to deficient individuals. However, neither reflect dietary intake of copper unless it is very low. Both copper and ceruloplasmin levels increase during pregnancy and in a number of infectious and inflammatory conditions and illnesses. In these cases, copper deficiency cannot be diagnosed by either of these tests.

The IOM also considered the concentration of copper in platelets (very tiny blood cells that help the blood clot), as well as cytochrome c oxidase activity in platelets, but there are not enough measurements of these yet. Levels of urinary copper have been considered, as have measurements of the activity of many of the enzymes containing copper as described above and levels of copper in hair. The IOM also looked at studies of copper balance, as well as analysis of amounts needed to replace daily copper losses.

The IOM used all available data to arrive at recommendations.

As has been stated above, there is no definitive test to determine copper deficiency or excess.[20]

For infants, the adequate intake levels (AI) were based on usual intake from human milk in healthy infants up to six months old. For 6- to 12-month-olds, the amount consumed in milk and usual food was considered. The AI for infants 0 to 6 months old is 200 µg a day of copper, or 30 µg/kg per day. For infants 6 to 12 months old, it is 220 µg a day of copper, or 24 µg/kg per day.

For children and adolescents, both the EAR (Estimated Average Requirement) and RDA (Recommended Dietary Allowances) were arrived at by using adult data. The EAR for children 1 to 3 years of age is 260 µg/day of copper. For those 4 to 8 years of age, the EAR is 340 µg/day of copper. The EAR for boys and girls 9 to 13 years old is 540 µg/day of copper. For boys and girls 14 to 18 years old, the EAR is 685 µg/day of copper.

The RDA is higher, because it is estimated to be enough to apply to 97 to 98 percent of individuals, as opposed to being the average requirement. The RDAs are as follows:

Recommended Daily Allowances of Copper

1 to 3 years of age	340 µg/day of copper
4 to 8 years of age	440 685 µg/day of copper
Boys and girls 9 to 13 years of age	700 µg/day of copper
Boys and girls 14 to 18 years of age	890 µg/day of copper

The adult values, from which the childhood recommendations were extrapolated, used data from trials in which healthy individuals were given low copper diets, and then normal copper diets. There were only 32 people tested in all three trials together. Various copper indicators were measured to verify results, as described previously.

The EAR was established for men and women of all ages at 700 µg of copper a day. The RDA was established for men and women of all ages at 900 µg of copper a day.

The EAR and RDA for pregnancy were calculated to meet the needs of the mother and growing fetus. The EAR for pregnancy in a 14- to 18-year-old is 785 µg of copper a day. For older pregnant women, the EAR is 800 µg of copper a day. The RDAs are the same for all pregnant women, 1,000 µg of copper a day.

For breast-feeding women, values include what the women themselves needed, plus enough copper to replace the amount secreted in human milk. The EAR for lactating females 14 to 18 years of age is 985 µg of copper a day. For other ages, it is 1,000 µg of copper a day. The RDA for lactating women of all ages is 1,300 µg of copper a day.[10]

Considering that most people in the United States get enough copper in the diet, supplements are usually unnecessary.

Treating copper deficiency involves much more copper. Severe copper deficiency, enough to cause serious symptoms, will usually be treated in the hospital with intravenous copper, especially in patients who may have trouble absorbing oral copper. This is the case in many patients with copper deficiency. An example is 2.4 mg of intravenous copper a day for about a week. This would be followed by 8 mg of copper by mouth a day plus 2.4 mg intravenously once a week for as long as three months, followed by continued oral copper. These patients often also have other vitamin deficiencies.[18]

POTENTIAL SIDE EFFECTS

The immediate side effects of taking too much copper over the short term are in the gastrointestinal tract, and include nausea, vomiting, stomach cramps, abdominal pain, and diarrhea. If the level of copper is not very high, people can get used to it, and symptoms disappear. These side effects have been used by the EPA and WHO to set safe copper levels for drinking water.[23] There are groups of people known who consumed anywhere from around 3 to 10 mg a day from their water supplies without any symptoms.[10]

There are no good studies of long-term copper toxicity from too much copper intake. There have been some studies of excess copper intake, for example, during a five-month period. One study showed that there might be a detrimental effect to some parts of the immune system when too much copper is taken, 7 to 7.8 mg a day of added copper. The authors of this study also stated that based on their previous work, low copper intake has similar effects on the immune system.[13]

The long-term effects of excess copper are known from cases of hereditary defects in some part of the system of copper regulation in the body. There are three of these—Wilson's disease, Indian childhood cirrhosis, and idiopathic copper toxicosis. With Indian childhood cirrhosis and idiopathic copper toxicosis, both high copper intake along with the genetic factors are necessary for damage to occur. In these three conditions, copper damages the liver. It can also damage the nervous system and kidneys.

People consuming 10 mg of copper a day do not demonstrate liver damage. The World Health Organization considers the upper safe limit of copper to be 10 to 12 mg a day. The IOM set the upper limit at 10 mg of copper a day in adults. Infants should not get more iron than this in their diet. Children's safe upper limit is decreased in the same proportion as the RDA. The UL for 1 to 3 years of age is 1 mg a day, between 9 to 13 years it is 5 mg a day.

People known to have one of the inherited defects should not take copper supplements. The only group that may get more than the UL from food and drinking water in the United States is young children, but this is unlikely.[10]

Interactions

Many metals interact with each other. Too much zinc and too much iron can cause copper deficiency. Other metals as well as other micronutrients can interact with copper.[6]

Antacids may decrease copper absorption.

Copper can be bound by penicillamine and trientine, both of which are used in treating Wilson's disease.

Ethambutol can also bind or chelate copper. This may occur in the retina at the back of the eye.

Copper levels have been noted to be affected by a number of anticonvulsants, antipsychotics, water pills, nifedipine, and birth control pills. AZT may lower copper levels.[6]

There are other potential interactions that have not been well documented or studied.

FACT VERSUS FICTION

The human body regulates copper metabolism very tightly. There are multiple ways that copper is maintained in a specific range. It is unusual for people to become copper deficient or accumulate excess copper enough to cause any damage under normal conditions. Because of this tight control, it is unlikely that copper supplementation will change the amount of copper available in the body.

The evidence for many conditions seems to show that too much copper is more of a problem than too little. Excess copper is implicated in many neuro-degenerative disorders, for example, like Alzheimer's disease and Parkinson's disease.

People with inborn genetic defects in the copper regulatory system can have either excess or deficiency, both with serious if not lethal effects.

Individuals who have difficulty with absorption of nutrients can become copper deficient. Anyone in that category should be under medical supervision, because multiple vitamin and mineral deficiencies are common.

The intense interest in copper metabolism in the body and inside cells is leading to new ways to look at this metal. Future therapies involving copper may be based more on regulating copper than just taking it as a supplement.

REFERENCES

1. Houwen, RHJ. Copper: Two sides of the same coin. *Neth J Med.* 2008;66(8): 325–326.
2. Field, LS, Luk, E, Culotta, VC. Copper chaperones: Personal escorts for metal ions. *J Bioenerg Biomembr.* 2002;34(5):373–379.
3. Prohaska, JR. Role of copper transporters in copper homeostasis. *Am J Clin Nutr.* 2008;88(3):826S–829S.
4. Easter, RN, Chan, Q, Lai, B, et al. Vascular metallomics: Copper in the vasculature. *Vasc Med.* 2010;15(1):61–69.
5. Desai, V, Kaler, SG. Role of copper in human neurological disorders. *Am J Clin Nutr.* 2008;88:855S–858S.
6. Natural Standard Research Collaboration. Medline Plus. Copper. 2009. http://www.nlm.nih.gov/medlineplus/druginfo/natural/patient-copper.html. Accessed March 2, 2010.
7. Kessler, H, Pajonk, FG, Bach, D, et al. Effect of copper intake on CSF parameters in patients with mild Alzheimer's disease: A pilot phase 2 clinical trial. *J Neural Transm.* 2008;115:1651–1659.
8. Arnesano, F, Scintilla, S, Calo, V, et al. Copper-triggered aggregation of ubiquitin. *PLoS ONE.* 2009;4(9):e7052. doi:10.1371/journal.pone.0007052.
9. Lee, JC, Gray, HB, Winkler, JR. Copper (II) binding to r-Synuclein, the Parkinson's protein. *J Am Chem Soc.* 2008;130:6898–6899.
10. Institute of Medicine. Food and Nutrition Board. *Dietary reference intakes for vitamin A, vitamin K, arsenic, boron, chromium, copper, iodine, iron, manganese, molybdenum, nickel, silicon, vanadium, and zinc.* Washington, DC: National Academies Press, 2001.
11. Zheng, Y, Li, XK, Wang, Y, Cai, L. The role of zinc, copper and iron in the pathogenesis of diabetes and diabetic complications: Therapeutic effects by chelators. *Hemoglobin.* 2008;32(1–2):135–145.
12. Cooper, GJ, Young, AA, Gamble, GD, et al. A copper (II)-selective chelator ameliorates left-ventricular hypertrophy in type 2 diabetic patients: A randomised placebo-controlled study. *Diabetologia.* 2009;52(4):715–722.

13. Turnlund, JR, Jacob, RA, Keen, CL, et al. Long-term high copper intake: Effects on indexes of copper status, antioxidant status, and immune function in young men. *Am J Clin Nutr.* 2004;79:1037–1044.
14. Herman, CJ, Allen, P, Hunt, WC, et al. Use of complementary therapies among primary care clinic patients with arthritis. *Preventing Chronic Disease.* 2004;1(4):1–15.
15. Zoli, A, Altomonte, L, Caricchio, R, et al. Serum zinc and copper in active rheumatoid arthritis: Correlation with interleukin 1 beta and tumour necrosis factor alpha. *Clin Rheumatol.* 1998;17(5):378–382.
16. Omoto, A, Kuwahito, Y, Prudovksy, I, et al. Copper chelation with tetrathiomolybdate suppresses adjuvant-induced arthritis and inflammation-associated cachexia in rats. *Arthritis Res Ther.* 2005;7(6):R1174–R1182.
17. Redman, BG, Esper, P, Pan, Q, et al. Phase II trial of tetrathiomolybdate in patients with advanced kidney cancer. *Clin Cancer Res.* 2003;9(5):1666–1672.
18. Griffith, DP, Liff, D, Ziegler, TR, et al. Acquired copper deficiency: A potentially serious and preventable complication following gastric bypass surgery. *Obesity (Silver Spring).* 2009;17(4):827–831.
19. Kumar, N. Copper deficiency myelopathy (human swayback). *Mayo Clin Proc.* 2006;81(10):1371–1384.
20. Olivares, M, Mendez, MA, Astudillo, PA, Pizarro, F. Present situation of biomarkers for copper status. *Am J Clin Nutr.* 2008;88(Suppl):859S–862S.
21. Kaler, SG, Holmes, CS, Goldstein, DS, et al. Neonatal diagnosis and treatment of Menkes' disease. *N Engl J Med.* 2008;358:605–614.
22. Shim, H, Harris, ZL. Genetic defects in copper metabolism. *J. Nutr.* 2003; 133:1527S–1531S.
23. Araya, M, Olivares, M, Pizarro, F. Community-based randomized double-blind study of gastrointestinal effects and copper exposure in drinking water. *Environ Health Perspect.* 2004;112:1068–1073.

9

Creatine

BRIEF OVERVIEW

Creatine is a "nonprotein nitrogen" molecule that is produced by the body and also consumed in a normal diet. It is found mainly in skeletal muscle where it helps generate energy for cells.

As such, it is used by athletes and bodybuilders who want to produce stronger muscles and improve their performance. Creatine is being used in hopes of increasing lean muscle mass and exercise capacity. It is one of the most commonly used supplements, accounting for hundreds of millions of dollars in sales every year.

Creatine has been used to prevent weak muscles and frailty in older people. It may also be beneficial in certain hereditary diseases that cause muscle wasting.

Creatine has not been banned for competitive athletes, so it is not on the latest World Anti-Doping Agency (WADA) Prohibited List.[1] The International Society of Sports Nutrition reviewed the literature on creatine extensively and came to conclusions on the safety and efficacy of creatine. Its official position has included the following statements:

"Creatine monohydrate is the most effective ergogenic nutritional supplement currently available to athletes."

"There is no scientific evidence that the short- or longterm use of creatine monohydrate has any detrimental effects on otherwise healthy individuals."

"If proper precautions and supervision are provided, supplementation in young athletes is acceptable."[2]

THE HYPE

Creatine Is a Performance Enhancer

Creatine increases high-intensity training capacity as well as increasing lean body mass when it is taken during training. There is very good evidence that creatine improves the ability to do high-intensity exercise when it is of short duration.[3] This is anaerobic exercise. Creatine increases stored glycogen, at least during loading.[3]

When creatine is taken in conjunction with an exercise regimen, significant increases in lean muscle mass occur. A meta-analysis of 96 studies demonstrated an average increase of 2.2 kg of lean body mass over 12 weeks. This does not occur in the absence of exercise.[3]

Greater muscle retention of creatine may occur if carbohydrates and/or protein are added; it is not clear if this will improve performance. No form of creatine has been proven more effective than creatine monohydrate.[2]

Hundreds of studies have shown the improvement in anaerobic capacity and increase in lean muscle mass that occurs when supplementation with creatine occurs during training. The average performance gain is between 10 and 15 percent. This includes improvements in power/strength, maximal effort muscle contractions, and single sprint performance. The increases in strength and performance have been seen in cycling, bench press, jump squat, sprinting, swimming, and soccer.

Over the long term, muscle creatine and phosphocreatine content increase; lean body mass increases; strength, power, and muscle diameter increase. Athletes taking creatine usually gain 2 to 4 pounds more muscle mass when training for anywhere from 4 to 12 weeks, compared to the athletes training but not taking creatine.[2]

Creatine Helps Reduce Frailty

Frailty syndrome in the elderly is marked by weakness, a feeling of exhaustion, slow walking, limited physical activity, and weight loss (unintentional). Frail elderly are at risk for falls, fractures, disability, and death. Another related condition is called sarcopenia, which is a decrease in skeletal muscle mass due to aging.

Some small, short-term studies have shown increase in strength and lean body mass in elderly given creatine, usually along with an exercise program. The subjects of most studies have been healthy. More studies are definitely warranted.[4] Although trials are ongoing, results continue to be mixed.[5]

Is Usage in Child and Teenage Athletes Safe?

There are not really any studies examining the safety of creatine for child or teenage athletes. Children with various inherited disorders (see below) have been treated with creatine for many years without any harmful effects.[2]

Young athletes do take creatine, sometimes in higher than recommended doses. Surveys have shown that children as young as 10 years old may already be taking creatine. Use of creatine goes up with age. Between 25 and 78 percent of college athletes take creatine. It is important for athletes to know how much creatine to take, and to make sure they are taking creatine only and not a mixture with other unsafe ingredients.[6]

Creatine Helps Treat Certain Inherited Disorders of the Nervous System and Muscular System

Huntington's disease is a genetic disorder leading to extensive nervous system damage. Cellular energy metabolism is definitely abnormal in this condition, which may involve the creatine and creatine kinase system (see "Mechanism of Action"). It has been hypothesized that creatine supplementation might improve the energy metabolism in this disease. In lab animals with models of Huntington's disease, this is very successful. Few trials have been carried out in humans. However, there is enough information that some believe a large-scale trial in humans is warranted.[3]

Problems with the creatine/creatine kinase system have also been found in animal models of amyotrophic lateral sclerosis (ALS) and Alzheimer's disease.

There are a number of inherited diseases that cause muscle wasting or dysfunction, including Duchenne muscular dystrophy. There is some evidence that creatine supplementation can improve muscular strength in these diseases.[3]

There are other inherited disorders of mitochondrial function that might respond to creatine supplementation.

Inborn Errors of Creatine Synthesis and Transport

There are two proteins that catalyze the synthesis of creatine, and one transport protein. There are a number of rare, genetic defects in these proteins needed for creatine synthesis. In these conditions, the deficiency of creatine in the brain is marked and probably causes the majority of symptoms, which can include mental retardation, developmental delay, seizures, and movement disorders.

There is no treatment for the defect in the transporter protein. The disorders of synthesis can be improved by supplemental creatine. However, since time elapses after birth, before the symptoms appear and the diagnosis is made, treated children still have significant neurologic impairment. Recently, in two cases, siblings of children already diagnosed with the deficiency were themselves diagnosed at birth and treated immediately. These two children seem to be developing normally.[3]

Inflammatory Muscle Diseases

Dermatomyositis and polymyositis are inflammatory, autoimmune diseases; people with these conditions have muscular weakness. The weakness may be due to abnormal phosphocreatine levels and abnormal energy metabolism. Patients who have been treated with corticosteroids and other medicines can improve their strength by exercising. There is also evidence to show that creatine may be helpful in these disorders.

In one double-blind, randomized, controlled trial of 29 patients with dermatomyositis or polymyositis, six months of creatine therapy (20 g per day for eight days then 3 g per day) improved functional performance with no adverse effects.[7]

DEFICIENCY

Children with the above genetic defects manifest a type of creatine deficiency that seems to mainly affect the brain. The major neurologic deficits that occur with these genetic defects demonstrate the importance of creatine.

Vegetarians and the elderly can become relatively deficient in creatine; supplementation might improve their lean muscle mass and strength.

FOOD SOURCES

Creatine is abundant in meats and fish. It is very well absorbed from the diet. There is essentially no creatine in plant-derived food. Vegetarians ingest very little creatine; vegans get almost none.

For creatine to be made from the diet, three amino acids (glycine, arginine, methionine) must be present in large enough amounts. Vegetarians need to be sure to eat enough protein so they can synthesize creatine.

MECHANISM OF ACTION: HOW DOES IT WORK?

Creatine is a major contributor to energy metabolism in the human body. It is used by the enzyme creatine kinase to rephosphorylate ADP, making it ATP. These nucleotides (ADP, ATP) are the sources of energy for cells. Ninety-five percent of the creatine is found in skeletal muscle. The rest of the creatine is found in the testes, heart, and brain.[2,6]

People eating a normal diet ingest large amounts of creatine. It is also made by the liver, kidneys, and pancreas from the amino acids glycine, arginine, and methionine. Free creatine can be stored in muscle; two-thirds of the creatine is stored as phosphocreatine.

What is known as the "creatine pool" is usually around 120 g, although more can be stored.

The creatine pool is in equilibrium between creatine and phosphocreatine. Creatine kinase interconverts the two forms. It is phosphocreatine that donates its phosphate to ADP to make ATP. Creatine and phosphocreatine help move energy from ATP in the mitochondria (the cells' powerhouse) to the parts of the cells where energy is needed. This is how creatine gives energy to muscles during anaerobic activity.[3]

During muscle recovery, when exercise is done aerobically, creatine receives a new phosphate group. For brief, intense bursts of activity, phosphocreatine is the rate-limiting component. ATP is used up during the first second of anaerobic activity. Phosphocreatine can provide nine more seconds-worth of energy via its phosphate group.

Hydrogen ions are used when phosphocreatine gives up its phosphate. This eventually leads to the accumulation of lactic acid in the muscle. Lactic acid is responsible for the feelings of fatigue experienced during intense exercise.[6]

One to two percent of the creatine in the creatine pool is broken down every day; the end products leave the body via the urine. What is lost will be replaced by dietary creatine or manufactured from amino acids. The daily requirement is about 2 g half of which is ingested and half synthesized in the body.

Creatine and phosphocreatine are both broken down to creatinine. This is the form that is lost in the urine. It is important to understand what happens to creatine and creatinine. The excretion of creatinine in the urine is also a way to measure/ estimate kidney function. When the kidneys stop working well, less creatinine goes out in the urine, and the level of creatinine in the blood goes up. Many people see creatinine simply as a measure of kidney function.

However, the total amount of creatine in the body depends on age and sex. Young men ages 19 to 29 years old have the most skeletal muscle, the most creatine, and excrete the most creatinine in their urine, if they have normal kidney function. In general, women excrete 80 percent of what men excrete. Creatine declines with age, as does creatinine loss in the urine, not necessarily because of kidney dysfunction. This is why creatinine in the blood and urine, and the clearance of creatinine from the body, have to be evaluated along with what is normal for a person's age and gender.[3]

Creatine is synthesized from three amino acids—glycine, arginine, and methionine. It is not entirely clear where all the steps in the synthesis occur. They may take place in multiple locations. It is believed that most take place in the liver and kidney. There is essentially no synthesis of creatine in muscle where it is needed. There is a transporter that moves creatinine into muscle, brain, and other parts of the body.[3]

PRIMARY USES

Athletes and Bodybuilders

- Athletes usually start with a loading dose for 5 days, followed by a maintenance dose.[2] There may be ways to increase the amount of creatine that gets into muscle. Increasing carbohydrate intake may do that, but a large amount is needed. Exercise is a much better way to increase creatine uptake into muscles.[3]

To Prevent Deficiency or Normalize Muscle Mass

- Vegetarians can take creatine. Older people trying to maintain muscle mass can also take creatine. It is so safe that it is reasonable to try as a way to build muscle.

COMMON DOSAGES

The daily requirement for creatine is about 2 g, with half coming from dietary sources and half made in the body.

The protocol for athletes is 0.3 g of creatine/kg/day of creatine monophosphate for five to seven days, then 3 to 5 g a day.[2] This usually means a loading dose of 20 g per day (in four divided doses) for five days, and then the maintenance dose of anywhere from 2 to 5 g a day. Five days of creatine loading are needed to get the desired improvement in anaerobic power and muscle strength.[8]

Most of the studies on the effects of creatine have used creatine monophosphate. It is also available in formulations with other added ingredients that are said to increase the effect of creatine. Some examples are creatine plus glycerol plus glutamine, creatine plus beta-alanine, and creatine plus beta-hydroxy-beta-methylbutyrate. It is possible that any of these as well as other formulations may turn out to be more effective in increasing lean body mass. However, at the current time, there is not enough information to recommend them; they are also more costly.[2]

There is another form, creatine ethyl ester, said to increase the bioavailability of creatine. In at least one study, the opposite appeared to be true, since the ester was less effective than the monohydrate.[9]

Caffeine as well as carbohydrates may increase tissue uptake of creatine.[10]

POTENTIAL SIDE EFFECTS

The main side effects of creatine consumption are gastrointestinal, including diarrhea, which may be dependent on dose.[11] Stomach pain and nausea are also reported, as are muscle cramps. Dividing the dose helps reduce these symptoms.

There have been anecdotal reports of serious reactions to creatine. In 1998 there was a case of one person with kidney disease whose kidney function may have worsened due to creatine. However, during hundreds of studies there has been no indication of kidney damage or dysfunction due to creatine supplementation.[2]

There has also been speculation that creatine may alter thermoregulation adversely. A number of deaths of athletes (wrestlers) during the 1990s due to heat exhaustion were attributed to creatine. Investigation (by the Centers for Disease Control) indicated that creatine was not a causative factor in the deaths.[12]

Since that time there have been many studies that show creatine does not alter thermoregulatory performance, including regulation of body temperature or hydration. For example, 12 active males, in a double-blind, randomized, crossover-design study took creatine or placebo for a week. They then exercised until they lost 2 percent of body mass (dehydration), followed by an exercise heat-tolerance test in a hot, humid room. After a wash-out period the placebo and creatine group were switched. There were no subjective or objective signs of compromised hydration or thermoregulation from the creatine.[13]

A subsequent meta-analysis of available studies on creatine and thermoregulation, performed in 2009, found no evidence that creatine alters thermoregulation in the short term, although there were no trials that included exercise of long duration. It was suggested that studies of athletes in game-simulation situations might be appropriate.[14]

Some side effects may be due to taking an excessive amount of creatine, and/or the concurrent use of other performance-enhancing supplements. Athletes are encouraged not to take more than the usual amounts of creatine.[12]

In one study of college football players taking creatine and followed for 21 months, there were no significant changes in laboratory tests (blood and urine) that are markers of health.[15] Most follow-up has only been for between two and five years. However, there is one group of patients that has been receiving creatine for atrophy of parts of the eye since 1981, with no long-term adverse effects.[2]

FACT VERSUS FICTION

Creatine is a safe and effective ergogenic nutritional supplement. Athletes looking to increase their lean body mass and improve their performance can take it in recommended doses with few side effects. It is not prohibited at any level of competition. Some believe it is similar to carbohydrate loading or hydration.

There are many trials looking at the therapeutic benefits of creatine in a number of rare conditions. It certainly appears safe, but it is unclear how much help it can be.

Anyone with a serious medical problem who wants to try creatine supplements should discuss this with his or her doctor.

REFERENCES

1. World Anti-Doping Agency Prohibited List 2010. http://www.wadaama.org/Documents/World_Anti-Doping_Program/WADP-Prohibited-list/WADA_Prohibited_List_2010_EN.pdf. Accessed April 30, 2010.
2. Buford, TW, Kreider, RB, Stout, JR, et al. International Society of Sports Nutrition position stand: Creatine supplementation and exercise. *Journal of the International Society of Sports Nutrition.* 2007;4:6.
3. Brosnan, JT, Brosnan, ME. Creatine: Endogenous metabolite, dietary, and therapeutic supplement. *Annu Rev Nutr.* 2007;27:241–261.
4. Cherniack, EP, Florez, HJ, Troen, BR. Emerging therapies to treat frailty syndrome in the elderly. *Altern Med Rev.* 2007;12(3):246–258.
5. Dalbo, VJ, Roberts, MD, Lockwood, CM, et al. The effects of age on skeletal muscle and the phosphocreatine energy system: Can creatine supplementation help older adults? *Dynamic Medicine.* 2009;8:6.
6. Calfee, R, Fadale, P. Popular ergogenic drugs and supplements in young athletes. *Pediatrics.* 2006;117:e577–e589.
7. Chung, Y-L, Alexanderson, H, Pipitone, N, et al. Creatine supplements in patients with idiopathic inflammatory myopathies who are clinically weak after conventional pharmacologic treatment: Six-month, double-blind, randomized, placebo-controlled trial. *Arthritis & Rheumatism (Arthritis Care & Research).* 2007;57(4):694–702.
8. Law, YL, Ong, WS, GillianYap, TL, Lim, SC, Von Chia, E. Effects of two and five days of creatine loading on muscular strength and anaerobic power in trained athletes. *J Strength Cond Res.* 2009;23(3):906–914.
9. Spillane, M, Schoch, R, Cooke, M, et al. The effects of creatine ethyl ester supplementation combined with heavy resistance training on body composition, muscle performance, and serum and muscle creatine levels. *Journal of the International Society of Sports Nutrition.* 2009;6:6.
10. Salomons, GS, Wyss, M, Jakobs, C. Creatine. In: Coates, PM. (Ed). *Encyclopedia of dietary supplements.* New York: Marcel Dekker, 2005, 151–158.

11. Ostojic, SM, Ahmetovic, Z. Gastrointestinal distress after creatine supplementation in athletes: Are side effects dose dependent? *Res Sports Med.* 2008; 16(1):15–22.
12. Sarubin-Fragakis, A, Thomson, C. Creatine. *The health professional's guide to popular dietary supplements.* 3rd edition. Chicago: American Dietetic Association, 2007.
13. Watson, G, Casa, DJ, Fiala, KA, et al. Creatine use and exercise heat tolerance in dehydrated men. *Journal of Athletic Training.* 2006;41(1):18–29.
14. Lopez, RM, Casa, DJ, McDermott, BP, et al. Does creatine supplementation hinder exercise heat tolerance or hydration status? A systematic review with meta-analyses. *Journal of Athletic Training.* 2009;44(2):215–223.
15. Kreider, RB, Melton, C, Rasmussen, CJ, et al. Long-term creatine supplementation does not significantly affect clinical markers of health in athletes. *Molecular and Cellular Biochemistry.* 2003;244:95–104.

10

D-Ribose

BRIEF OVERVIEW

D-ribose is a simple sugar that can be found in all living things. It is a key part of ribonucleic acid (RNA), a polymer responsible for transcribing DNA, the genetic blueprint. Transcription means translating DNA into actual proteins and other cellular components.

D-ribose can be phosphorylated, and then become part of ATP and other compounds that transport energy. It is also part of a number of coenzymes and vitamins, such as riboflavin.

It is hard to overstate how important D-ribose is in the body. Every cell needs it to function.

However, it is not hard to find. Not only does it occur in basically everything that humans eat, it can also be made from glucose and other compounds in the body. D-ribose itself can be used and recycled.

THE HYPE

Most of the news about D-ribose has to do with the way it brings energy to a cell, muscle, heart, or person. As a supply of energy, it could theoretically be useful for many conditions. To understand how D-ribose works, a person needs to know a little bit of biochemistry. If the following seems difficult to understand, skip the parts in italics. Anyone who wants to understand more can read the whole chapter (please see "Mechanism of Action" for more information). When looking at an advertisement for D-ribose as an energy enhancer, you will see some of these terms in use.

Since ribose becomes part of ATP, and ATP is the energy carrier of the cell, extra ribose might translate into extra energy. *However, the way energy is extracted from ATP is by breaking the bond between two phosphate groups. The part of the molecule containing ribose is inert. Therefore, ribose does not directly contribute energy.* The question is whether or not extra ribose will somehow cause more ATP to be produced.

How would extra ribose work? In some situations, such as impaired blood supply to the heart muscle, ATP levels decline. *ATP can be degraded. In that case, many of its constituent parts can be washed out of the cell. It then becomes more difficult to regenerate* ATP. ATP levels also decline in muscle cells with strenuous activity.

Can Large Doses of D-Ribose Be Safe?

Giving supplements of D-ribose has been shown under laboratory conditions to help regenerate ATP in both cardiac muscle and skeletal muscle. There has been some concern that using ribose in this way might lead to unwanted metabolic results, such as a decrease in glucose or an increase in purine metabolites. Purine metabolites are byproducts of ATP generation. The best known is probably uric acid.

To look at the metabolism of extra D-ribose, a study was done giving D-ribose to healthy volunteers, 10 in total, of varying ages. They received oral doses of ribose, 0, 2, 5, and 10 g dissolved in water. There were 24 hours in between each dose.

After the ribose was ingested, blood levels of insulin, glucose, lactate, and uric acid were measured at various intervals, from 0 to 120 minutes later. These particular substances could be affected by increasing ribose levels.

The subjects experienced no adverse effects. Glucose levels fell in all cases and then returned to baseline. *Insulin rose a little corresponding to the decrease in glucose values. The older age group (40 to 50 years of age) had slightly higher increases of insulin. Lactate both rose and fell differently in each age group, but these levels were all normal.* Uric acid levels did increase in all cases, but they were still within normal limits.

The investigators concluded that the doses of D-ribose they tested were safe and well tolerated in healthy people.[1]

Another study looked at the effects of D-ribose ingestion over a 14-day period. Nineteen healthy adults took in 20 g of D-ribose a day. *There were no adverse effects seen in blood cells at 7 or 14 days.* Glucose trended slightly down. Uric acid went up slightly, and back down by day 14, *as did certain liver function tests. Slight abnormalities observed on day 7 were either back to pretest levels or close to that on day 14. None were in the abnormal range.* The researchers noted that other investigators have also found the trend toward low blood sugar values (hypoglycemia) and slightly elevated uric acid levels.[2] None of the volunteers experienced side effects.

Ischemic Heart Disease and Congestive Heart Failure

D-ribose has been shown in animal studies to help the heart recover from lack of oxygen (ischemia). In this situation, where the blood flow has been decreased to the heart, ATP levels plummet. Giving the animals D-ribose helps the heart muscle recover more quickly.[3]

The heart goes through two phases, systole and diastole. The contraction in systole is followed by a relaxation during diastole. Although D-ribose helps ischemic heart muscle recovery, ATP does not need to be completely returned to normal for systolic heart function. Diastole, even though it is a relaxation, is energy dependent and ATP is needed for this as well. Depending on the length of time that the heart muscle is deprived of oxygen, as ATP drops, damage goes from reversible to irreversible. Systolic function can be reversed more easily than diastolic function. However, when ischemia lasts long enough, no recovery is possible and the heart muscle dies.

D-ribose is not used directly by the heart. However, it can help replenish ATP. Tests on humans with severe coronary artery disease who show signs of ischemia on cardiograms during treadmill exercise can walk farther without chest pain or cardiogram changes if they are given D-ribose.

In humans with cardiomyopathy, the heart muscle does not work well. In a rat model of cardiomyopathy, D-ribose improves the heart muscle's ability to work. D-ribose can also help living heart muscle work better after the recent death of adjacent heart muscle.

From a variety of animal and human tests, D-ribose shows promise in limiting damage and aiding recovery of heart muscle that has had a lack of oxygen supply.[3]

A key study published in 2003 showed that D-ribose improved both diastolic function and quality of life in patients with congestive heart failure. This study included 15 patients with coronary heart disease and congestive heart failure. It was a double-blind, randomized trial with crossover, so that both groups eventually received the D-ribose. Improvements in heart function were seen on echocardiography, a test with sound waves like a sonogram. In this study, 5 g of D-ribose was given three times a day and there were no adverse effects.[4]

While it seems clear that D-ribose can improve ATP stores that may be depleted in ischemic myocardium, it is not equally clear how much actual improvement is made in the cardiac muscle. In one study, investigators stressed myocardium with a drug called dobutamine, to see if D-ribose would improve the contraction of healthy myocardium when given dobutamine. They also looked at whether or not intravenous D-ribose could reduce ischemia of the cardiac muscle under the dobutamine stress.

This was a randomized, double-blind, crossover trial comparing the effects of D-ribose on cardiac wall movement in 26 patients with ischemic cardiomyopathy, which means damaged heart muscle due to insufficient blood supply. These patients already had damaged hearts. Echocardiograms (using sound, like sonograms) were checked before treatment, after D-ribose or placebo injection, and during each increasing dose of dobutamine. Patients were watched overnight and switched into the other group on day two. The result showed that intravenous D-ribose was able to improve the contraction of some of the heart muscle segments that were already abnormal when stressed with dobutamine. These are called "hibernating" areas that are alive but damaged.

Dobutamine testing is often done to decide if patients have enough healthy heart muscle to benefit from having coronary bypass or other procedures to improve blood supply. Dobutamine alone may miss the hibernating areas. D-ribose can be used as a diagnostic aid to help find these areas. Dobutamine is also used to help a damaged heart pump more blood, at some risk. D-ribose may minimize the risk by keeping ATP levels high. Although D-ribose did not reduce stress-induced ischemia in this study, the length of time that D-ribose was administered was short, 4.5 hours. Giving D-ribose over a longer period might have a different result. This indicates the need for further testing.[5]

D-Ribose Is Used by Bodybuilders for Extra Energy and Endurance

Studies of D-ribose use for energy and/or endurance have had mixed results. Although a number of studies in animals and humans have indicated that administering ribose allows muscle to regain high levels of ATP after the levels have been lowered during exercise, there is very little proof that this translates into extra strength, energy, or endurance. There are minimal concerns about D-ribose lowering glucose, which it does to a small degree, and raising uric acid, which it also does to some degree.

D-ribose has been tested in many animals and shown to increase the rates of ATP recovery after muscular effort. In one study of rat muscle, perfusing the skeletal muscle with ribose allows ATP levels to recover quickly after exercise.[6] However, even very high concentrations of ribose did not translate into increased muscular strength.

One placebo-controlled study of healthy male volunteers doing maximal exercise (dynamic knee extensions) was undertaken to investigate the effect of ribose ingestion. The participants took 16 g of ribose (four doses of 4 g) a day or placebo. They were tested before and after a variety of repeated knee extensions and rest periods. The participants given ribose did not perform in any way different from the volunteers who got the placebo. Under these conditions there were no differences in blood values of uric acid between those who got the ribose and those who did not. In a separate part of the study, the volunteers did similar exercise with and without ribose and had muscle biopsies done. There was no significant difference between ATP or other related chemicals between the subjects who took ribose before exercise and those who did not. However, there was proof that the exercise was exhaustive and repetitive enough to raise levels of lactate and ammonia. These indicate that ATP was broken down. Extra ribose did not change any parameter that would be expected if it was increasing ATP synthesis. It also did not change the muscle power production of the subjects that took it. These investigators did not find an elevation of uric acid. There were no side effects due to the ribose.

These investigators stated, "In conclusion, oral ribose supplementation at 16 g (4 doses at 4 g each) per day does not beneficially impact muscle ATP recovery and muscle force and power output during repeated days of maximal intermittent exercise training." They suggested a much higher dose might be beneficial, but that it would be hard to get ribose levels as high as those in test animals using oral ribose.[7]

A study after this one had volunteers cycling for multiple training sessions over two seven-day periods. The ribose was administered after a training session, 200 mg/kg after the session and then with each meal for three days, for a total of nine times. These investigators found increased levels of ATP in muscle biopsies. They stated that, "oral intake of ribose in humans after 1 wk of high-intensity training leads to an enhanced resynthesis of ATP, suggesting that a limiting factor for the rate of resynthesis of ATP is the availability of ribose." These investigators found the increased ATP 72 hours after exercise, whereas the previous investigators only biopsied at 24 hours. However, there was still no improvement in muscle performance.[8]

One placebo-controlled study of 16 healthy young men given ribose or placebo while doing high-intensity cycle sprints showed an increase in power in the men given ribose. This study suggested that D-ribose may provide an ergogenic effect.[9] Studies like this one are the reason that bodybuilders and athletes take D-ribose. It is also very safe, and not off limits for athletes.

Another study found that D-ribose offered no improvement in anaerobic exercise capacity or metabolic markers in highly trained athletes. These subjects took 5 g of D-ribose twice a day. There was also no change in uric acid and glucose.[10]

Other investigators in 2006 used the dose of D-ribose suggested by the distributor (625 mg in this case) and found no change in performance.[11] Studies to date have fairly consistently showed an increase in ATP levels that do not translate into improved performance.

Chronic Fatigue Syndrome and Fibromyalgia

There has been one open study, as well as one case report that indicate D-ribose may help for either or both of these conditions.

The first was a case study of an individual patient in 2004, who suffered from fibromyalgia. D-ribose was added to her treatment with a decrease in her symptoms. It was postulated that the extra ATP that might be made could help increase her energy reserves and lessen symptoms.[12]

There has also been one open-label, uncontrolled pilot study of D-ribose in treating both fibromyalgia (FMS) and chronic fatigue syndrome (CFS). Both conditions may be associated with decreased energy metabolism at a cellular level. Forty-one patients were given D-ribose. The dose was 5 g, three times a day until a total of 280 g was taken.

Patients were assessed with questionnaires. Subjects were recruited by e-mail, from Web sites, and other sites with sources of information on FMS and CFS. Their diagnoses were self-reported. They were mailed the ribose with instructions. At the beginning and end of the study they were asked to rate themselves on a visual analog scale that included energy, sleep, mental clarity, pain, and sense of well-being. Thirty-six people completed the study. They reported significant improvements in energy levels, sleep patterns, pain, mental clarity, and state of well-being. They reported a positive feeling about the experiment.

There were a few nonspecific complaints. Three patients (not counted in the above) stopped the D-ribose because of anxiety, lightheadedness, and increased appetite. Of the 36 participants, one experienced brief nausea and another mild anxiety. Lowering the ribose dose relieved these symptoms.[13]

The authors of this study, while finding the results promising, did not see the need for randomized, controlled studies, and stated that such a study was underway. However, there has not yet been such a study published.

This kind of study is filled with bias, subject to the placebo effect. The patients were self-selected and never even met face-to-face with the researchers. This is not the kind of data that can be used to draw any conclusions about the usefulness of D-ribose.

Skin

ATP levels decline in aging skin. The levels drop in fibroblasts, which are important to maintaining youthful tone. It has been postulated that the decline in ATP may contribute to the appearance of aging. In culture, skin fibroblasts regenerate ATP and have increased rate of energy production when given D-ribose.

In a clinical study, 20 adult women used a facial lotion with 0.5 percent D-ribose. There was a reduction in the appearance of wrinkles at 14 days and further reduction at 28 days. This was said to be evaluated both subjectively, by the women using the lotion, and objectively by the investigators. No adverse effects were noted.[14]

DEFICIENCY

There is no deficiency disease involving D-ribose. Since it occurs in all foods and is manufactured in the human body, there cannot be a deficiency. The question is, are there circumstances when the body can use more than usual?

FOOD SOURCES

D-ribose exists in all living things. It is therefore in all plants and animals. It is also made in the human body.

MECHANISM OF ACTION: HOW DOES IT WORK?

D-ribose is a five-carbon sugar. It is a basic structure, a kind of building block, for every living cell and is involved in many critical cellular processes, from translating the genetic code to making energy.

Before it can be used, it must gain a phosphate group, a process called phosphorylation. It is then called D-ribose 5-phosphate. This can be used to make the amino acids tryptophan and histidine. It can also be used to make ATP. ATP transports energy around every cell. It has been called "the molecular unit of currency" in terms of energy transfer.

D-ribose becomes the backbone of RNA, ribonucleic acid. In all cells, DNA contains the genes, the code for everything in the cell. RNA helps translate the commands in the DNA into the actual molecules needed in the cells. Being part of RNA is one extremely important action of D-ribose.

RNA is made up of a chain of nucleotides. Each nucleotide has a unit of ribose, a phosphate group, and a nitrogenous base. Many units are strung together, usually into a single strand. DNA is the cell blueprint. It is transcribed, which can be thought of as a kind of translation, into RNA. RNA takes the information to the parts of the cell that make protein. The RNA can be read and the information will be translated into proteins. That is RNA's main role, to make sure DNA is translated correctly into the cell's needed proteins. RNA can also regulate DNA to a certain extent and influence which genes are actually translated.

An alternate pathway for glucose metabolism is the hexose monophosphate shunt. Glucose is converted into D-ribose-5-phosphate, and then into PPRP (1-phospho-D-ribose 1-pyrophosphate). Purine nucleotides are built onto PPRP. This is how they become nucleotides, including ATP and ADP as well as others. A number of the nucleotides are needed for RNA and others for DNA.

However, the heart muscle does not have an active hexose monophosphate shunt. It salvages degraded nucleotides and recycles them. Degraded nucleotides release free purines, which are reused.

When heart muscle is low on blood flow (ischemic), ATP is shuttled in the cells to help the contractile proteins. The oxygen deficit limits the electron transport chain. AMP and ADP rise because they cannot be rephosphorylated to ATP. AMP is degraded to inosine and hypoxanthine. These diffuse into the blood and are washed out when more blood flows to the heart. They are lost to the cells. Not only ATP is lost, but the amounts of other nucleotides, including GTP, CTP, UDP, and NAD are lowered. NAD and the triphosphates can be depressed even 60 minutes after blood flow returns. Hypoxanthine is metabolized to uric acid, which also takes energy from NADH. With ischemia it is reduced by xanthine oxidase (to uric acid), which produces oxygen free radicals and more damage. This leads to accumulation of fatty acids and other chemical shifts that cause more damage. Eventually it is irreversible. There are many strategies to try and replenish ADP and ATP and other nucleotides. The administration of D-ribose bypasses the hexose monophosphate shunt and gives the cells a new source for PPRP for AMP synthesis.

This idea has been tested with rat heart muscle and been successful. After moderate periods of ischemia (low blood flow and oxygen), there is a 50 to70 percent decrease in myocardial ATP. This stays depressed for hours to days after reperfusion. With supplemental D-ribose, ATP levels can return to normal in 12 hours instead of 72 hours. This has also been tested in dog hearts. Not only are ATP levels normal, but the heart muscle becomes functional again.[3]

PRIMARY USES

- At the current time, D-ribose is being used to treat certain patients with heart failure and ischemic heart disease due to coronary vascular disease. It is being used in clinical trials. People also take it on their own for heart health.
- It is being used to treat fibromyalgia and chronic fatigue syndrome.
- Athletes are taking supplements to improve their performance. D-ribose is marketed to bodybuilders and others looking to improve strength or endurance.
- D-ribose is also marketed for heart health and energy in generally healthy people.

COMMON DOSAGES

A commonly used dose is 5 g given two to three times a day used for mild heart failure as well as to improve athletic performance. Some trials have used less, some more, up to 20 g a day.

For energy in healthy people, 5 g is probably enough.

It has been suggested that 15 to 30 g is a good dose for people awaiting heart transplant in advanced heart failure, as well as patients with fibromyalgia.[15]

It is sold as a powder, capsule, bar, and chewable tablet. One supplement has 2,200 mg in a scoop. Another is a capsule with 850 mg and the directions to take two or three times a day. Yet another powder is to be dissolved in liquid and taken twice a day; each dose (scoop) has 4.5 g of D-ribose.

One company sells 850-mg capsules on sale at 100 capsules for $39.58, which is just under 40 cents a pill. The directions are to take two to six capsules a day, which would cost around 80 cents to $2.40. Other brands can cost twice that much.

POTENTIAL SIDE EFFECTS

There are no known serious side effects of D-ribose. In one study, participants took 5 g three times a day. Out of 36 individuals, one reported some anxiety and another reported some nausea. Both symptoms went away with a slight decrease in dose. People have reported lightheadedness with large doses.[15]

As has been noted, there can be a slight increase in uric acid with the use of D-ribose. This could be of concern in patients with gout, which is caused by elevated uric acid.

D-ribose does lower blood sugar. This needs to be kept in mind if used for diabetic patients, who can become hypoglycemic due to insulin or other medications. While the hypoglycemia from D-ribose is asymptomatic, if added to that caused by diabetic treatment, it could be potentially dangerous. For most people, taking it with fruit juice can help prevent the hypoglycemia.[15]

FACT VERSUS FICTION

D-ribose is a naturally occurring sugar with multiple important biological functions. It is critical to many bodily processes. It can be ingested in just about any food source. The body can also make D-ribose as well as recycle D-ribose.

It may be useful in treating patients with heart failure or with coronary vascular disease and impaired blood supply to the heart. In these cases it should be added to a regular medical regimen and not substituted. It should also be discussed with the health care provider.

It can also be used to treat fibromyalgia and chronic fatigue syndrome. It is extremely safe and may help relieve symptoms.

Athletes can certainly take it. It is not prohibited by any group. There are no conclusive studies about its effects. Any athlete that wants to try it can be assured that it is safe but cannot be told that it will definitely improve performance.

It may also help reduce wrinkles when used on the skin. Very little research has been done about this possibility.

REFERENCES

1. Fenstad, ER, Gazal, O, Shecterle, LM, et al. Dose effects of D-ribose on glucose and purine metabolites. *The Internet Journal of Nutrition and Wellness.* 2008;5(1):1–4.

2. Seifert, J, Frelich, A, Shecterle, L, St. Cyr, J. Assessment of hematological and biochemical parameters with extended D-ribose ingestion. *Journal of the International Society of Sports Nutrition.* 2008;5:13:1–5.

3. Pauly, DF, Pepine, CJ. D-Ribose as a supplement for cardiac energy metabolism. *J Cardiovasc Pharmacol Ther* 2000;5:249–258.

4. Omran, H, Illien, S, MacCarter, D, et al. D-ribose improves diastolic function and quality of life in congestive heart failure patients: A prospective feasibility study. *The European Journal of Heart Failure.* 2003;5:615–619.

5. Sawada, SG, Lewis, S, Kovaks, R, et al. Evaluation of the anti-ischemic effects of D-ribose during dobutamine stress echocardiography: A pilot study. *Cardiovascular Ultrasound* 2009;7:5. doi:10.1186/1476–7120–7–5.

6. Zarzeczny, R, Brault, JJ, Abraham, KA. Influence of ribose on adenine salvage after intense muscle contractions. *J Appl Physiol.* 2001;91:1775–1781.

7. Op't Eijnde, B, Van Leemputte, M, Brouns, F, et al. No effects of oral ribose supplementation on repeated maximal exercise and de novo ATP resynthesis. *J Appl Physiol.* 2001;91:2275–2281.

8. Hellsten, Y, Skadhauge, L, Bangsbo, J. Effect of ribose supplementation on resynthesis of adenine nucleotides after intense intermittent training in humans. *Am J Physiol Regul Integr Comp Physiol.* 2004;286:R182–R188.

9. Raue, U, Gallagher, PM, Williamson, DL, Godard, MP, Trappe, SW. Effects of ribose supplementation on performance during repeated high-intensity cycle sprints. *Medicine & Science in Sports & Exercise.* 2001;33(5):S44.

10. Kreider, RB, Melton, C, Greenwood, M, et al. Effects of oral D-ribose supplementation on anaerobic capacity and selected metabolic markers in healthy males. *Int J Sport Nutr Exerc Metab.* 2003;13(1):76–86.

11. Peveler, WW, Bishop, PA, Whitehorn, EJ. Effects of ribose as an ergogenic aid. *J Strength Cond Res.* 2006;20(3):519–522.

12. Gebhart, B, Jorgenson, JA. Benefit of ribose in a patient with fibromyalgia. *Pharmacotherapy.* 2004;24(11):1646–1648.

13. Teitelbaum, JE, Johnson, C, St. Cyr, J. The use of D-ribose in chronic fatigue syndrome and fibromyalgia: A pilot study. *The Journal of Alternative and Complementary Medicine.* 2006;12(9):857–862.

14. Shecterle, LM, St. Cyr, JA. Dermal benefits of topical D-ribose. *Clinical, Cosmetic and Investigational Dermatology.* 2009;2:151–152.

15. Sinatra, ST, Roberts, JC, Zucker, M. *Reverse heart disease now.* Hoboken, NJ: John Wiley & Sons, 2007.

11

Folic Acid

BRIEF OVERVIEW

Folic acid is the name given to the synthetic form of folate, one of the water-soluble B vitamins. It was identified some 70 years ago as a substance that could prevent anemia during pregnancy. Folate was ultimately extracted from spinach leaves, and its chemical structure identified.

Folate is essential for normal cellular growth because it has an indispensable role in DNA synthesis. When cells are growing and dividing quickly, such as during pregnancy, folate is even more important. Folate also helps maintain normal levels of the amino acid homocysteine. While homocysteine is needed in order to make proteins, elevated levels of homocysteine have been implicated in a wide variety of disease processes, from cardiovascular disease to cancer.

Many of folic acid's actions are well understood, and indications for its use are clear. An example of this is the anemia caused by low folate levels. In other disease states, the role of folic acid has not yet been proven.

THE HYPE

The Homocysteine Hypothesis

In many studies, elevated blood levels of homocysteine have consistently been observed in patients with cardiovascular disease. This includes coronary artery disease leading to heart attacks and disease of the blood vessels to the brain, which can cause a stroke. This raises the question, is homocysteine causing any of these problems?

Many other conditions have been associated with cardiovascular disease and have been found to contribute to the damage. High blood pressure, for example, is not only associated with cardiovascular disease but also worsens it. Controlling high blood pressure can reduce the injury to blood vessels. In the same way, lowering

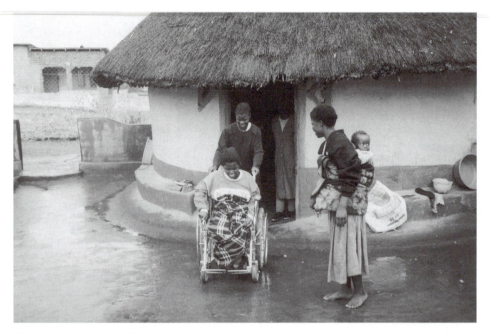

This photo taken in 2003 provided by the March of Dimes shows a young woman with spina bifida living in a rural village in South Africa. The child on the woman's back at right belongs to the woman in the wheelchair. That child was helped to be born healthy because the woman with spina bifida took the B vitamin folic acid beginning before pregnancy. About 8 million children worldwide are born every year with a serious birth defect, many of whom die or are disabled—a stunning and largely hidden toll, says research released by the March of Dimes. The report found that while birth defects are underappreciated globally, most occur in poor countries, where babies can languish with problems easily fixed or even prevented in wealthier nations. (AP Photo/March of Dimes)

elevated cholesterol can prevent or even help decrease existing fatty plaques that are clogging blood vessels.

However, it is not clear if homocysteine is just a marker for cardiovascular disease or is actually a risk factor that actually contributes to it. Most of the evidence is observational only—people with higher homocysteine levels have higher rates of cardiovascular disease.

Homocysteine could actually cause vascular injury in a number of ways. It has been observed that homocysteine can reduce the normal vasomotor function of the vascular endothelial cells that line the blood vessels, which would affect blood flow. Homocysteine may cause damage to coronary arteries directly and may cause platelets to clump, which can cause a clot.

Folate deficiency causes higher homocysteine levels. Administering folate, with or without other B vitamins, lowers homocysteine levels. The question then becomes, does lowering homocysteine levels actually decrease the risk of cardiovascular disease? This has to be decided by clinical trials.[1]

It must be kept in mind that different countries implemented folic acid fortification of grains and cereals at different times during the last 10 to 20 years. In the United States, fortification was in place by 1998. Most people eat enough grains and cereals that the average amount of folic acid ingested in this country significantly increased. Most of the observational studies were finished and reported in the mid- to late 1990s before fortification programs were started.

Cardiovascular Disease and Homocysteine

There have been studies using folate together with other B vitamins to lower homocysteine levels, in an attempt to decrease cardiovascular disease. In one trial (the NORVIT trial), 3,749 people who had just suffered heart attacks were randomized to receive vitamins—either 0.8 mg of folic acid, 0.4 mg B12, and 40 mg B6; 0.8 mg folic acid and 0.4 mg B12; 40 mg of B6; or placebo. They were followed for 40 months, looking for reoccurrence of a heart attack, a stroke, or sudden death from heart disease. Although homocysteine levels were lowered by an average of 27 percent in the patients given folic acid plus B12, there was no observed benefit. In the group given all three vitamins, there was a slightly increased risk of heart attack.[2]

The HOPE trial published results at the same time in 2006. More than 5,000 patients age 55 or older with vascular disease or diabetes received 2.5 mg of folic acid, 50 mg of B6, and 1 mg of vitamin B12, or placebo for five years. Investigators were looking for death from cardiovascular disease, heart attack, or stroke. Again, homocysteine levels were lowered, but the risk of major cardiovascular events was not.[3]

In 2008, the results were published of a trial involving more than 8,000 female health professionals at high risk for cardiovascular disease, called the Women's Antioxidant and Folic Acid Cardiovascular Study (WAFACS). The results were similar to those found in the HOPE study.[4]

Other studies were continuing during this time period. The SEARCH trial used 2 mg of folic acid plus 1 mg of vitamin B12 in a randomized, placebo-controlled trial involving more than 12,000 patients followed for 10 years. Homocysteine levels were lowered, but there were no observed benefits in terms of cardiovascular disease. These patients were also followed for cancer incidence, and it was not any higher in the treatment group than placebo group. The researchers in this study stated unequivocally that folic acid does not produce any beneficial effects as far as cardiovascular disease is concerned.[5]

It is possible that baseline folate levels in some of these studies could have been higher because of folic acid fortification of grains. Perhaps homocysteine levels and cardiovascular risk are only related when people are relatively deficient in folate.

Folic acid does not improve cardiovascular risk in subgroups of patients, such as those with chronic kidney failure. High-dose folic acid reduces homocysteine but not adverse cardiovascular events in this group.[6]

In at least one study, folate was found to act directly on the blood vessels (veins and arteries) to improve function. This was observed giving participants an amount of folate similar to what is found in normal dietary intake including fortified foods, with no increase in function found by giving higher levels of folic acid. This could

be an explanation for the observation that people with higher dietary intake of folate have lower incidence of cardiovascular disease, but high doses of folic acid do
not seem to affect risk.[7]

Stroke

The homocysteine hypothesis also applies to stroke. There are researchers who
believe that lowering homocysteine with folic acid supplements does lower the risk
of stroke. This is based on analysis of studies in which folic acid was given, and
stroke was one of the reported endpoints, for example, the HOPE trial.[3] Looking
just at stroke and not all cardiovascular events, some evidence in the studies does
seem to indicate folic acid may lower the risk of stroke. More research needs to
be done.[8,9]

Cancer

The relationship between folate and cancer has been called the "dual effect of
folate." Folate has been called a "dual modulator." This is because folate is needed
for both normal cell growth and cancer cell growth. While there is evidence that
higher folate levels can lower the incidence of cancer, there is also evidence that
supplemental folate can cause increased incidence of cancer. It has been suggested
that folate may be useful if there are absolutely no precancerous cells in the body,
but that if any precancerous lesions are there, excess folate may increase the incidence of cancer and the growth of cancer.[10]

There has been at least limited evidence found for a protective effect of folate,
possibly decreasing the incidence of breast, lung, pancreas, mouth, esophagus,
stomach, cervix, ovary, and certain other cancers. There have been a number of
good-quality studies allowing for larger analysis that seem to confirm the protective effect of folate against esophagus, stomach, and gastrointestinal cancers, and
to a lesser extent, breast cancer.[10]

Colorectal cancer has been studied the most. There had been consensus from
many trials, both case-control studies and prospective cohort studies, that higher
levels of folate consumption and higher levels of blood folate are associated with
lower risk of both colorectal cancer and the precancerous adenomatous polyp. The
scientific explanation is thought to be that folate is critical to cellular processes
like normal DNA synthesis; abnormalities of these processes can lead to cells becoming malignant.[10] The decrease in risk is not always apparent unless the study
follows participants at least 10 to 15 years.

However, some prospective studies have found a surprising increase in adenomas
(polyps) in patients given folic acid after detection and removal of a first polyp.
This takes some 6 to 8 years to be apparent.

It is possible that the dual effect, possible protection versus increasing incidence,
may have to do with timing as well as baseline folate levels. People free of any
cancerous or precancerous cells may gain protection from folate. Folic acid may
cause even tiny amounts of cancerous cells to grow and therefore folate supplements may increase the incidence of cancer in some groups. There may be factors

such as genetic variations in various enzymes and whether or not a person smokes, as well as many others factors that contribute to the dual outcomes.[10]

One 10-year trial showed no decrease in the incidence of colorectal polyps but rather a possible increase.[11]

It has been suggested that folic acid, which is not the natural form of folate, may be responsible for some of the negative effects of folate supplementation, like the increased risk of cancer. At high doses, folic acid itself appears in the blood, because the large amounts overwhelm the conversion of folic acid to 5-methyltetrahydrofolate.[10]

Looking at the larger population, the incidence of colorectal cancer in the United States, which was decreasing, started to rise again after the introduction of mandatory grain fortification that began in 1996 and was fully implemented by 1998. There is informed speculation that there may be a relationship between these two things.[12]

It is not yet possible to say whether or not folic acid can protect against colon cancer. It probably depends to some degree on individual, genetic factors and whether or not there are any small loci of early cancer already present.[13]

In one trial designed to evaluate the effect of folic supplementation on colon polyps, the data were also analyzed in regard to prostate cancer. In this study of approximately 700 men, folic acid supplementation was associated with a higher risk of prostate cancer, while higher dietary intake of folate as well as higher measured folate levels showed a possible association with a lower risk of prostate cancer.[14] However, this trial was not designed to evaluate prostate cancer risk.

In at least one study, there was an increased risk of breast cancer found in women taking folic acid supplements.[10]

A recent study showed that 40 percent of older adults in the United States have unmetabolized folic acid in their blood, considered a possible cancer risk.[15]

Alzheimer's Disease

The homocysteine hypothesis also applies to central nervous system functions. Most studies have not shown an improvement in cognitive function with folate supplementation, even when homocysteine levels are lowered. However, an analysis of cognitive function as a secondary endpoint in the FACIT trial, which was set up to evaluate the effects of folic acid on cardiovascular endpoints, did find a beneficial effect of folate on sensitive cognitive function tests. In this study, approximately 800 people were randomized to take either 800 μg of folic acid or placebo for three years, and those who took folic acid performed better on a number of tests.[16]

In some studies, a low folate level has been a risk factor for dementia. On the other hand, elderly patients given folic acid who are low in B12 can manifest a number of neurologic abnormalities (see "Cautions" below). These include problems with memory and cognition.[9] On an individual level, knowing B12 and folate levels and taking both supplements if needed is best. But in terms of fortifying food and recommending general supplementation, it is impossible to know who might need B12.

Depression

There is some evidence that low folate levels are associated with depression, and that administration of folic acid or other forms of folate may improve treatment results with antidepressants, or even mitigate the need for antidepressants in some individuals.[17]

Pregnancy

There is no question that low folate levels are related to fetal neural tube defects (see "Deficiency"). Low folate levels may also cause other problems during pregnancy. These may include other birth defects. Low folate has also been linked premature birth and low birth weight. There may also be a relationship between low folate levels and miscarriages, preeclampsia, and abruption of the placenta (detachment of the placenta).

While the risk of neural tube defects is specific to early pregnancy, many believe that folate intake should remain high because of the other possible risks.[18]

DEFICIENCY

In general terms, folate deficiency usually is the result of inadequate intake, or the inability of the intestine to absorb folate. It can also occur as the result of increased demand without increased intake, for example, during pregnancy and breast-feeding.[1]

Inadequate intake was common before the FDA mandated enriching grains with folic acid.

Certain individuals are more likely to have folate deficiency. This can be because of decreased intake, decreased absorption, or increased need. They include:

- Alcoholics (alcohol reduces the absorption of folate; also alcoholics often do not ingest enough folate)
- People with kidney failure getting dialysis (which causes a loss of folate)
- People with other liver diseases (which cause a loss of folate)
- People with intestinal diseases that interfere with folate absorption
- People taking medications that interfere with folate metabolism including (but not limited to):

  - Anticonvulsants (Dilantin, phenytoin, and primidone)
  - Metformin (for diabetes)
  - Sulfasalazine (for inflammatory intestinal diseases)
  - Triamterene (a diuretic)
  - Barbiturates (sedatives)
  - Methotrexate

As an example, methotrexate can be taken for cancer or autoimmune diseases and interferes significantly with folate metabolism. People taking methotrexate need to ask their physicians exactly what form of folic acid that they can take without causing the methotrexate to be less effective.[1]

Mild folate deficiency causes few symptoms. Babies and children who don't get enough folate will not grow at a normal rate. Adults who are folate deficient develop a specific kind of anemia. The babies born to folate-deficient pregnant women are more likely to be preterm, low birth weight, and/or have a congenital anomaly called a neural tube defect.

While the anemia is the best-known abnormality associated with low folate levels, other symptoms in adults include loss of appetite, diarrhea, weight loss, and a sore, smooth tongue. With progressive folate deficiency, weakness, fatigue, shortness of breath, headaches, irregular heart rhythms can also occur. A change in behavior may be observed by others, as can irritability and worsening memory.

The anemia is called "megaloblastic" or "macrocytic" because the immature red blood cells produced are larger than normal. There can also be abnormalities seen in certain types of white blood cells. Since the life of a red blood cell is usually four months, individuals deficient in folate will not become anemic for a number of months. Deficiency of vitamin B12 presents a similar picture.

Some with low folate, such as people with celiac disease, also have elevated homocysteine levels that can be corrected with treatment of the underlying disease. This is another reason to take extra folate. Some have suggested that 5-methyltetrahydrofolate (5-MTHF) might be a better replacement than folic acid.[19]

Many of these symptoms can be caused by other diseases or nutritional deficits, so a physician needs to make the diagnosis. Folic acid levels can be measured, along with other tests that can help confirm the deficiency. B12 levels must be evaluated in folate deficient individuals.

Neural Tube Defects

During pregnancy, the fetus is rapidly growing and needs a lot of folate for DNA and RNA synthesis. Neural tube defects in newborns have been noted as a result of inadequate maternal folate consumption. These defects involve the brain and spinal column. Babies can be born with anencephaly, which is the absence of most of the brain, and is essentially always fatal.

They can also be born with spina bifida. In this case, the fetus' neural tube does not completely close. This means that the baby's spinal cord is not protected by linings and bones as it should be. There can be varying amounts of open area. Babies with spina bifida are paralyzed because of the open spinal cord. The paralysis can be partial or complete.[18]

This part of the fetus' development occurs early, before many women even know they are pregnant, before the first missed menstrual period. Because of this, women who can become pregnant are advised to take at least 400 µg of folic acid a day. The U.S. Preventive Services Task Force continues to monitor this advice and outcomes of supplementation. It currently suggests 400 to 800 µg of folic acid for women of childbearing age.[19,20] This should be continued for the first two to three months of pregnancy to prevent neural tube defects.

Women with a history of babies born with neural tube defects are recommended to take 4 mg of folic acid a day.

Women taking medicine for seizures (epilepsy) may need more folate (see "Deficiency").

The risk of a neural tube defect used to be 1 in every 1,000 pregnancies. This has been reduced by 60 percent or more, as shown in many randomized trials. Larger reductions in the number of babies with neural tube defects can be achieved by supplementation rather than just with food fortification.

For women who have already had a baby with a neural tube defect, supplementation can reduce the risk of reoccurrence by 70 percent.[21] Since some 29 percent of neonatal deaths are due to neural tube defects in low-income countries, reducing the incidence of the defects also lowers the neonatal death rate.

Since all women of childbearing age do not take the recommended folic acid supplements, the FDA embarked on the program of fortifying grains, which may increase the amount of folate most people get by at least 100 µg. Since this fortification began, estimates of the reduction of neural tube defects range from 26 to 50 percent.[18]

It is also possible that folic acid supplements reduce the risk of congenital cleft lip, with or without cleft palate.[22]

FOOD SOURCES

As implied by its name, folate is found in green, leafy vegetables (foliage = green leaves). It is also found in citrus fruits and legumes.[18]

In the United States, grains have been supplemented with folic acid since 1998 when the FDA started requiring supplementation. This is also called fortification, and it applies to refined grain products.

Some examples of foods with naturally occurring folate, approximate amount per serving:

- Beef liver (185 µg)
- Spinach, cooked (100 µg)
- Asparagus, four spears (85 µg)
- Frozen then cooked broccoli or green peas (50 µg)
- Romaine lettuce (40 µg)
- Tomato or orange juice (35 µg)
- Cantaloupe or papaya (25 µg)

Some examples of foods supplemented with folic acid, per serving:[18]

- Breakfast cereals—fortified with 25 (100 µg) to 100 percent of the DV (400 µg)
- Bread (20 µg)
- Pasta and rice, cooked (60 µg)

MECHANISM OF ACTION: HOW DOES IT WORK?

Folate is a coenzyme for single carbon transfers (addition or subtraction of a single carbon molecule). This is critical for DNA metabolism. A folate coenzyme is necessary to synthesize nucleotides from their components, in order to make DNA as well as RNA. A folate coenzyme is also necessary for the synthesis of the amino acid methionine. Methionine is part of the chain of reactions leading to the production of S-adenosylmethionine (SAMe; see Chapter 28). SAMe is a methyl donor. Folate is therefore necessary for reactions that involve methylation, many of which are critical to cell function and survival.

Folate's contributions to methylation reactions as well as nucleotide synthesis may both be important in regard to the prevention of cancer.

As noted, folate coenzymes are necessary for the synthesis of methionine from homocysteine. This reaction also needs vitamin B12. Without folate (or B12), homocysteine builds up. High levels of homocysteine have been found in many chronic diseases (see "The Hype" above).

Folate is especially important for cells that are rapidly dividing and growing, such as red blood cells.[18]

Folic acid is the synthetic form of folate used for most supplementation. It is the oxidized state of folate and not the reduced form; it also has a single glutamate residue as opposed to the many glutamates attached to folate normally in the body. This means it is quite different from the natural form.

Folic acid is more rapidly absorbed than other folates, and with food fortification, most people have unmetabolized folic acid in their bodies. It is possible that this folic acid might compete with natural folates and actually cause a decrease in the normal folate metabolism. The significance of this is not yet completely clear.[9]

PRIMARY USES

- Folic acid supplementation is given to anyone with deficiency due to any of the above causes. Folic acid must be given along with B12 if a person is deficient in both.
- All women of childbearing age should be taking folic acid to prevent neural tube defects.
- Folic acid supplementation to reduce the risk of cardiovascular disease, cancer, or Alzheimer's disease has not been proven to work. In some cases, folic acid supplementation can cause increased risk of cancer and possibly other conditions.
- Before taking additional folic acid, it is important to estimate how much is being consumed from fortified grains and cereals. These amounts will be noted on packaging.

COMMON DOSAGES

Folic acid and folate are not exactly equivalent. The Food and Nutrition Board of the Institute of Medicine created a new unit called the Dietary Folate Equivalent

(DFE) in 1998. Synthetic folic acid is more bioavailable, that is, more easily absorbed and used by the body, than is natural folate. Therefore, if 1 μg of folate is 1 μg DFE, 1 μg of folic acid taken with meals would be 1.7 μg DFE. A 1 μg supplement of folic acid taken on an empty stomach would be 2 μg DFE.[1]

In general terms, folic acid supplements are more effectively used than natural folate; they are even more absorbed and used when taken on an empty stomach as opposed to in a meal.

The DFE is only used for children and adults, and not infants, because it has not been evaluated in infants.

The RDA for pregnant women was not based on prevention of neural tube defects. That has been considered separately.

The Average Intake recommended for infants 0 to 6 months old, both male and female, is 65 μg of folate. Infants 7–12 months of age need 80 μg.

The RDA (Recommended Dietary Allowance) for Folate in Dietary Folate Equivalents (DFE) is as follows:[1,23]

- Boys and girls ages 1 to 3 years need 150 μg/day.
- Boys and girls 4 to 8 years old need 200 μg/day.
- Children 9 to 13 years old need 300 μg/day.
- Adolescents 14 to 18 years old need 400 μg/day.
- Adults 19 years of age and older need 400 μg/day, except pregnant women, who need 600 μg a day, and breast-feeding women, who need 500 μg a day. This does not address prevention of neural tube defects (see above).

Folic acid can be taken as a single supplement or together with other vitamins. Amounts of 1 mg or more need a doctor's prescription.

All of the above recommendations assume that folic acid will be functionally the same as folate. There is some evidence that folic acid in the body cannot always be metabolized to an active folate form and may not be the best way to supplement folate.[9]

Because folic acid is not the form of folate in the body, some have suggested that 5-methyltetrahydrofolate (5-MTHF) might be a better way to supplement folate.[24] This is available as a dietary supplement.

POTENTIAL SIDE EFFECTS

There are no problems associated with folate intake from food. There is also very little risk from fortified foods. Since folate is a water-soluble vitamin, extra folate can be eliminated in the urine.

Important to take note of folate's dual relationship with cancer. Please see above, under "The Hype." Cancer, therefore, can be considered a potential side effect.

In one study, side effects of very large doses of folic acid (15 mg a day) included gastrointestinal distress, trouble sleeping, and mental changes. Other studies have not been able to reproduce these findings.

Allergy to folic acid is rare, but can occur.[23]

Cautions: Folic Acid and B12

Deficiency of both vitamin B12 and folate cause similar types of anemia. If folic acid is given to a person who is deficient in both, and the person is not given B12, this can correct the anemia but not the damage to the nervous system caused by low B12 levels. If this is not treated with B12, damage can be permanent. Anyone with anemia and low folate levels must have vitamin B12 levels checked. They may both be low, especially in the elderly.[1]

There is an upper limit intake level set by the Institute of Medicine for folate from supplements and fortified foods. By definition, this would be folic acid, because that is what folate is in fortified foods. The UL is the level at which neurologic complications can occur because of insufficient B12. Low B12 levels are often not recognized.[23]

The Upper Limits are:

- Age 1 to 3 years old—300 µg a day
- Age 4 to 8 years old—400 µg a day
- Age 9 to 13 years old—600 µg a day
- Age 14 to 18 years old—800 µg a day (including pregnant and breast-feeding women
- 19 years of age and older—1,000 µg a day

These are very conservative safety limits. Higher levels may be prescribed by physicians. For example, as stated previously, women who might become pregnant who have had a baby with a neural tube defect are advised to take 4 mg of folic acid a day, which is the same as 4,000 µg.

Cautions: Seizures and Other Medical Conditions

High levels of folic acid supplements can precipitate seizures in people who take anticonvulsant medicine. This needs to be done under medical supervision.[1]

The UL set are not applicable to patients taking medications that interfere with the metabolism of folate, like methotrexate. Appropriate folate supplementation needs to be individualized in these cases.[23]

It is possible that folic acid supplementation may make methotrexate and other drugs that interfere with folate metabolism less efficacious.[9]

FACT VERSUS FICTION

Folate is an absolutely necessary vitamin. People can develop folate deficiency despite fortification of grains with folic acid. Anyone with symptoms or signs of folate deficiency, measured by blood tests, should take folic acid or other supplementary folate.

Women who can become pregnant should take folic acid to prevent neural tube defects in their babies.

While folic acid administration can lower elevated homocysteine levels, it has not been shown to reduce cardiovascular disease or prevent cancer. In fact, it may raise the risk of cancer in some people.

The conflicting results of tests with folates may be related to the fact that folic acid is not the form of folate active in the body. In high doses, it is absorbed as is, instead of being converted to a folate. In the future, tests with 5-methyltetrahydrofolate (5-MTHF) may or may not have other outcomes.

The dual nature of folic acid in regard to cancer may be related to the presence or absence of precancerous or early cancerous cells in the body. Since no one can know if they have unknown precancerous cells, taking folic acid or other folates to prevent cancer does not seem reasonable at the current time, since it is possible folates will increase the risk of cancer.

Much more research must be done to answer the bigger questions.

REFERENCES

1. Dietary Supplement Fact Sheet: Folate. Office of Dietary Supplements. National Institutes of Health. Updated April 15, 2009. http://ods.od.nih.gov/factsheets/folate.asp. Accessed June 25, 2010.
2. Bønaa, KH, Njølstad, I, Ueland, PM, et al. Homocysteine lowering and cardiovascular events after acute myocardial infarction. *N Engl J Med.* 2006;354:1578–1588.
3. The Heart Outcomes Prevention Evaluation (HOPE) 2 Investigators. Homocysteine lowering with folic acid and B vitamins in vascular disease. *N Engl J Med.* 2006;354:1567–1577.
4. Albert, CM, Cook, NR, Gaziano, JM, et al. Effect of folic acid and B-vitamins on risk of cardiovascular events and total mortality among women at high risk for cardiovascular disease: A randomized trial. *JAMA.* 2008;299(17):2027–2036.
5. Study of the Effectiveness of Additional Reductions in Cholesterol and Homocysteine (SEARCH) Collaborative Group Authors: Armitage, JM, Bowman, L, Clarke, RJ, et al. Effects of homocysteine-lowering with folic acid plus vitamin B12 vs. placebo on mortality and major morbidity in myocardial infarction survivors. *JAMA.* 2010;303(24):2486–2494.
6. Zoungas, S, McGrath, BP, Branley, P, et al. Cardiovascular morbidity and mortality in the Atherosclerosis and Folic Acid Supplementation Trial (ASFAST) in chronic renal failure. *J Am Coll Cardiol.* 2006;47:1108–1116.
7. Shirodaria, C, Antoniades, C, Lee, J, et al. Global improvement of vascular function and redox state with low-dose folic acid. Implications for folate therapy in patients with coronary artery disease. *Circulation.* 2007;115:2262–2270.
8. Wang, X, Qin, X, Demirtas, H, et al. Efficacy of folic acid supplementation in stroke prevention: A meta-analysis. *Lancet.* 2007;369:1876–1882.
9. Smith, AD, Kim, Y-I, Refsum, H. Is folic acid good for everyone? *Am J Clin Nutr.* 2008;87:517–533.
10. Mason, JB. Folate, cancer risk, and the Greek god, Proteus: A tale of two chameleons. *Nutr Rev.* 2009;67(4):206–212.

11. Cole, BF, Baron, JA, Sandler, RS, et al. Folic acid for the prevention of colorectal adenomas. *JAMA.* 2007;297:2351–2359.

12. Mason, JB, Dickstein, A, Jacques, PF, et al. A temporal association between folic acid fortification and an increase in colorectal cancer rates may be illuminating important biological principles: A hypothesis. *Cancer Epidemiol Biomarkers Prev.* 2007;16(7):1325–1329.

13. Hubner, RA, Houlston, RS. Folate and colorectal cancer prevention. *British Journal of Cancer.* 2009;100:233–239.

14. Figueiredo, JC, Grau, MV, Haile, RW, et al. Folic acid and risk of prostate cancer: Results from a randomized clinical trial. *J Natl Cancer Inst.* 2009;101:432–435.

15. Bailey, RL, Mills, JL, Yetley, EA, et al. Unmetabolized serum folic acid and its relation to folic acid intake from diet and supplements in a nationally representative sample of adults aged ≥60 y in the United States. *Am J Clin Nutr.* 2010. http://www.ajcn.org/content/92/2/383.abstract. Accessed August 8, 2010.

16. Durga, J, van Boxtel, MPJ, Schouten, EG, et al. Effect of 3-year folic acid supplementation on cognitive function in older adults in the FACIT Trial: A randomised, double blind, controlled trial. *Lancet.* 2007;369:208–216.

17. Miller, AL. The methylation, neurotransmitter, and antioxidant connections between folate and depression. *Altern Med Rev.* 2008;13:216–226.

18. Higdon, J. Folic acid. Micronutrient Information Center. Linus Pauling Institute. April 2002; updated and reviewed September 2007. http://lpi.oregonstate.edu/infocenter/vitamins/fa/index.html. Accessed June 25, 2010.

19. Wolff, T, Witkop, CT, Miller, T, Syed, SB, et al. Folic acid supplementation for the prevention of neural tube defects: An update of the evidence for the U.S. Preventive Services Task Force. *Ann Intern Med.* 2009;150:632–639.

20. Folic Acid for the Prevention of Neural Tube Defects: U.S. Preventive Services Task Force Recommendation Statement. *Ann Intern Med.* 2009;150:626–631.

21. Blencowe, H, Cousens, S, Modell, B, Lawn, J. Folic acid to reduce neonatal mortality from neural tube disorders. *International Journal of Epidemiology.* 2010;39:i110–i121.

22. Wilcox, AJ, Lie, RT, Solvoll, K, et al. Folic acid supplements and risk of facial clefts: National population based case-control study. *BMJ.* 2007 doi:10.1136/bmj.39079.618287.0B.

23. Institute of Medicine. Food and Nutrition Board. *Dietary reference intakes: Thiamin, riboflavin, niacin, vitamin B6, folate, vitamin B12, pantothenic acid, biotin, and choline.* Washington, DC: National Academies Press, 1998.

24. Malterre, T. Digestive and nutritional considerations in celiac disease: Could supplementation help? *Altern Med Rev.* 2009;14(3):247–257.

12

Glucosamine

Glucosamine is a carbohydrate-like substance and is known as an amino sugar. It acts as a precursor in the synthesis of glycosylated (or sugar-linked) proteins and lipids. Glucosamine is part of the structure of the polysaccharides chitosan and chitin, which compose the exoskeletons of crustaceans (shellfish) and other arthropods and is produced commercially most commonly by the hydrolysis of these exoskeletons.

Glucosamine is crucial for the construction of glycosaminoglycans in articular cartilage, which help cushion our joints from wear and tear.[1] For this reason, oral glucosamine is commonly used for the treatment of pain and inflammation associated with osteoarthritis (OA). It is often found in supplement form together with chondroitin sulfate, a glycosaminoglycan, which is an important competent of cartilage, which gives joints their stability.

Glucosamine is not a naturally occurring dietary nutrient, but D-glucosamine is made naturally in the form of glucosamine-6-phosphate and is the biochemical precursor of all nitrogen-containing sugars. In the body, glucosamine-6-phosphate is synthesized from fructose-6-phosphate and glutamine.[1]

THE HYPE

Arthritis, the predominant reason why glucosamine chondroitin supplements came about, is one of the most common chronic complaints in adults. An estimated 46 million adults in the United States reported being told by a doctor that they have some form of arthritis, rheumatoid arthritis, gout, lupus, or fibromyalgia.[2] Glucosamine is popular both as a complement to and an alternative for conventional pain medications, like NSAIDS (nonsteroidal anti-inflammatory drugs) and COX-2 inhibitors. In the United States, glucosamine is one of the most commonly used nonvitamin, nonmineral, natural products taken by adults as a complementary

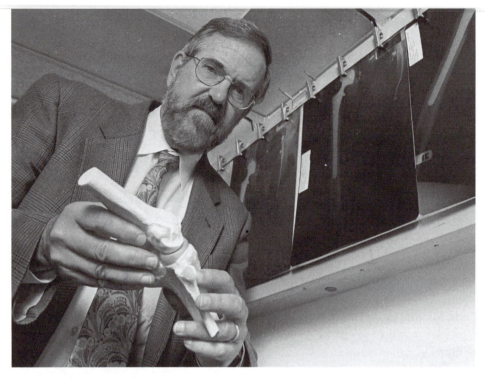

Orthopedic surgeon David S. Hungerford, head of arthritis surgery at Johns Hopkins University, poses in front of an X-ray light table holding a model of a knee joint in his Baltimore office in 1998. Dr. Hungerford is among a small group of doctors who offer their patients dietary supplements for the treatment of arthritis. He has proscribed two supplements, glucosamine sulfate and chondroitin sulfate, to treat his own bad knee and fingers. (AP Photo/Gail Burton)

or alternative medicine. According to the *Nutrition Business Journal,* U.S. sales for these combined supplements were $810 million in 2005.[3]

Oral glucosamine is a therapy for pain, inflammation, and joint damage associated with arthritis. It appears safe, but there is conflicting evidence as to its effectiveness, depending on the type of glucosamine used. Glucosamine supplements appear to be more effective in the sulfate form and when combined with chondroitin sulfate.

DEFICIENCY

Glucosamine is not present in many food sources and is not considered an essential nutrient in the diet. No deficiency symptoms have ever been reported in the literature for glucosamine. A rare disorder of *N*-acetyl-glucosamine-6-sulfatase enzyme, which helps manufacture glucosamine in the body, leads to a syndrome called Sanfilippo syndrome, characterized by a delay in rising and walking in neonates, ataxia, bowing of front limbs, clouding of the cornea, dwarfism, and cartilaginous and bony deformities.[4]

MECHANISMS OF ACTION AND PRIMARY USES

The mechanism of action of glucosamine remains to be fully elucidated, but one of the major effects seems to be that of an anti-inflammatory. The pro-inflammatory cytokine, Interleukin-1 (IL-1), can lead to the degeneration of joint cartilage. Studies have shown that glucosamine and chondroitin sulfate are able to abrogate IL-1-induced gene expression of COX-2, thereby exhibiting anti-inflammatory effects.

In one study of osteoarthritis joint cartilage cells (called chondrocytes) stimulated with the pro-inflammatory cytokine IL-1 (which can degrade joint cartilage), glucosamine sulfate was able to modify the NFkappaB (nuclear factor-kB) activity and the expression of COX-2, an NFkappaB-dependent gene.[5] In another study of bovine cartilage stimulated with IL-1, a glucosamine and chondroitin sulfate combination abrogated IL-1-induced gene expression COX-2 and NF-kB, thereby exhibiting anti-inflammatory effects.[6]

Glucosamine may also act by stimulating the chondrocytes to synthesize proteoglycans, which are glycoproteins covalently attached to glycosaminoglycan, and which influence joint stability.[7] In addition, glucosamine may directly inhibit the synthesis of proteolytic enzymes and other substances that can damage the joint cartilage matrix and destroy the joint chondrocytes.[8,9,10]

Glucosamine Sulfate May Decrease Pain and Inflammation Associated with Osteoarthritis

Glucosamine supplements are often sold in the form of glucosamine hydrochloride. A 2007 review study demonstrated that, although some clinical trials showed modest improvement in the symptoms of osteoarthritis with glucosamine hydrochloride combined with other agents, glucosamine hydrochloride by itself appears to offer little benefit to those suffering from osteoarthritis.[11] Supplements in the form of glucosamine sulfate may have more value in osteoarthritis treatment.

The first impressive trials that sparked much of the interest in glucosamine supplements were sponsored in the 1980s and 1990s by a European patent holder, Rattapharm, who used a crystalline glucosamine in the form of glucosamine sulfate in its product, known as Rotta. A Cochrane Database Review in 2005 looked at all randomized control trials evaluating the effectiveness of glucosamine in osteoarthritis, which included 10 Rotta and 10 non-Rotta trials (2,570 patents in total). Collectively, the 20 analyzed trials found glucosamine favored placebo with a 28 percent (change from baseline) improvement in pain and a 21 percent improvement in joint function, using a 10-question index called the Lequesne Index, but these results were not significant when looking at just the non-Rotta group. When using another measure of pain and stiffness, the WOMAC, there was no difference between glucosamine and placebo groups. This led the authors to conclude that only some brands of supplements may be effective in actually reducing arthritic pain and that glucosamine sulfate may be more effective than glucosamine in other forms.[12]

Results for studies using glucosamine seem to offer very conflicting results. One report lists potential explanations that include different glucosamine preparations, inadequate allocation concealment, and industry bias.[13]

Glucosamine in Combination with Chondroitin May Decrease Pain and Inflammation Associated with Osteoarthritis to a Better Degree Than Glucosamine Alone

Studies using a combination of glucosamine and chondroitin seem to show more promise in arthritis treatment than stand-alone glucosamine preparations. A meta-analysis of chondroitin sulfate trials has also been published. Seven randomized double-blind placebo-controlled trials were entered into the meta-analysis. Following patients for 120 days or more, chondroitin sulfate was shown to be significantly superior to placebo with respect to the Lequesne Index and pain visual analog scale. All patients in the study were also concurrently given NSAID drugs. Pooled data demonstrated at least 50 percent improvement in the study variables in the chondroitin-treated group.[14]

Another study of double-blind placebo-controlled trials of greater than four weeks' duration. It looked at oral or parenteral glucosamine or chondroitin for treatment of hip or knee osteoarthritis. Thirteen trials (six with glucosamine, seven with chondroitin) met eligibility criteria. The authors used the global pain score or the Lequesne Index in the index joint as the primary outcome measure and considered the trial positive if improvement in the treatment group was equal to or greater than 25 percent compared with the placebo group and was significant. All 13 studies reviewed were classified as positive, demonstrating large effects, compared with placebo (39.5% for glucosamine and 40.2% for chondroitin).[15]

The National Institutes of Health later funded a large multicenter clinical trial (the GAIT trial), comparing groups treated with chondroitin sulfate, glucosamine hydrochloride, and the combination, as well as both placebo and celecobix (an NSAID drug). The results of this six-month trial found that patients taking glucosamine hydrochloride, chondroitin sulfate, or a combination of the two had no statistically significant improvement in their symptoms compared to patients taking a placebo.[16] The group of patients who took celecoxib did have a statistically significant improvement in their symptoms. Analysis of a small subgroup of patients suggested that combination glucosamine hydrochoride and chondroitin sulfate may be significantly more effective than placebo. The problem with this study is that it used glucosamine hydrochoride, instead of glucosamine sulfate (which has been proven more effective) in its analysis.

However, according to a 2007 review study, several randomized controlled studies have assessed the structure-modifying effect of glucosamine sulfate and chondroitin sulfate using plain radiography to measure joint space narrowing over years. With respect to the structure-modifying effect, there is compelling evidence that glucosamine sulfate and chondroitin sulfate may interfere with progression of OA.[17]

One study showed that glucosamine and chondroitin sulfate may delay radiological progression of OA of the knee after daily administration for more than two or three years, but no results were seen at one year.[18]

Type II Collagen (COL II) is a new natural therapy for osteoarthritis, which may reduce pain, stiffness, and immobility associated with osteoarthritis to an even greater extent than glucosamine and chondroitin. A recent study looked at different markers in the structural progression of osteoarthritis in 104 patients given glucosamine chondroitin alone and in combination with COL II. After one year it was evident from the study that glucosamine and chondroitin helped delay the progression of osteoarthritis, and the effects were enhanced with the addition of COL II.[19]

COMMON DOSAGES

The amounts generally administered to produce desired effects are glucosamine sulfate, 1,500 mg, and chondroitin sulfate, 1,200 mg, daily.[12,14,15] Although glucosamine has been described as effective when used alone, it is probably reasonable to use the combination pending further studies.

TOXICITY

Clinical trials involving glucosamine and/or chondroitin supplements generally report high safety and minimal side effects.[12,14,15] The LD50 (or the lethal dose that would kill 50% of animals in a study group) for glucosamine is high, at 8,000 mg/kg.[20] One side effect that does stand out as a concern is glucosamine's potential effects on blood sugar. Altered glucose metabolism can be associated with parenteral administration of large doses of glucosamine.[21] A review of studies involving 3,063 human subjects receiving oral dosages of glucosamine failed to show any significant blood sugar modulating effects.[20] Animal studies demonstrating effects of glucosamine on glucose metabolism have used concentrations that are 100 to 200 times higher than tissue levels expected with oral glucosamine administration in humans.[20] Glucosamine supplements should still be used with caution in patients taking diabetes medications, as well as in patients on blood-thinning medication, due to glucosamine's potential to thin the blood.[22]

FACT VERSUS FICTION

Glucosamine appears to be a safe, well-tolerated supplement that, with long-term use, may help reduce pain and inflammation associated with osteoarthritis, although studies involving its use are still delivering conflicting results. Supplements in the form of glucosamine sulfate appear to be more effective than glucosamine hydrochloride and are especially effective when used in combination with chondroitin sulfate. In addition, glucosamine and chondroitin supplements may offer a structure-modifying effect, which would not be seen with conventional NSAID and COX II drugs, which work primarily as anti-inflammatory and pain medications.

REFERENCES

1. Ghosh, S, Blumenthal, HJ, Davidson, E, Roseman, S. Glucosamine metabolism. V. Enzymatic synthesis of glucosamine-6-phosphate. *J Biol Chem.* May 1960;235(5):1265.
2. National Center for Health Statistics. *Complementary and alternative medicine use among adults and children: United States, 2007.* December 10, 2008.

3. *Nutrition Business Journal.* http://nutritionbusinessjournal.com/supplements/news/10–07-glucosamine-chondroitin-efficacy-concerns-surface/. Accessed October 2009.

4. Valstar, MJ, Ruijter, GJ, van Diggelen, OP, Poorthuis, BJ, Wijburg, FA. Sanfilippo syndrome: A mini-review. *J Inherit Metab Dis.* 2008 Apr. http://www.ncbi.nlm.nih.gov/pubmed/18392742. (Epup ahead of print).

5. Largo, R, et al. Glucosamine inhibits IL-1beta-induced NFkappaB activation in human osteoarthritic chondrocytes. *Osteoarthritis Cartilage.* 2003 Apr;11(4):290–298.

6. Chan, PS, et al. Short-term gene expression changes in cartilage explants stimulated with interleukin beta plus glucosamine and chondroitin sulfate. *J Rheumatol.* 2006;33(7):1329–1340.

7. Bassleer, C, et al. Stimulation of proteoglycan production by glucosamine sulfate in chondrocytes isolated from human osteoarthritic articular cartilage in vitro. *Osteoarthritis Cartilage.* 1998 Nov;6(6):427–434.

8. Dodge, GR, et al. Glucosamine sulfate modulates the levels of aggrecan and matrix metalloproteinase-3 synthesized by cultured human osteoarthritis articular chondrocytes. *Osteoarthritis Cart.* 2003 Jun;11(6):424–432.

9. Chan, PS, et al. Effect of glucosamine and chondroitin sulfate on regulation of gene expression of proteolytic enzymes and their inhibitors in interleukin-1-challenged bovine articular cartilage explants. *Am J Vet Res.* 2005;66(11):1870–1876.

10. Uitterlinden, EJ, et al. Glucosamine decreases expression of anabolic and catabolic genes in human osteoarthritic cartilage explants. *Osteoarthritis Cartilage.* 2006 Mar;14(3):250–257.

11. Fox, BA, Stephens, MM. Glucosamine hydrochloride for the treatment of osteoarthritis symptoms. *Clin Interv Aging.* 2007;2(4):599–604.

12. Towheed, TE, Maxwell, L, Anastassiades, TP, Shea, B, Houpt, J, Robinson, V, Hochberg, MC, Wells, G. Glucosamine therapy for treating osteoarthritis. *Cochrane Database of Systematic Reviews.* 2005 Apr 18;(2):CD002946.

13. Vlad, SC, LaValley, MP, McAlindon, TE, Felson, DT. Glucosamine for pain in osteoarthritis: Why do trial results differ? *Arthritis Rheum.* 2007 Jul;56(7):2267–2277.

14. Leeb, BF, Schweitzer, H, Montag, K, Smolen, JS. A meta-analysis of chondroitin sulfate in the treatment of osteoarthritis. *J Rheumatol.* 2000 Jan; 27(1):205–211.

15. McAlindon, TE, LaValley, MP, Gulin, JP, Felson, DT. Glucosamine and chondroitin for treatment of osteoarthritis: A systematic quality assessment and meta-analysis. *JAMA.* 2000 Mar 15;283(11):1469–1475.

16. National Center for Complimentary and Alternative Medicine. The NIH Glucosamine/Chondroitin Arthritis Intervention Trial (GAIT). *J Pain Palliat Care Pharmacother.* 2008;22(1):39–43.

17. Bruyere, O, Reginster, JY. Glucosamine and chondroitin sulfate as therapeutic agents for knee and hip osteoarthritis. *Drugs Aging.* 2007;24(7):573–580.

18. Lee, YH, Woo, JH, Choi, SJ, Ji, JD, Song, GG. Effect of glucosamine or chondroitin sulfate on the osteoarthritis progression: A meta-analysis. *Rheumatol Int.* 2009 Jun 21. http://www.ncbi.nlm.nih.gov/pubmed/19544061. [Epub ahead of print]

19. Scarpellini, M, Lurati, A, Vignati, G, Marrazza, MG, Telese, F, Re, K, Bellistri, A. Biomarkers, type II collagen, glucosamine and chondroitin sulfate in osteoarthritis follow-up: The "Magenta Osteoarthritis Study." *J Orthop Traumatol.* 2008 Jun;9(2):81–87.

20. Anderson, JW, Nicolosi, RJ, Borzelleca, JF. Glucosamine effects in humans: A review of effects on glucose metabolism, side effects, safety considerations and efficacy. *Food Chem Toxicol.* 2005 Feb;43(2):187–201.

21. Hawkins, M, Hu, M, Yu, J, Eder, H, Vuguin, P, She, L, Barzilai, N, Leiser, M, Backer, JM, Rossetti, L. Discordant effects of glucosamine on insulin-stimulated glucose metabolism and phosphatidylinositol 3-kinase activity. *J Biol Chem.* 1999 Oct 29;274(44):312–319.

22. *Physicians' Desk Reference.* http://www.pdrhealth.com/drugs/altmed. Accessed October 2009.

13

Glutathione (GSH)

BRIEF OVERVIEW

Glutathione (γ-glutamyl-cysteinyl-glycine, or GSH) is a tripeptide with many important actions throughout the human body. It is an antioxidant and can prevent cellular damage. When glutathione levels are low, the body is more susceptible to oxidative stress, which may contribute to the development of cancer, Alzheimer's disease, Parkinson's disease, and more.

Glutathione plays a role in many cellular processes. Much research is ongoing to define all of its activities. Glutathione has so many actions that it has been difficult to determine whether or not it is causative in any specific disease.

Decreased glutathione, or dysregulation of its synthesis, may cause or worsen cancer and cystic fibrosis, as well as metabolic, cardiovascular, inflammatory, immune, metabolic, and neurodegenerative diseases. It may contribute to aging.

While glutathione would be an ideal supplement in many ways, it appears that it cannot be absorbed by the gastrointestinal tract. The only dietary way to increase levels is to take the precursors of glutathione, including sulfur-containing molecules like N-acetylcysteine and S-adenosyl-l-methionine (SAMe). Glutathione can be well absorbed when given intravenously.

THE HYPE

Since glutathione is an antioxidant, it may help treat a multitude of diseases and disorders that may involve oxidative stress, which occurs when there is an imbalance between reactive oxygen molecules and the mechanisms the body has to remove them. Many of the associations between low glutathione levels and disease are just being uncovered. In many cases, there is no good data yet on treatment with GSH.

Most research has shown that oral supplements with glutathione are not effective. There has been research that shows the glutathione precursor N-acetylcysteine can get into cells, where it is eventually metabolized to glutathione. Alpha lipoic acid also raises the levels of glutathione. SAMe can also be used as a glutathione precursor. Even companies that sell oral glutathione encourage consumption of precursors.[1]

As of now, the consensus seems to be that oral glutathione cannot be absorbed. Some evidence suggests that even if glutathione is absorbed, it does not get inside cells where it is needed. It may have to be synthesized inside cells to be of use.[2] This may be why precursors are effective.

Liver

Many substances that damage the liver lower GSH levels. These include ethanol and acetaminophen.[3] Glutathione helps protect the liver. Raising levels can be beneficial for liver disease and/or liver failure. SAMe is sometimes used, which will increase glutathione in the liver. It seems to be particularly useful in alcoholic liver disease.[4]

When the liver is already stressed by a toxic substance, and GSH levels are low, it is even more sensitive to acetaminophen (paracetamol) overdose.[5]

NEURODEGENERATIVE DISEASES

Alzheimer's Disease

Glutathione may be a key to protecting the brain from oxidative damage. Low levels of GSH may contribute to the development of Parkinson's disease and Alzheimer's disease. The evidence is not clear as it relates to Alzheimer's disease. Different investigators have found normal and low levels of GSH in some people with the disease. Examinations of the brain at autopsy have also yielded conflicting results.[3]

Parkinson's Disease

Measurements of GSH in the brains of patients with Parkinson's disease have been consistently low. It is not known if this is cause or effect. Low GSH is probably one of the many factors involved in the disease. There has been difficulty getting supplemental glutathione or its precursors successfully into the brain. It could be expected to help Parkinson's patients.[3]

It is still not completely clear whether or not glutathione crosses the human blood-brain barrier. It crosses in the rat and guinea pig and human cerebrovascular cells (brain blood cells) in a laboratory setting.[6]

An early study of intravenous glutathione for Parkinson's disease was done in 1996. Nine patients were given 600 mg of intravenous glutathione twice daily for a month. These patients improved symptomatically during the treatment and for a few months thereafter.[7]

Dr. David Perlmutter has been treating patients with Parkinson's disease with intravenous glutathione for many years, since 1998. His Web site contains many testimonials from patients who believe they have benefitted from this therapy.

He describes his results as "miraculous." While he believes glutathione is very beneficial, he also encourages the use of glutathione precursors.[8]

As far as published clinical trials, one preliminary study done to assess the tolerability of glutathione over the short term in patients with Parkinson's disease, as well as its safety, and preliminary idea of efficacy, was successful. It was a double-blind, randomized, placebo-controlled trial. Intravenous glutathione, given 1,400 mg three times a week, was well tolerated, and patients showed some improvement compared with those who got placebo, although the trial was not set up to determine effectiveness.[6]

Multiple Sclerosis

Sulfur-containing antioxidants like glutathione may help patients with multiple sclerosis. Usually a GSH precursor is used, such as N-acetylcysteine.[9]

Aging

GSH levels decrease with age. These lower GSH levels may contribute to many of the disorders associated with aging. In the eye, this includes macular degeneration, cataracts, and glaucoma. Antioxidant supplementation is already known to protect eye health.

Hearing loss and osteoporosis are also both associated with oxidative stress; there is no evidence as yet that increasing glutathione levels would benefit people with these problems.[3]

Cancer

It is well known that oxidative and other damage can occur to DNA; this damage can cause cancer. GSH can protect against this type of injury. However, cancerous cells often have high levels of GSH.[3]

Cardiovascular Disease

There is an oxidative imbalance in hypertension (high blood pressure) and atherosclerosis. In atherosclerosis, there is damage to the vascular wall, which glutathione could prevent. It has been suggested that little pouches of fat (liposomes) might be able to deliver glutathione to the atheromatous lesions. This has been done in animals.[3]

Cystic Fibrosis

GSH status may be very important in the development of cystic fibrosis. A genetic mutation found in the disease may alter where glutathione concentrates. GSH is abnormally low in the lining of the lung epithelium as well as a particular kind of white blood cell in patients with cystic fibrosis. This increases the lungs susceptibility to oxidative damage. N-acetylcysteine has been used to thin the mucous in patients with this disease for many years, in an inhaled form. Oral N-acetylcysteine has been shown to raise GSH levels, but this has not been proven to improve lung function. Further studies are underway, including the use of inhaled glutathione.[3]

Inflammatory and Immune System

GSH may play an important role in immune function. There is a depletion of sulfur-containing compounds in many diseases involving the immune system, which means that more sulfur-containing molecules are needed. These could include cysteine, N-acetylcysteine, and others.

GSH affects the correct responses of T helper cells, key cells in the immune response. If this regulation is off, T cell overactivity may result, which is associated with rheumatoid arthritis, and other autoimmune diseases. GSH levels are low in many of these diseases, including RA, systemic lupus erythematosus, and Crohn's disease.

GSH levels are low in patients with HIV, and decreasing levels are associated with decreased survival. In addition to its protective function of an antioxidant, it is thought that GSH may be involved in signaling cells as part of the immune response.[3]

Diabetes

Oxidative stress definitely plays a role in diabetes. Evidence exists of abnormal GSH regulation in diabetes mellitus. The activity of glutathione synthetase is decreased (see "Mechanism of Action,") and the glutathione pool is smaller. High glucose levels themselves cause oxidative stress. This includes potential damage to the cells that produce insulin, the beta cells of the pancreas. Reactive oxygen molecules may also help make other cells more resistant to insulin. The two hallmarks of type 2 diabetes are decreased insulin levels and less sensitivity to the insulin that is produced. This seems to be somewhat of an explanation for how elevated blood sugar levels eventually lead to frank diabetes.

GSH and oxidative stress are also partly responsible for many of the complications of diabetes. The concentration of GSH in the eye is abnormally low in diabetes, and this may affect the lens and retina, which can be damaged. Abnormal glutathione metabolism may contribute to diabetic neuropathy—damage to peripheral nerves with elevated blood sugar. The same may be true of some damage to the kidney.

Much of the evidence for the role of abnormal GSH metabolism in diabetics has been in vitro and observational. Clinical studies are needed.[2]

While most believe that oral glutathione is not effectively absorbed, there has been some research that topical application of esters of glutathione may help protect the eye in diabetics. This treatment has been shown effective in animal models of diabetes.[2] Both esters of glutathione and n-acetylcysteine have been used with some success as eye drops in preventing rat cataracts.[10]

Peripheral Neuropathy

Oxidative damage is thought to be partially responsible for peripheral neuropathy in some cases. This type of nerve damage can be caused by the chemotherapy agent, cisplatin. Intravenous glutathione may prevent damage to the peripheral nerves that cisplatin and other related chemotherapeutic agents can cause.

However, in diabetic neuropathy, glutathione precursor ALA (alpha lipoic acid) but not glutathione works in rat models to protect against peripheral neuropathy.[11]

Miscellaneous

GSH has been used to help treat male infertility and HIV.[2]

Glutathione may also be useful for asthma and other lung problems, including COPD (chronic obstructive pulmonary disease), environmental lung disease, acute respiratory distress syndrome, and idiopathic pulmonary fibrosis. Glutathione precursors such as N-acetylcysteine may be useful.[3,13]

DEFICIENCY

Low levels of glutathione in specific organs are associated with a number of diseases. Glutathione deficiency is suspected as contributing to or causing, among other illnesses, kwashiorkor (protein malnutrition illness), seizures, Alzheimer's disease, Parkinson's disease, liver disease, cystic fibrosis, sickle cell anemia, HIV/AIDS, cancer, heart disease, stroke, diabetes, and aging.[14]

Defects in the many enzymes catalyzing synthesis of GSH cause serious diseases. There are five enzymes involved in glutathione synthesis and reuse, the gamma-glutamyl cycle (see "Mechanism of Action"). The first two enzymes are necessary to make glutathione. Defects in these enzymes cause anemia and neurologic problems.[3]

Common problems in all the genetic defects of GSH metabolism are neurologic deficits, particularly in the central nervous system. GSH levels in the brain are low relative to other organs, but there is a lot of oxidative stress in the brain. Insufficient GSH may lead to diseases like Parkinson's disease.[3]

Overtraining in athletes and other stress such as trauma can lower glutathione levels. Athletes often take whey protein, which has a large amount of cysteine; the cysteine can be converted to GSH.[12]

FOOD SOURCES

There is glutathione in food. Fruits and vegetables contain some 50 percent of glutathione in the diet; less than 25 percent comes from meat. It seems that glutathione is not absorbed intact, but broken down into its constituents. It is then made into glutathione again in the body.

Whey protein, from milk, is an excellent source of cysteine that can be converted into GSH.[12]

Most or all of the glutathione in the body has been synthesized and not ingested.

MECHANISM OF ACTION: HOW DOES IT WORK?

Glutathione is a free radical scavenger and also detoxifies peroxide. It helps to regulate cell growth and the function of proteins; it also helps maintain immune function. The body's glutathione exists in a pool, called the glutathione pool.[12]

GSH is an essential part of a complex system that protects cells against oxidative damage. An enzyme called glutathione peroxidase prevents the accumulation of reactive oxygen molecules and protects cells from peroxide damage. GSH is a cofactor for glutathione peroxidase; the reaction produces oxidized glutathione. Glutathione reductase converts the oxidized form back to glutathione, which is in its reduced form. Glutathione in cells is almost all reduced and ready to defend against potential damage.

Glutathione is a cofactor for the enzyme that keeps vitamins C and E in their active form. It also is a cofactor in reactions that modify potential toxins such as drugs or cancer-inducing compounds. GSH has an effect on thiol (sulfur) groups in signaling proteins. These proteins have a variety of functions including how genes are expressed, how cells proliferate, and also how cells are programmed to die. How glutathione does this is not completely understood. It can get into the cell nucleus, where the DNA and genes are.

When glutathione is used by the body under conditions of significant oxidative stress, its levels can be lowered significantly. There is a significant amount of evidence linking low levels of GSH with chronic disease and high levels with good health.[2]

Decreased levels of GSH cause increased susceptibility to oxidative stress, and this may initiate or worsen many disease processes. If there is oxidative stress along with protein-energy malnutrition, GSH may be depleted. This can occur with AIDS, cancer, alcoholism, malnutrition, burns, and chronic digestive diseases.[12]

Maintaining the GSH pool with the proper level, turnover rate, and state of oxidation is critical for many important cell functions. When there is not enough GSH, there will be increased susceptibility to oxidative stress and increased damage. The converse is also true. Elevated levels of GSH can be protective. It is important to note that some cancer cells maintain high GSH levels. This has made developing ways to use glutathione to help cancer patients more complicated.[3]

The three components of glutathione are glutamate, cysteine, and glycine. Glutathione (GSH) is synthesized via two enzymes, gamma-glutamylcysteine synthetase (or ligase) and GSH synthetase. GSH synthesis is regulated by the first enzyme, the availability of cysteine, and how much GSH is already present. In the two-step process, cysteine is converted to gamma-glutamylcysteine, and then to glutathione.[14] Glutathione is eventually metabolized into other components. The rest of this gamma-glutamyl cycle helps recycle parts of the metabolites back into glutathione.

There are a number of inborn errors of GSH metabolism, where babies are born with defects in GSH synthesis or recycling. Five of the six enzymes that catalyze the cycle producing and/or recycling GSH can be defective. These genetic conditions can lead to severely decreased GSH levels and even early death. Those with defects leading to diminished GSH levels have anemia and neurological disorders.[3] These are very rare conditions.[15]

Most of the GSH in the GSH pool is synthesized by the liver and distributed to the rest of the body.[16] It may be broken back into its constituent amino acids in order to enter other cells. Presumably, these cells then synthesize GSH from the amino acids.

PRIMARY USES

• Because glutathione is not absorbed intact, there are really no good uses for the supplement in oral form. It can supply the molecules needed to resynthesize itself, but other ways to increase glutathione in the body may turn out to be just as good or better.

• Precursors, or glutathione boosters, may be used in any of the chronic diseases noted in "The Hype."

• Intravenous glutathione is being used to treat Parkinson's disease, as well as an energy booster for people whose body has been under significant stress.

• It is also given with cisplatin and similar cancer chemotherapy to reduce the risk of peripheral neuropathy.

COMMON DOSAGES

Cysteine, methionine, N-acetylcysteine and SAMe can be used by the body to synthesize glutathione (see other chapters). Supplemental alpha lipoic acid can raise GSH levels.

When given with cisplatin to cancer patients, an intravenous dose of 1.5–2.5 g/m^2 has been used. Alternatively, 600 mg can be given intramuscularly. The same IM dose has been given to treat male infertility.[12]

One protocol for Parkinson's disease uses 1,400 mg of glutathione by vein three times a week.[6]

POTENTIAL SIDE EFFECTS

Glutathione is known to be very well tolerated. So are precursors like N-acetylcysteine.[13] There do, however, appear to be anecdotal reports of allergic reaction to intravenous glutathione treatment, especially in asthma patients.

In one pilot study for Parkinson's disease, two patients reported mild, transient nausea, not on the day they were given the glutathione intravenously, but the next day.[6]

In the same study, other side effects, such as headache and dizziness, were very similar, with no statistically significant difference between the group getting placebo and the group getting glutathione.[6]

FACT VERSUS FICTION

There is no question of the importance of glutathione to a healthy body. There are questions in regard to specific diseases. Do low levels of glutathione cause specific diseases? Or are the diseases causing the lower levels? Either way, will providing supplemental glutathione to people with these diseases improve their condition? What is the best way to do that?

Glutathione may turn out to be a very important supplement, but right now, in itself, it is not of great use in its oral form.

Intravenous glutathione may indeed help patients with Parkinson's disease. Since it seems to be very safe, it seems reasonable to try under the care of a physician.

REFERENCES

1. LifeExtension. Immune system strengthening. http://www.lef.org/. Accessed May 17, 2010.
2. Livingstone, C, Davis, J. Review: Targeting therapeutics against glutathione depletion in diabetes and its complications. *British Journal of Diabetes & Vascular Disease*. 2007;7:258–265.
3. Ballatori, N, Krance, SM, Notenboom, S, et al. Glutathione dysregulation and the etiology and progression of human diseases. *Biol Chem*. 2009;390(3): 191–214.
4. Purohit, V, Abdelmalek, MF, Barve, S, et al. Role of *S*-adenosylmethionine, folate, and betaine in the treatment of alcoholic liver disease: Summary of a symposium. *Am J Clin Nutr*. 2007;86:14–24.
5. Lauterburg, BH, Velez, ME. Glutathione deficiency in alcoholics: Risk factor for paracetamol hepatotoxicity. *Gut*. 1988;29:1153–1157.
6. Hauser, RA, Lyons, KE, McClain, T, et al. Randomized, double-blind, pilot evaluation of intravenous glutathione in Parkinson's disease. *Movement Disorders*. 2009;24(7):979–983.
7. Sechi, G, Deledda, MG, Bua, G, et al. Reduced intravenous glutathione in the treatment of early Parkinson's disease. *Prog Neuropsychopharmacol Biol Psychiatry*. 1996;20(7):1159–1170.
8. Perlmutter, D. New advances in Parkinson's disease. BrainRecovery.com. Last updated 2004, currently unavailable. Chapter found at http://www.inutrition als.com/healthy-living/neurodegenerative-conditions/parkinsons-disease/glu tathione/glutathione-8. Accessed December 29, 2010.
9. Kidd, PM. Multiple sclerosis, an autoimmune inflammatory disease: Prospects for its integrative management. *Altern Med Rev*. 2001;6(6):540–566.
10. Zhang, S, C, Yan, H, et al. Effects of N-acetylcysteine and glutathione ethyl ester drops on streptozotocin-induced diabetic cataracts in rats. *Molecular Vision*. 2008;14:862–870.
11. Head, KA. Peripheral neuropathy: Pathogenic mechanisms and alternative therapies. *Altern Med Rev*. 2006;11(4):294–329.
12. Parcell, S. Sulfur in human nutrition and applications in medicine. *Altern Med Rev*. 2002;7(1):22–24.
13. Hunninghake, GW. Antioxidant therapy for idiopathic pulmonary fibrosis. *N Engl J Med*. 2005;353(21):2285–2287.
14. Wu, G, Fang, Y-Z, Yang, S, et al. Glutathione metabolism and its implications for health. *J Nutr*. 2004;134:489–492.
15. Ristoff, E, Larsson, A. Inborn errors in the metabolism of glutathione. *Orphanet Journal of Rare Diseases*. 2007;2:16–19.
16. Lu, S. Regulation of hepatic glutathione synthesis: Current concepts and controversies. *Faseb J*. 1999;13:1169–1183.

14

L-Carnitine

BRIEF OVERVIEW

Carnitine is an amino acid–like substance involved in cellular metabolism. Carnitine is not an amino acid in the strictest sense (it is actually a substance related to the B vitamins), but its chemical structure is similar to an amino acid. Unlike the amino acids, it is not used for protein synthesis or hormone production. Its main function is transporting long-chain fatty acids into the mitochondria (the fat incinerators of the cells), where they are oxidized into energy. It also facilitates the transport of intermediate toxic compounds out of the mitochondria preventing their accumulation. Carnitine has been coined a "conditionally essential" nutrient by National Institutes of Health,[1] which means that although our bodies can synthesize it, requirements for carnitine may exceed this ability under certain circumstances. Carnitine is the generic term for a number of compounds that include L-carnitine, acetyl-L-carnitine, and propionyl-L-carnitine.[2]

THE HYPE

Much of the hype around the use of carnitine as a supplement is related to its proposed ability to induce weight loss through accelerated fat burning. Carnitine supplements are also widely used by sportsmen wanting to boost athletic performance. The evidence linking carnitine supplements to weight loss or boosted athletic performance is sketchy; and according to the National Institutes of Health's Office of Dietary Supplements Review, it is not generally an effective supplement in this regard.[3] However, carnitine does have roles in protecting the heart muscle and has promise in the treatment of type II diabetes.

DEFICIENCY

Carnitine deficiencies may be caused by genetic disorders, liver or kidney problems, high-fat diets, certain medications, and low dietary levels of the amino acids lysine and methionine or vitamin B1, B6, or iron (substances needed to make carnitine).[1,4] The genetic disorder that affects the cellular carnitine-transporter system is a congenital disorder that usually manifests by five years of age and includes symptoms of cardiomyopathy, skeletal muscle weakness, and hypoglycemia.[4] Carnitine supplements can help to treat symptoms during times when carnitine becomes conditionally essential, and it is valued as a prescription drug in this regard.[2]

FOOD SOURCES

Healthy children and adults do not need to consume carnitine from food or supplements, as the liver and kidneys produce sufficient amounts from the amino acids lysine and methionine to meet daily needs.[2,3] Red meat (particularly lamb and beef) and the whey fraction of dairy products are the primary source. Carnitine can also be found in fish, poultry, tofu, tempeh, mushrooms, bread, rice, asparagus, avocados, and peanut butter.[2,3] Red meat is by far the richest source, with beef steak containing 56–162 mg carnitine per 4-ounce portion; the same portion of chicken or fish or a cup of milk contains only 3–8 mg carnitine in comparison.[3]

Carnitine occurs in two forms, known as D and L, that are mirror images (isomers) of each other. Only L-carnitine is active in the body and is the form found in food.[3,5]

MECHANISMS OF ACTION AND PRIMARY USES

Since carnitine has functions related to cellular metabolism and energy production, its primary uses are mostly related to weight loss and athletic performance, but carnitine also has potential uses in improving cardiac function and boosting brainpower.

Carnitine May Aid Weight Loss and Associated Metabolic Abnormalities

The importance and function of the carnitine system relates not only to the metabolism of fatty acids, but also to systemic fat balance and insulin resistance. The carnitine system is shown to be a determinant in insulin regulation of fat and glucose metabolism in skeletal muscle, which is critical to determining body composition and relevant risk factors for cardiovascular disease, obesity, hypertension, and type II diabetes.[6] There are quite a few studies that do not show any significant link between L-carnitine supplementation and weight loss. One study using 3g L-carnitine for 10 days in slightly overweight subjects showed no change in body composition when compared to a placebo.[7] A study using 36 rats divided into either a treatment group (receiving 5 g/kg L-carnitine supplementation) or control group (no supplementation) and all put onto a calorie-restricted diet showed that weight loss was apparent in both groups but the difference in weight loss was not significant.[8] In contrast, another study of obese cats showed that when cats were supplemented with 250 mg L-carnitine, weight reduction on a calorie-restricted diet was significantly faster than that of cats given a placebo.[9] In a randomized, double-blind, placebo-controlled study of 36 moderately obese women given either 2 g L-carnitine per day or a placebo and who were made to walk for 30 minutes 4 days a week, no significant changes in mean total body mass (TBM), fat mass FM, and resting lipid utilization occurred over time, nor were there any significant differences between groups for any variable.[10]

Still, there seems to be a lack of well-designed clinical trials investigating the role of L-carnitine in weight loss. There are some studies that point toward a weight loss benefit when L-carnitine is used together with other weight loss aids, like choline and caffeine.[11,12]

Although the evidence linking L-carnitine and weight loss is still sketchy, L-carnitine supplementation helps offset some of the negative consequences of being overweight. Obesity results in an increase in circulating levels of free fatty acids, which in turn impair endothelial function. Endothelial dysfunction is a serious consequence of being overweight as it leads to an increased cardiovascular mortality. One study showed that L-carnitine supplementation helped attenuate free fatty acid–induced and obesity-related endothelial dysfunction in obese subjects.[13]

Obesity is also associated with an increase in plasma cholesterol levels and an abnormal blood lipid profile. In several studies, people who took L-carnitine supplements had a significant lowering of their total cholesterol and triglycerides and an increase in HDL levels.[14,15] L-carnitine supplementation has also been shown to reduce levels of lipoprotein in patients with type II diabetes mellitus.[16]

Carnitine Helps in Type II Diabetes

Type II diabetes, another serious consequence of obesity, is also helped by L-carnitine supplementation, primarily through carnitine's ability to improve insulin sensitivity. Another theory is that diabetes may be associated with a defect in fatty acid oxidation in muscle.[17] In one study, 35 type II diabetics were randomly allocated to receive either 1 g L-carnitine or a placebo for a 12-week period. Fasting blood glucose decreased significantly in the group receiving L-carnitine supplementation. Plasma triglycerides did, however, increase in the treatment group.[18] Early research suggests that supplementation with L-carnitine intravenously may improve insulin sensitivity in diabetics by decreasing fat levels in muscle and may lower glucose levels in the blood by more promptly increasing its oxidation in cells.[18,19,20]

Carnitine May Aid Athletic Performance

Animal studies suggest that L-carnitine supplementation decreases lactic acid accumulation and spares glycogen, therefore playing a role in delaying fatigue during exercise.[21] Other animal studies point toward carnitine reducing muscle pain and muscle damage post exercise.[22,23]

A double-blind placebo-controlled study published in *Physiologie*[24] looked at chronic and acute effects of L-carnitine on 110 top athletes (including swimmers and long-distance runners). Significant changes were noted after single dose and after three weeks of treatment. The L-carnitine group showed higher blood carnitine levels, less lactic acid buildup after exercise, and greater muscular potential.

Another double-blind placebo-controlled trial looked at the chronic and acute effects of 3 g L-carnitine administered over three weeks in 40 top athletes (rowers and weightlifters). Significant changes were noted in the treated group for triglycerides, free fatty acids, strength index, and VO_2 max, indicating a positive effect. Administration of an acute 4 g dose of L-carnitine in 18 top weightlifters registered a significant change in triglycerides and free fatty acids.[21]

A review of studies done on carnitine supplementation in athletes in 2004, after looking at the evidence, reported that L-carnitine supplementation increases maximal oxygen consumption and can speed up recovery from exercise stress.[25]

However, despite some studies pointing toward benefits, the National Institutes of Health's Office of Dietary Supplements states that after 20 years of research, it finds no consistent evidence that carnitine supplements can improve exercise or physical performance in healthy subjects.[3,26,27,28] However, all the studies it bases this finding on were conducted by the same research team.

Carnitine Improves Heart Health

The heart receives 70 percent of its energy from fat breakdown, making L-carnitine a crucial energy provider for the heart. Studies using carnitine for vascular problems use it in the form of levocarnitine or propionyl-L-carnitine. Studies suggest that people who take L-carnitine supplements soon after suffering a heart attack may be less likely to suffer a subsequent heart attack, die of heart disease, experience chest pain and abnormal heart rhythms, or develop congestive heart failure.[29] In a randomized multicenter trial performed on 472 patients, levocarnitine treatment (9 g/day by intravenous infusion for 5 initial days and 6 g/day orally for the next 12 months), when initiated early after acute myocardial infarction, attenuated left ventricular dilatation and prevented ventricular remodeling. In treated patients, there was a trend toward a reduction in the combined incidence of death and CHF after discharge.[30]

The results of studies in chronic heart failure patients showed that long-term oral treatment with propionyl-L-carnitine improves maximum exercise duration and maximum oxygen consumption over placebo and indicated a specific propionyl-L-carnitine effect on peripheral muscle metabolism. A multicenter trial showed that propionyl-L-carnitine improves exercise capacity in patients with heart failure, but preserved cardiac function.[30]

Carnitine for Peripheral Arterial Disease

Some research exists that enables specialists to recommend L-carnitine as a treatment for intermittent claudication (IC)—a condition that causes great pain in the legs during exercise because of a lack of oxygen flow to the muscles.

In a randomized, double-blind placebo-controlled trial of 155 patients suffering from claudication, a form of carnitine, propionyl-L-carnitine, safely improved treadmill exercise performance and enhanced the functional status of patients.[31]

In a review of the pharmacological treatment of IC in 2001, it was reported that propionyl-L-carnitine might eventually lead to significant benefit in lessening the symptoms of IC.[32]

COMMON DOSAGES

The FNB has not established dietary reference intakes for carnitine.[3] Most studies pointing toward carnitine benefits use carnitine at dosages of between 1 and 3 g per day.

TOXICITY

Carnitine supplements are relatively safe, even at very high doses, with very little in the way of toxicity symptoms being reported.[2,3] At doses of approximately 3 g/day, carnitine supplements may cause nausea, vomiting, abdominal cramps, diarrhea, and a "fishy" body odor. More rare side effects include muscle weakness in uremic patients and seizures in those with seizure disorders.[3]

FACT VERSUS FICTION

Carnitine may play a small role in weight loss, but only when used in conjunction with other weight loss aids. With all weight loss supplements, a good diet and exercise program must be followed in order to achieve results. There may be some benefit of carnitine supplements for athletes, but the effects, if any, would probably be minimal. However, because carnitine is a safe and well-tolerated supplement that benefits the heart and circulatory system, it may still provide benefits other than weight loss or enhanced exercise performance in people using it for these purposes. Carnitine does show promise as a useful supplement for diabetes.

REFERENCES

1. National Institutes of Health Office of Dietary Supplements. Carnitine: The science behind a conditionally essential nutrient. 2004. http://ods.od.nih.gov/News/Carnitine_Conference_Summary.aspx. Accessed October 14, 2009.
2. Institute of Medicine. Food and Nutrition Board. *Recommended dietary allowances.* 10th edition. Washington, DC: National Academies Press, 1989.
3. National Institutes of Health Office of Dietary Supplements. Carnitine. http://ods.od.nih.gov. Accessed October 14, 2009.
4. Stanley, CA. Carnitine deficiency disorders in children. *Ann NY Acad Sci.* 2004;1033:42–51.
5. Rebouche, CJ. Kinetics, pharmacokinetics, and regulation of L-carnitine and acetyl-L-carnitine metabolism. *Ann NY Acad Sci.* 2004;1033:30–41.
6. Reda, E, et al. The carnitine system and body composition. *Acta Diabetol.* 2003 Oct;40(Suppl 1):S106–S113.
7. Wutzke, KD, et al. The effect of L-carnitine on fat oxidation, protein turnover, and body composition in slightly overweight subjects. *Metabolism.* 2004 Aug;53(8):1002–1006.

8. Brandsch, C, et al. Effect of L-carnitine on weight loss and body composition of rats fed a hypocaloric diet. *Ann Nutr Metab*. 2002;46(5):205–210.

9. Center, SA, et al. The clinical and metabolic effects of rapid weight loss in obese pet cats and the influence of supplemental oral L-carnitine. *J Vet Intern Med*. 2000 Nov–Dec;14(6):598–608.

10. Villani, RG, et al. L-carnitine supplementation combined with aerobic training does not promote weight loss in moderately obese women. *Int J Sport Nutr Exerc Metab*. 2000 Jun;10(2):199–207.

11. Hongu, N, et al. Caffeine, carnitine and choline supplementation of rats decreases body fat and serum leptin concentrations as does exercise. *J Nutr*. 2000 Feb;13(2):152–157.

12. Zhi-Qian, He, et al. Body weight reduction in adolescents by a combination of measures including using L-carnitine. *Acta Nutrimenta Sinica*. 1997;19(2).

13. Sudha, S, et al. L-carnitine may attenuate free fatty acid-induced endothelial dysfunction. Article first published online January 12, 2006.

14. Pola, P, et al. Carnitine in the therapy of dyslipidemic patients. *Curr Ther Res Clin Exp*. 1980;27(2):208–216.

15. Pola, P, et al. Statistical evaluation of long term L-carnitinetherapy in hyperlipo proteinemias. *Drugs under Exp Clin Res*. 1983;9(12):925–934.

16. Derosa G, Cicero AF, Gaddi A, et al. The effect of L-carnitine on plasma lipoprotein(a) levels in hypercholesterolemic patients with type 2 diabetes mellitus. *Clin Ther*. 2003;25:1429–1439.

17. Mingrone, G. Carnitine in type 2 diabetes. *Ann NY Acad Sci*. 2004;1033: 99–107.

18. Rahbar, AR. Effect of L-carnitine on plasma glycemic and lipidemic profile in patients with type II diabetes mellitus. *Eur J Clin Nutr*. 2005 Apr;59(4):592–596.

19. De Gaetano, A, Mingrone, G, Castagneto, M, Calvani, M. Carnitine increases glucose disposal in humans. *J Am Coll Nutr*. 1999;18:289–295.

20. Mingrone, G, Greco, AV, Capristo, E, Benedetti, G, Giancaterini, A, De Gaetano, A, Gasbarrini, G. L-carnitine improves glucose disposal in type 2 diabetic patients. *J Am Coll Nutr*. 1999 Feb;18(1):77–82.

21. Dragan, IG, Vasiliu, A, et al. Studies concerning chronic and acute effects of L-carnitine in elite athletes. *Physiologie*. 1989 Apr–Jun;26(2):111–129.

22. Kraemer WJ, et al. The effects of L-carnitine L-tartrate supplementation on hormonal responses to resistance exercise and recovery. *J Strength Cond Res*. 2003 Aug;17(3):455–462.

23. Volek, JS, et al. L-carnitine and L-tartrate supplementation favourably affects markers of recovery from exercise stress. *Am J Physiol Endocrinol Metab*. 2002 Feb;282(2):E474–E482.

24. Dragan, IG, Vasiliu, A, et al. Studies concerning chronic and acute effects of L-carnitine in elite athletes. *Physiologie*. 1989 Apr–Jun;26(2):111–129.

25. Karlic, H, Lohninger, A. Supplementation of L-carnitine in athletes: Does it make sense? *Nutrition*. 2004 Jul–Aug;20(7–8):709–715.

26. Brass, EP, Hiatt, WR. The role of carnitine and carnitine supplementation during exercise in men and in individuals with special needs. *J Am Coll Nutr.* 1998;17:207–215.

27. Brass, EP. Supplemental carnitine and exercise. *Am J Clin Nutr.* 2000; 72:618S–623S.

28. Brass, EP. Carnitine and sports medicine: Use or abuse? *Ann NY Acad Sci.* 2004;1033:67–78.

29. Rizzon, P, et al. High doses of L-carnitine in acute myocardial infarction: Metabolic and antiarrythmic effects. *European Heart Journal.* 1989;10:502–508.

30. Ferrari, R, et al. Therapeutic effects of L-carnitine and propionyl-L-carnitine on cardiovascular diseases: A review. *Ann NY Acad Sci.* 2004 Nov;1033:79–91.

31. Dean, SM. Pharmacological treatment for intermittent claudication. *Vasc Med.* 2002;7(4):301–309.

32. Hiatt, WR, et al. Propionyl-L-carnitine improves exercise performance and functional status in patients with claudication. *Am J Med.* 2001;110:616–622.

15

L-Arginine

BRIEF OVERVIEW

Arginine is a conditionally essential amino acid, which means that under most circumstances, the human body synthesizes its own arginine as needed. Arginine's first function was identified as its ability to create urea, a waste product that clears ammonia, a toxin, from the body.[1] Arginine is also a precursor for nitric oxide (NO), a simple gas made up of nitrogen and oxygen that penetrates and crosses the membranes of almost all cells in the human body and helps regulate many cellular functions.[2] Arginine also helps the body to manufacture protein and is needed for the production of certain hormones, including growth hormone.[1,2]

THE HYPE

L-arginine supplements are common among bodybuilders and athletes who use them to enhance endurance as well as to stimulate growth hormone production in an attempt to build muscle mass. Arginine's role as a precursor for NO synthesis has made it a popular supplement for the treatment of circulatory disorders, like erectile dysfunction and cardiovascular disease. There is also some hype around L-arginine in diabetes management due to its ability to augment insulin sensitivity.

DEFICIENCY

Arginine is a conditionally essential amino acid, so deficiency is rare. It can become essential in certain people; for example, people with protein malnutrition, excessive ammonia production, burns, infections, rapid growth, urea synthesis disorders, or sepsis may not have enough arginine. Symptoms of arginine deficiency include poor wound healing, muscular weakness, impotence, hair loss, skin rash, constipation, and fatty liver.[3,4]

FOOD SOURCES

The average American generally ingests up to 5.4 g (5,400 mg) of L-arginine per day through foods. This amount is generally more than adequate to serve as a substrate for nitric oxide synthesis. The richest sources of arginine are found in vegetable proteins. Nuts, and especially peanuts, are particularly high in arginine (3 g arginine per 100 g). Other nuts and seeds range between 2–3 g arginine per 100 g of product. Legumes, like soybeans, chickpeas, and kidney beans, as well as chicken and fish contain between 1–2 g arginine per 100 g.[5]

MECHANISMS OF ACTION AND PRIMARY USES

L-Arginine Enhances Growth Hormone Production and May Prevent Low HGH Related Symptoms

Human growth hormone (HGH) promotes a healthy metabolism and a more ideal ratio of lean muscle tissue to body fat. As we age, HGH levels begin to decline and age-associated decreases in muscle mass and increases in body fat become noticeable. Naturally, stimulating HGH has therefore become quite a buzz. Since arginine is a precursor for HGH synthesis, arginine supplements have become popular with athletes, people wanting to lose body fat, and bodybuilders. Low HGH levels also lead to low levels of insulin-like growth factor 1 (IGF-1). Diminishing GH/IGF-1 has been shown to reflect disordered sleeping patterns, bone frailty, increases in central adiposity (fat accumulation around the middle of the body including the abdomen), as well as decreases in cognition and muscle mass, strength, and conditioning.[6,7,8] Whether or not L-arginine supplements can raise HGH and IGF-1 levels in humans and impact on any of the deficiency symptoms is a contentious issue. While studies have demonstrated that L-arginine supplementation of 5–9 g can augment HGH secretion at rest significantly,[9,10] others have shown L-arginine to be ineffective in augmenting both GH and IGF-I release in adults.[11] However, the latter study used a dosage of only 7 g L-arginine.

L-Arginine Aids Sports Performance

Arginine has proposed ergogenic potential and supplements have been used in an attempt to boost athletic performance. Athletes have taken arginine for three main reasons: (1) its role in the secretion of endogenous growth hormone (HGH), (2) its involvement in the synthesis of creatine (a metabolite of arginine that has ergogenic potential), and (3) its role in augmenting nitric oxide.[12]

Studies have demonstrated that L-arginine supplementation can augment HGH secretion at rest by 100 percent,[9] which seems like a great feat but exercise alone can augment HGH production by as much as 300–500 percent, with the combination of L-arginine and exercise offering no additional benefits.[9] A study using arginine aspartate supplements found no influence on performance, selected metabolic or endocrine parameters, including the stimulation of HGH.[13] A 2007 review argues that, although there is some evidence linking L-arginine supplements to enhanced endurance, studies are lacking. The review notes that there is preliminary evidence that L-arginine infusion enhances exercise performance, probably mostly via increases in nitric oxide (NO) and an altered skeletal-muscle metabolism during exercise.[14]

Another form of arginine, in the form of arginine alpha-ketoglutarate (AAKG), seems to offer more promise as a sports enhancement supplement. A randomized, double-blind, controlled study showed that AAKG supplementation of 4 g per day appeared to be safe and well tolerated and positively influenced bench press ability and Wingate peak power performance. AAKG did not influence body composition or aerobic capacity, however.[15] Another study showed that AAKG in combination with creatine improves upper body muscle endurance, and Cr + AAKG supplementation improves peak power output on repeated Wingate tests.[16]

L-Arginine Helps Produce Nitric Oxide (NO)

Attention has focused on endothelial production of nitric oxide as a key element in many of the processes associated with the development of atherosclerosis. Arginine is the substrate for the enzyme nitric oxide synthase (NOS), which is responsible for the endothelial production of nitric oxide. Arginine is thought to work through its ability to produce nitric oxide (NO), a simple gas made up of nitrogen and oxygen that penetrates and crosses the membranes of almost all cells in the human body and helps regulate many cellular functions. In blood vessels, NO is extremely important because it regulates the tone of the layer of cells known as endothelial cells that line the inside of blood vessels.[17,18] If these endothelial cells become dysfunctional, they can cause spasms or constrictions of the blood vessels that can then lead to hypertension (high blood pressure), which can cause heart disease on its own and worsen atherosclerosis.[17,18]

L-Arginine Helps Prevent Vascular Disease

Results of studies from animals with hypercholesterolemia show that L-arginine supplementation has a beneficial effect on markers of endothelial function (including vasodilatation ability), macrophage function, and platelet aggregation and adhesion, which all help reduce atherosclerotic plaque formation.[19] Human studies are lacking, however, and no conclusive evidence of benefit can be given.

A study from Italy examined blood pressure changes among six male volunteers who were placed on three different diets.[20] The first diet consisted of foods that contained 3–4 g of arginine. The second diet was high in arginine-rich foods so that these volunteers consumed about 10 g of arginine daily. People in diet three ate the same foods as people in diet one but took 10 g of arginine supplements daily. After only one week on either diet two or diet three (the arginine-rich/ supplementation diets), significant decreases in blood pressure were observed in the volunteers on those diets, as compared to those on diet one. One study done on preeclamptic pregnant women showed that L-arginine supplementation raised NO levels and lowered systolic and diastolic blood pressure within three weeks.[21]

A large trial of 153 post–myocardial infarction patients, randomized to receive either L-arginine supplements or a placebo, found no evidence that L-arginine supplementation reduces vascular stiffness measurements or left ventricular ejection fraction after six months of supplementation.[22]

However, a more recent review of 13 trials on L-arginine and endothelial function showed that when flow-mediated dilation is low, oral L-arginine supplementation increases vascular endothelial function.[23]

L-Arginine Helps Maintain Healthy Erectile Function

Erectile dysfunction is essentially a vascular disorder, which is why NO-enhancing therapies have received quite a lot of press when it comes to this topic. NO from nerves and possibly endothelia plays a crucial role in initiating and maintaining intracavernous pressure increase, penile vasodilatation, and penile erection that are dependent on cyclic GMP synthesized with activation of soluble guanylyl cyclase by NO in smooth muscle cells.[24,25]

The Massachusetts Male Aging Study of 1,290 men, aged 40–70 years, has documented the extraordinarily high prevalence of erectile dysfunction among aging men: 50 percent of men at 50 years of age, and 70 percent by age 70 have erectile dysfunction.[26] What is interesting to note is that in a recent Italian study of men with severe heart disease, an astounding 93 percent had some form of erectile dysfunction 24 months before their heart attack or onset of heart disease symptoms, highlighting the link between heart disease and erectile dysfunction.[27]

Using L–arginine supplementation on its own has shown no real benefit in improving erectile function in impotent men, using a dose of 1.5 g/day for four weeks.[28] Another study did show some positive effects on erectile function with l-arginine supplementation in men with existing defects in NO excretion or production. This study used six weeks of a much higher dose (5 g/day) L-arginine therapy.[29]

Using L-arginine in combination with other supplements for erectile dysfunction, like pycnogenol, has demonstrated more impressive results than using L-arginine on its own.[30]

L-Arginine and Cancer: A Double-Edged Sword

Arginine is an amino acid that is converted two different ways: it can become L-ornithine, or it can become nitric oxide. Each has different actions with regard to cancer. If it's converted to nitric oxide, it helps the type of immune cells that attack cancer. If it's converted to L-ornithine, it can help cancer grow.[31]

Melanoma and hepatocellular (liver) cancer require arginine for growth, and arginine depletion via arginine deiminase (ADI), an arginine-metabolizing enzyme, has been used to retard cancer cell growth.[32] Liver cancer patients treated with plasma arginine depletion therapy demonstrated a complete tumor response in one study.[33]

In contrast to arginine depletion, arginine supplementation augments both specific and nonspecific antitumor mechanisms, retards tumor growth, and prolongs

survival in some animal tumor models.[34] Breast cancer patients undergoing chemotherapy have benefitted from arginine. In one study, women who took 30 g/day
for three days prior to each chemo treatment had stronger immunity.[35] L-arginine
supplementation may also limit the progression of colon cancer, as seen in some
studies.[36,37]

COMMON DOSAGES

There is a lack of standard or well-established doses of arginine, and many different doses have been used and studied. A therapeutic dose of 2–3 g taken by mouth
three times daily, equivalent to 6–9 g per day, seems to offer benefits.[9,10,20,29]

TOXICITY

In studies, up to 16 g of arginine have been taken daily by mouth for up to six
months, with minimal side effects.[1] Stomach discomfort, including nausea, stomach cramps, or an increased number of stools, may occur with larger dosages. One
study found that 13 g arginine per day caused stomach upsets.[10] Arginine allergy
and anaphylaxis has been reported in some cases where arginine injections were
used. Other potential side effects include low blood pressure and changes in nu-
merous chemicals and electrolytes in the blood.

FACT VERSUS FICTION

Arginine can augment HGH levels, which may have implications for improving
body composition and slowing the aging process, but these effects are still uncon-
firmed. L-arginine supplements may improve exercise performance through this
mechanism of increased HGH production but also through its role in increasing NO
levels. L-arginine taken in the form of AAKG has been shown to boost endurance
and exercise performance. L-arginine supplements do hold some promise in maintaining a healthy vascular endothelium and helping to reduce blood pressure, through
its effects on NO production. Its role in helping with erectile dysfunction is probably small, but L-arginine combined with other supplements may work well in this
regard. L-arginine's role in cancer is too controversial, and because of its attenuating
effects on some cancers, it is generally not recommended as a suitable therapy.

REFERENCES

1. National Institute of Health. *Medline Plus supplement review.* http://www.nlm.
   nih.gov/medlineplus/druginfo/natural/patient-arginine.html. Accessed October 23, 2009.
2. Wu, G, Morris, SM, Jr. Arginine metabolism: Nitric oxide and beyond. *Biochem J.* 1998 Nov 15;336(1):1–17.
3. Braverman, MD, ER, *The healing nutrients within.* New Canaan, CT: Keats
   Publishing, 1997, 18, 21–23, 212, 214, 219–221, 223, 228–229.
4. Balch, MD, JF, Balch, CNC, PA. *Prescription for nutritional healing.* 2nd edition. Garden City Park, NY: Avery Publishing Group, 1997, 35–36.

5. USDA Nutrient Database for Standard References, Release 22 (2009). http://www.ars.usda.gov/ba/bhnrc/ndl. Accessed October 27, 2009.

6. de Boer, H, Blok, GJ, Van der Veen, EA. Clinical aspects of growth hormone deficiency in adults. *Endocr Rev*. 1995 Feb;16(1):63–86.

7. Aleman, A, de Vries, WR, de Haan, EH, et al. Age-sensitive cognitive function, growth hormone and insulin-like growth factor 1 plasma levels in healthy older men. *Neuropsychobiology*. 2000 Jan;41(2):73–78.

8. Toogood, AA, Shalet, SM. Ageing and growth hormone status. *Baillieres Clin Endocrinol Metab*. 1998 Jul;12(2):281–296.

9. Kanaley, JA. Growth hormone, arginine and exercise. *Curr Opion Clin Nutr Metab Care*. 2008 Jan;11(1):50–54.

10. Collier, SR, Casey, DP, Kanaley, JA. Growth hormone responses to varying doses of oral arginine. *Growth Horm IGF Res*. 2005 Apr;15(2):136–139.

11. Fayh, AP, Friedman, R, Sapata, KB, Oliveira, AR. Effect of L-arginine supplementation on secretion of human growth hormone and insulin-like growth factor in adults. *Arg Bras Endocrinol Metabol*. 2007 Jun;51(4):587–592.

12. Campbell, BI, La Bounty, PM, Roberts, M. The ergogenic potential of arginine. *Int Soc Sports Nutr*. 2004 Dec 31;1(2):35–38.

13. Abel, T, Knechtle, B, Perret, C, Eser, P, von Arx, P, Knecht, H. Influence of chronic supplementation of arginine aspartate in endurance athletes on performance and substrate metabolism—a randomized, double-blind, placebo-controlled study. *Int J Sports Med*. 2005 Jun;26(5):344–349.

14. McConell, GK. Effects of L-arginine supplementation on exercise metabolism. *Curr Opin Clin Nutr Metab Care*. 2007 Jan;10(1):46–51.

15. Campbell, B, Roberts, M, Kerksick, C, Wilborn, C, Marcello, B, Taylor, L, Nassar, E, Leutholtz, B, Bowden, R, Rasmussen, C, Greenwood, M, Kreider, R. Pharmacokinetics, safety, and effects on exercise performance of L-arginine alpha-ketoglutarate in trained adult men. *Nutrition*. 2006 Sep;22(9):872–881.

16. Little, JP, Forbes, SC, Candow, DG, Cornish, SM, Chilibeck, PD. Creatine, arginine alpha-ketoglutarate, amino acids, and medium-chain triglycerides and endurance and performance. *Int J Sport Nutr Exerc Metab*. 2008 Oct;18(5):493–508.

17. Furchgott, RF, Zawadzki, JV. The obligatory role of endothelial cells in the relaxation of arterial smooth muscle by acetylcholine. *Nature*. 1980 Nov 27;288(5789):373–376.

18. Desjardins, F, Balligand, JL. Nitric oxide-dependent endothelial function and cardiovascular disease. *Acta Clin Belg*. 2006 Nov–Dec;61(6):326–334.

19. Preli, RB, Klein, KP, Herrington, DM. Vascular effects of dietary L-arginine supplementation. *Atherosclerosis*. 2002 May;162(1):1–15.

20. Siani, A, Pagano, E, Iacone, R, et al. Blood pressure and metabolic changes during dietary L-arginine supplementation in humans. *American Journal of Hypertension*. 2000;13:547–551.

21. Rytlewski, K, Olszanecki, R, Korbut, R, Zdebski, Z. Effects of prolonged oral supplementation with l-arginine on blood pressure and nitric oxide synthesis in preeclampsia. *Eur J Clin Invest*. 2005 Jan;35(1):32–37.

22. Schulman, SP, Becker, LC, Kass, DA, Champion, HC, Terrin, ML, Forman, S, Ernst, KV, Kelemen, MD, Townsend, SN, Capriotti, A, Hare, JM, Gerstenblith, G. L-arginine therapy in acute myocardial infarction: The Vascular Interaction with Age in Myocardial Infarction (VINTAGE MI) randomized clinical trial. *JAMA*. 2006 May 10;295(18):2138–2139.

23. Bai, Y, Sun, L, Yang, T, Sun, K, Chen, J, Hui, R. Increase in fasting vascular endothelial function after short-term oral L-arginine is effective when baseline flow-mediated dilation is low: A meta-analysis of randomized controlled trials. *Am J Clin Nutr*. 2009 Jan;89(1):77–84.

24. Toda, N, Ayajiki, K, Okamura, T. Nitric oxide and penile erectile function. *Pharmacol Ther*. 2005 May;106(2):233–266.

25. Burnett, AL. The role of nitric oxide in erectile dysfunction: Implications for medical therapy. *J Clin Hypertens (Greenwich)*. 2006 Dec;8(12 Suppl 4):53–62.

26. Feldman, HA, Goldstein, I, Hatzichristou, DG, Krane, RJ, McKinlay, JB. Impotence and its medical and psychosocial correlates: Results of the Massachusetts Male Aging Study. *J Urol*. 1994 Jan;151(1):54–61.

27. Montorsi, P, Ravagnani, PM, Galli, S, et al. Association between erectile dysfunction and coronary artery disease. Role of coronary clinical presentation and extent of coronary vessels involvement: The COBRA Trial. *Eur Heart J*. 2006 Nov;27(22):2632–2639.

28. Klotz, T, Mathers, MJ, Braun, M, Bloch, W, Engelmann, U. Effectiveness of oral L-arginine in first-line treatment of erectile dysfunction in a controlled crossover study. *Urol Int*. 1999;63(4):220–223.

29. Chen, J, Wollman, Y, Chernichovsky, T, Iaina, A, Sofer, M, Matzkin, H. Effect of oral administration of high-dose nitric oxide donor L-arginine in men with organic erectile dysfunction: Results of a double-blind, randomized, placebo-controlled study. *BJU Int*. 1999 Feb;83(3):269–273.

30. Stanislavov, R, Nikolova, V. Treatment of erectile dysfunction with pycnogenol and L-arginine. *J Sex Marital Ther*. 2003 May–Jun;29(3):207–213.

31. Lind, DS. Supplement: Arginine metabolism: Enzymology, nutrition, and clinical significance. Arginine and cancer. *J Nutr*. 2004 Oct;134:2837S–2841S.

32. Ensor, CM, Holtsberg, FW, Bomalaski, JS, Clark, MA. Pegylated arginine deiminase (ADI-SS PEG20,000 mw) inhibits human melanomas and hepatocellular carcinomas in vitro and in vivo. *Cancer Res*. 2002;62:5443–5450.

33. Izzo, F, Marra, P, Beneduce, G, Castello, G, Vallone, P, De Rosa, V, Cremona, F, Ensor, CM, Holtsberg, FW, Bomalaski, JS, Clark, MA, Ng, C, Curley, SA. Pegylated arginine deiminase treatment of patients with unresectable hepatocellular carcinoma: Results from phase I/II studies. *J Clin Oncol*. 2004;22:1815–1822.

34. Stechmiller, JK, Childress, B, Porter, T. Arginine immunonutrition in critically ill patients: A clinical dilemma. *Am J Crit Care*. 2004;13:17–23.

35. Brittenden, J, et al. Natural cytotoxicity in breast cancer patients receiving neoadjuvant chemotherapy: Effects of L-arginine supplementation. *Eur J Surg Oncol*. 1994;20(4):467–472.

36. Yeh, CL, Pai, MH, Li, CC, Tsai, YL, Yeh, SL. Effect of arginine on angiogenesis induced by human colon cancer: In vitro and in vivo studies. *J Nurt Biochem*. 2009 May 14, http://www.jnutbio.com/article/S0955-2863(09)00058-8/abstract (Epub ahead of print).
37. Papadokostopoulou, A, Mathioudaki, K, Scorilas, A, Xynopoulos, D, Ardavanis, A, Kouroumalis, E, Talieri, M. Colon cancer and protein arginine methyltransferase 1 gene expression. *Anticancer Res*. 2009 Apr;29(4):1361–1366.

16

Vitamin C

BRIEF OVERVIEW

Vitamin C is one of the most popular stand-alone vitamin supplements in the world. A 2002 report showed that next to multivitamins, vitamin C was the most commonly used supplement in the United States.[1] Vitamin C is a water-soluble vitamin, which means it cannot be stored and humans need a constant, daily supply of it for normal growth and development. Vitamin C's primary function is that of an antioxidant and quencher of a variety of reactive oxygen species. It is necessary for the formation of skin, scar tissue, tendons, ligaments, and blood vessels. Vitamin C is essential for the healing of wounds and for the repair and maintenance of cartilage, bones, and teeth.

THE HYPE

The role of vitamin C (ascorbic acid) in the prevention and treatment of the common cold has been a subject of controversy for 60 years, but it is widely sold and used as both a preventive and therapeutic agent. While vitamin C supplements may play a role in

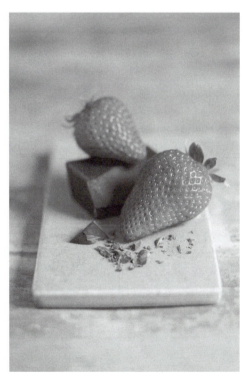

Packed with vitamin C, potassium, folate, and antioxidants, strawberries are a low carb/ low sugar treat that is heart-healthy, with potential memory-enhancing and cancer-preventing perks. (PRNewsFoto/California Strawberry Commission)

prevention as well as in shortening the duration of a cold, the effects on symptom severity are controversial. Vitamin C does show some promise in the prevention of heart disease as well as in heart attack recovery. Vitamin C may also play a role in HIV and cancer management.

DEFICIENCY

A severe form of vitamin C deficiency, known as scurvy, is characterized by general weakness, anemia, gum disease (gingivitis), and skin hemorrhage. Scurvy is seen more frequently in older, malnourished patients and is very rare in the United States.[2]

Information from the Third National Health and Nutrition Examination Survey (NHANES III) suggests that 13 percent of Americans are vitamin C deficient.[3] Smokers have higher vitamin C requirements because of smoking's ability to increase oxidative stress, and deficiencies are more common in smokers than in nonsmokers. Data from the NHANES III showed that smokers had one-third lower mean vitamin C concentrations than nonsmokers. Vitamin C deficiency was also directly related to low fruit and vegetable intakes.

Symptoms of vitamin C deficiency include dry and splitting hair, gingivitis, rough, dry skin, decreased wound healing rate, weakened tooth enamel, anemia, and a decreased ability to fight infections.[2]

FOOD SOURCES

Vitamin C is found in high concentration in fruits and vegetables. Excellent food sources of vitamin C include broccoli, bell peppers, kale, cauliflower, strawberries, lemons, mustard and turnip greens, brussels sprouts, papaya, chard, cabbage, spinach, kiwifruit, snow peas, cantaloupe, oranges, grapefruit, limes, tomatoes, zucchini, raspberries, asparagus, celery, pineapples, lettuce, watermelon, fennel, peppermint, and parsley.[2]

The United States Department of Agriculture (USDA) recommends five servings of fruit and vegetables per day, which should equate to 200–400 mg vitamin C per day, depending on the source and quality of the produce.[3] However, at least 20–30 percent of Americans ingest less than 60 mg vitamin C per day and are not nearly meeting their daily quota of fruit and vegetables.[4]

MECHANISMS OF ACTION AND PRIMARY USES

The production of reactive oxygen species by free radicals has been proven to damage bodily tissues.[5] Most of vitamin C's potential to prevent and fight disease is due to its effects as an antioxidant and free radical scavenger.

Vitamin C Helps Prevent and Fight Infections

Vitamin C has long been hailed as a prevention and treatment mechanism for all kinds of acute infections, including the common cold. In vitro studies have shown an antiviral effect of ascorbic acid, and especially dehydroascrobic acid (an oxidized form of the vitamin), on herpes simplex virus (HSV-1), influenza A virus, and poliovirus 1.[6]

Vitamin C may play a role in both the prevention and treatment of pneumonia. A 2007 Cochrane review found that trials showed as much as an 80 percent reduction in the incidence of pneumonia with vitamin C supplementation when compared to placebo groups.[7] However, most trials that showed a statistically significant prophylactic effect for pneumonia were carried out on groups likely to be consuming vitamin C deficient diets, like lower-income groups and military personnel.[7,8] In one study, elderly patients that were hospitalized with pneumonia or bronchitis showed improvement following supplementation with vitamin C;[9] however, the effects were restricted to the most ill patients.

Vitamin C supplementation may be particularly important to people in developing countries, who are highly vulnerable to developing life-threatening infections. In this at-risk population, daily supplementation with up to 1,000 mg of vitamin C, along with the mineral zinc, reduced the likelihood of developing potentially deadly pneumonia, malaria, and infection-related diarrhea.[10]

The role that vitamin C plays in the prevention and treatment of the common cold remains controversial. A recent Cochrane review looked at various studies using daily oral doses of 200 mg or more of vitamin C on the duration and severity of the common cold when used either as continuous prophylaxis or after the onset of symptoms.[11] A consistent benefit on common cold duration during prophylaxis with vitamin C was observed. The subgroup of six trials, however, was limited to athletes. Vitamin C administered after the onset of cold symptoms yielded no significant effects on cold duration. The review also reports no significant effects of vitamin C supplementation on cold symptom severity. A double-blind, five-year randomized controlled trial on elderly persons in Japan showed that high-dose (500 mg per day) vitamin C supplementation reduces the frequency of the common cold but had no apparent effect on the duration or severity of the common cold.[12] One study, conducted on younger persons, actually showed a decrease in cold and flu symptoms severity with very high dose vitamin C.[13] In this study, students who supplemented with hourly doses of 1,000 mg of vitamin C for six hours and then three times daily thereafter exhibited an 85 percent decrease in cold and flu symptoms compared to those who took pain relievers and decongestants for their infectious symptoms.

Vitamin C Improves Heart Health

Vitamin C may help support the heart and vascular system by protecting against endothelial dysfunction, preventing heart attacks, and countering the dangerous oxidation of blood lipids. In one trial, men in the highest third of vitamin C intake had a 66 percent lower risk of coronary heart disease than men in the lowest third, after controlling for various other cardiovascular risk factors.[14]

Moreover, in a meta-analysis of studies that followed subjects for more than 10 years, the use of vitamin C supplements at a dosage of at least 700 mg per day reduced risk of coronary artery disease by 25 percent.[15] In another study of vitamin C intake and heart disease risk, women who used vitamin C supplements had a 28 percent reduction in coronary heart disease compared to women who did not supplement with the vitamin.[16] The mechanisms through which vitamin C may improve heart health, include the following.

Improved Endothelial Function

The endothelium is the delicate lining of the blood vessels leading to and from the heart muscle. In endothelial dysfunction, the blood vessel walls become stiffer and their ability to dilate (or expand) to cope with an increase in blood flow is reduced. Vitamin C is thought to improve endothelial function possibly through its ability to reduce oxidative stress.[17,18] Researchers have found that while eating a meal high in fat temporarily impairs endothelial function for up to four hours in healthy individuals, pretreatment with the antioxidant vitamins C and E prevents this impairment.[19] In addition supplementation with 1,000 mg vitamin C per day protects the endothelium from the damaging effects of homocysteine (an amino acid like substance that can hasten endothelial dysfunction).[20]

Endothelial dysfunction is severely attenuated in smokers, and studies have shown that this can be surmounted by high-dose vitamin C supplementation.[21] One study using high-dose vitamin C (2,000 mg per day) in smokers showed a 59 percent reduction in endothelial dysfunction.[22] Authors warn, however, that high-dose vitamin C supplementation by no means cancels out the negative effects of smoking on heart disease risk.

Heart Attack Prevention and Protection

Vitamin C deficiency has been tied to heart attack risk. One study of middle-aged men without evidence of preexisting heart disease showed that men who were deficient in vitamin C were 3.5 times more likely to suffer heart attacks compared to those who were not deficient in the vitamin.[23] In another study, subjects in the highest quartile of vitamin C intake had 80 percent lower risk of heart attack compared to those in the lowest quartile.[24]

However, supplementing with vitamin C has not consistently shown to prevent heart attacks. Data from the Physicians' Health Study II, supplementing with 500 mg vitamin C per day, showed no significant risk reduction for cardiovascular events, including heart attacks.[25]

Vitamin C may, however, improve outcomes after suffering a heart attack. For example, in a large study of patients who had suffered an acute heart attack, supplementing with high doses of vitamin C (1,200 mg daily) for one month significantly reduced the combined rate of death, new heart attack, and other severe complications by about 20 percent. The participants also supplemented with 600 mg vitamin E in this study.[26]

Reduction in Lipid Peroxidation

It is not only the presence of LDL (low density lipoprotein), or "bad cholesterol," in the blood that affects heart disease risk, but also the oxidative state of these lipids.[27] While vitamin C has not consistently shown to be able to reduce cholesterol directly, it may help prevent the oxidation of bad cholesterol. Supplementation with 2,000 mg vitamin C per day for five days in smokers was associated with a significant reduction in markers for lipid peroxidation.[28]

Vitamin C May Be Useful in HIV Infection

It has been demonstrated that oxidative stress induced by the production of reactive oxygen species may play a critical role in the stimulation of HIV replication and the development of immunodeficiency.[29] Laboratory studies have shown that high doses of vitamin C could be toxic to HIV cells.[30,31] In a study of HIV-infected patients, subjects with advanced immune deficiency who supplemented with high doses of vitamin C together with the antioxidant N-acetylcysteine exhibited improvements in several measures of immune system function.[32]

Vitamin C May Be Useful in Cancer Prevention and Treatment

Vitamin C supplements have been used as a means to prevent and treat cancer, by virtue of their antioxidant effects. However, the U.S. Department of Health and Human Services released a summary report of studies relating to antioxidants (including vitamin C) and cancer and found no conclusive evidence that vitamin C can help either prevent or treat cancer.[33]

COMMON DOSAGES

The Food and Nutrition Board at the Institute of Medicine recommends a daily intake of 75 mg vitamin C for women and 90 mg for men, in contrast to the previous recommended daily allowance (RDA) of 60 mg per day.[34]

Many results pointing toward the benefits of vitamin C were achieved using high-dose supplementation.[3]

Dietary supplements typically contain vitamin C in the form of ascorbic acid and are often found together with bioflavonoids to enhance absorption. Also widely available is a metabolite complex form of vitamin C, sold commercially under the trade name Ester-C™, in which ascorbic acid is combined with several of its naturally occurring metabolites including dehydroascorbate, threonate, and aldonic acids.

TOXICITY

According to the Food and Nutrition Board, vitamin C toxicity is very rare, because the body cannot store the vitamin. However, amounts greater than 2,000 mg/day are not recommended because such high doses can lead to stomach upset and diarrhea.[33] There is some concern about the link between high-dose vitamin C supplementation to an increased risk of calcium oxalate kidney stones, but other studies have refuted this link.[35,36]

FACT VERSUS FICTION

Vitamin C deficiency can lower immunity and increase susceptibility to both acute infections and chronic conditions, through a decreased ability to neutralize reactive oxygen species. Using vitamin C supplements for acute upper respiratory infections may be useful as a prophylaxis or in reducing the duration of an illness, especially in people at high risk of vitamin C deficiency. The relationship between vitamin C supplements and symptom severity remains a sketchy area. Vitamin C supplements show promise in the prevention of heart disease, primarily through vitamin C's ability to improve endothelial dysfunction and reduce lipid peroxidation. The effects of vitamin C supplementation on attenuating the effects of cigarette smoking show great promise. Given that many Americans are not meeting their daily requirements of fruit and vegetables, vitamin C remains one of the most useful supplements for overall health and well-being. There may be some benefit in supplementing patients with immune deficiency symptoms with vitamin C, but its role in cancer management and prevention remains a grey area.

REFERENCES

1. Murphy, SP, Wilkens, LR, Hankin, JH, Foote, JA, Monroe, KR, Henderson, BE, Kolonel, LN. Comparison of two instruments for quantifying intake of vitamin and mineral supplements: A brief questionnaire versus three 24-hour recalls. *Am J Epidemiology*. 2002;156:669–675.
2. Mason, JB. Vitamins, trace minerals, and other micronutrients. Chapter 237 in: Goldman, L, Ausiello, D. (Eds). *Cecil medicine*. 23rd edition. Philadelphia: Saunders Elsevier, 2007.
3. Schleicher, RL, Carroll, MD, Ford, ES, Lacher, DA. Serum vitamin C and the prevalence of vitamin C deficiency in the United States: 2003–2004 National Health and Nutrition Examination Survey (NHANES). *American Journal of Clinical Nutrition*. 2009 Nov;90(5):1252–1263.
4. La Chace, P. To supplement or not to supplement: Is it a question? *Am Coil Nutr*. 1994;13:113–115.
5. Sureda, A, Batle, JM, Tauler, P, et al. Hypoxia/reoxygenation and vitamin C intake influence NO synthesis and antioxidant defenses of neutrophils. *Free Radic Biol Med*. 2004 Dec 1;37(11):1744–1755.
6. Furuya, A, Uozaki, M, Yamasaki, H, Arakawa, T, Arita, M, Koyama, AH. Antiviral effects of ascorbic and dehydroascorbic acids in vitro. *Int J Mol Medicine*. 2008 Oct;22(4):541–545.
7. Hemilä, H, Louhiala, P. Vitamin C for preventing and treating pneumonia. *Cochrane Database of Systematic Reviews*. 2007 Jan 24; (1). Art. No.: CD005532. doi: 10.1002/ 14651858.
8. Hemila, H. Vitamin C supplementation and respiratory infections: A systematic review. *Mil Med*. 2004 Nov;169(11):920–925.
9. Hemila, H, Douglas, RM. Vitamin C and acute respiratory infections. *Int J Tuberc Lung Dis*. 1999 Sep;3(9):756–761.
10. Wintergerst, ES, Maggini, S, Hornig, DH. Immune-enhancing role of vitamin C and zinc and effect on clinical conditions. *Ann Nutr Metab*. 2006; 50(2):85–94.

11. Douglas, RM, Hemilä, H, Chalker, E, Treacy, B. Vitamin C for preventing and treating the common cold. *Cochrane Database Syst Rev.* 2007 Jul 18;(3):CD000980.

12. Sasazuki, S, Sasaki, S, Tsubono, Y, Okubo, S, Hayashi, M, Tsugane, S. Effect of vitamin C on common cold: Randomized controlled trial. *Eur J Clin Nutr.* 2006 Jan;60(1):9–17.

13. Gorton, HC, Jarvis, K. The effectiveness of vitamin C in preventing and relieving the symptoms of virus-induced respiratory infections. *J Manipulative Physiol Ther.* 1999 Oct;22(8):530–533.

14. Nam, CM, Oh, KW, Lee, KH, et al. Vitamin C intake and risk of ischemic heart disease in a population with a high prevalence of smoking. *J Am Coll Nutr.* 2003 Oct;22(5):372–378.

15. Knekt, P, Ritz, J, Pereira, MA, et al. Antioxidant vitamins and coronary heart disease risk: A pooled analysis of 9 cohorts. *Am J Clin Nutr.* 2004 Dec;80(6):1508–1520.

16. Osganian, SK, Stampfer, MJ, Rimm, E, et al. Vitamin C and risk of coronary heart disease in women. *J Am Coll Cardiol.* 2003 Jul 16;42(2):246–252.

17. Kinugawa, S, Post, H, Kaminski, PM, et al. Coronary microvascular endothelial stunning after acute pressure overload in the conscious dog is caused by oxidant processes: The role of angiotensin II type 1 receptor and NAD(P)H oxidase. *Circulation.* 2003 Dec 9;108(23):2934–2940.

18. Varadharaj, S, Steinhour, E, Hunter, MG, et al. Vitamin C-induced activation of phospholipase D in lung microvascular endothelial cells: Regulation by MAP kinases. *Cell Signal.* 2006 Sep;18(9):1396–1407.

19. Plotnick, GD, Corretti, MC, Vogel, RA. Effect of antioxidant vitamins on the transient impairment of endothelium-dependent brachial artery vasoactivity following a single high-fat meal. *JAMA.* 1997 Nov 26;278(20):1682–1686.

20. Chambers, JC, McGregor, A, Jean-Marie, J, Obeid, OA, Kooner, JS. Demonstration of rapid onset vascular endothelial dysfunction after hyperhomocysteinemia: An effect reversible with vitamin C therapy. *Circulation.* 1999 Mar 9;99(9):1156–1160.

21. Stadler, N, Eggermann, J, Vöö, S, Kranz, A, Waltenberger, J. Smoking-induced monocyte dysfunction is reversed by vitamin C supplementation in vivo. *Arterioscler Thromb Vasc Biol.* 2007 Jan;27(1):120–126.

22. Katayama, Y, Shige, H, Yamamoto, A, Hirata, F, Yasuda, H. Oral vitamin C ameliorates smoking-induced arterial wall stiffness in healthy volunteers. *J Atheroscler Thromb.* 2004;11(6):354–357.

23. Nyyssonen, K, Parviainen, MT, Salonen, R, Tuomilehto, J, Salonen, JT. Vitamin C deficiency and risk of myocardial infarction: Prospective population study of men from eastern Finland. *BMJ.* 1997 Mar 1;314(7081): 634–638.

24. Lopes, C, Von, HP, Ramos, E, et al. Diet and risk of myocardial infarction. A case-control community-based study. *Acta Med Port.* 1998 Apr;11(4):311–317.

25. Sesso, HD, Buring, JE, Christen, WG, Kurth, T, Belanger, C, MacFadyen, J, Bubes, V, Manson, JE, Glynn, RJ, Gaziano, JM. Vitamins E and C in the

prevention of cardiovascular disease in men: The Physicians' Health Study II randomized controlled trial. *JAMA*. 2008 Nov 12;300(18):2123–2133.

26. Jaxa-Chamiec, T, Bednarz, B, Drozdowska, D, et al. Antioxidant effects of combined vitamins C and E in acute myocardial infarction. The randomized, double-blind, placebo controlled, multicenter pilot Myocardial Infarction and VITamins (MIVIT) Trial. *Kardiol Pol*. 2005 Apr;62(4):344–350.

27. Tsimikas, S, Brilakis, ES, Miller, ER, et al. Oxidized phospholipids, Lp(a) lipoprotein, and co. *N Engl J Med*. 2005;353:46–57.

28. Reilly, M, Delanty, N, Lawson, JA, FitzGerald, GA. Modulation of oxidant stress in vivo in chronic cigarette smokers. *Circulation*. 1996 Jul 1;94(1):19–25.

29. Suresh, DR, Annam, V, Pratibha, K, Prasad, BV. Total antioxidant capacity—a novel early bio-chemical marker of oxidative stress in HIV infected individuals. *J Biomed Sci*. 2009 Jul 7;16:61.

30. Harakeh, S, Jariwalla, RJ. Comparative study of the anti-HIV activities of ascorbate and thiol-containing reducing agents in chronically HIV-infected cells. *Am J Clin Nutr*. 1991 Dec;54(6 Suppl):1231S–1235S.

31. Rivas, CI, Vera, JC, Guaiquil, VH, et al. Increased uptake and accumulation of vitamin C in human immunodeficiency virus 1-infected hematopoietic cell lines. *J Biol Chem*. 1997 Feb 28;272(9):5814–5820.

32. Muller, F, Svardal, AM, Nordoy, I, et al. Virological and immunological effects of antioxidant treatment in patients with HIV infection. *Eur J Clin Invest*. 2000 Oct;30(10):905–914.

33. Coulter, I, Hardy, M, Shekelle, P, et al. *Effect of the supplemental use of antioxidants vitamin C, vitamin E, and the coenzyme Q_{10} for the prevention and treatment of cancer*. Summary, Evidence Report/Technology Assessment: Number 75. AHRQ Publication Number 04-E002, October 2003. Agency for Healthcare Research and Quality, Rockville, MD. http://www.ahrq.gov/clinic/epcsums/aoxcansum.htm. Accessed December 29, 2010.

34. Institute of Medicine. Food and Nutrition Board. *Dietary reference intakes for vitamin C, vitamin E, selenium and caretenoids*. Washington, DC: National Academies Press, 2000;Chapter 5: 95–167.

35. Auer, BL, Auer, D, Rodgers, AL. The effect of ascorbic acid ingestion on the biochemical and physicochemical risk factors associated with calcium oxalate kidney stone formation. *Clin Chem Lab Med*. 1998 Mar;36(3):143–147.

36. Gerster, H. No contribution of ascorbic acid to renal calcium oxalate stones. *Ann Nutr Metab*. 1997;41(5):269–282.

17

Iodine

BRIEF OVERVIEW

Human life is not possible without iodine. Iodine is an essential part of thyroid hormones, which regulate metabolism. Thyroid hormones affect essentially the entire body and must be in the correct range for good health. The same is true for iodine—it must be in the correct range for good health.

There are some indications that iodine has other specific functions. None of these can be as critical as the actions of thyroid hormones.

THE HYPE

There is no question that iodine is essential, primarily as a result of its contribution to thyroid hormone. However, evidence is accumulating that iodine may do other things. It concentrates not only in the thyroid gland, but also in the breast tissue, eye, stomach lining, uterine cervix, and salivary glands.[1]

Iodine may have a role in treating mammary dysplasia (abnormal breast tissue) and fibrocystic breast disease. It may be able to inactivate bacteria and increase the immune response. When levels are low, there may be a higher risk of stomach cancer.[2]

It seems possible that different forms of ingested iodine may preferentially go to different areas in the body. Molecular iodine (I_2) that is converted iodide (I) is most beneficial for the thyroid gland. I_2 may have more action on breast tissue that reduces atypical cells.[3,4]

In breast tissue, iodine actually reaches four times the concentration it does in the thyroid. The breast tissue has two enzymes to control the amount of free iodine, which is higher during puberty, pregnancy, and lactation.

There have been a number of studies using various forms of iodine to treat fibrocystic breast disease. Iodine seems to decrease the symptoms of fibrocystic breast disease without harming thyroid function.[1,4]

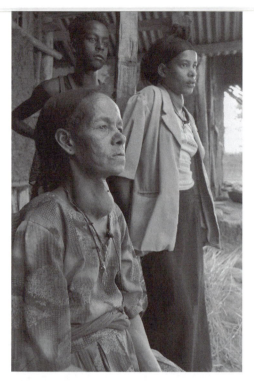

Dembele Terefe Gendo, 48, foreground, and her daughter Rome Berinhun, 16, right, sit outside their home in Nedjo, Ethiopia, in 2008. Gendo has had a goiter since she was a young girl. Her daughter has also developed one, and her son says he feels the beginning of one as well. The 16-year-old is among some 80 percent of Ethiopians suffering from an easily preventable deficiency of iodine, an essential nutrient that was readily available from Eritrea until the 1998–2000 war halted all trade between the countries. (AP Photo/ Anita Powell)

There is evidence that iodine plays a role in preventing breast cancer. In areas with high iodine consumption such as Japan, the incidence is much lower than in areas with low iodine intake. The breast tissue of women with breast cancer contains less iodine than women without cancer. It has also been hypothesized that the protective effect of multiple pregnancies on breast tissue (risk goes down with multiple pregnancies) may be because of the increased iodine in breast tissue during pregnancy and lactation.[4]

There has been much research on iodine levels and breast cancer in animals; iodine can inhibit mammary cancer in rats. Human trials will be needed to try and confirm iodine's effects on human breast cancer.[1] In one preliminary study, a small number of women with metastatic breast cancer, whose initial tumor expressed the sodium/iodine symporter (see "Mechanism of Action"), were given iodine radioisotopes, and in one patient, the radioisotope was concentrated in a metastatic lesion. This shows that it is possible that some breast cancer metastases could be treated with radioisotopes of iodine. Radioisotopes of iodine are already used as part of the treatment for thyroid cancer and metastases.[5]

Iodine is also an antioxidant. Iodine is converted to iodide using hydrogen peroxide, an oxidizing agent. When iodine is converted, it may decrease damage by free oxygen radicals in the area. This may play a role in immune function.[1]

DEFICIENCY

Abnormal growth and development are major manifestations of most iodine deficiency disorders (IDD). Problems include low thyroid hormone levels (hypothyroidism), goiter (an enlarged thyroid gland), mental retardation and cretinism. Childhood mortality is increased and normal reproduction is decreased.

Cretinism occurs when a growing fetus is low on thyroid hormone. In addition to severe mental retardation it also includes deafness, mutism, spasticity, and short stature. In some parts of the world, as many as 1 in 10 people are cretins. Groups with iodine deficiency have an average 13.5-point lower IQ score than that of populations with normal iodine intake.[2]

With insufficient iodine, the thyroid gland enlarges while trying to make more hormones. Over time it can develop nodules and even cancer.

Iodine deficiency can occur anywhere in the world. In the United States, some salt is iodized with potassium iodide, but the use of iodized salt is optional. In Canada, all salt is iodized.

There is iodine deficiency in Africa and Asia, and also in parts of Europe, such as Germany. In many countries it is a large public health problem; the World Health Organization makes recommendations and gives assistance to countries where needed.[6]

In the United States, it has been estimated that as many as 36 percent of women of childbearing age may have insufficiency, with 15 percent of these women having frank iodine deficiency. Furthermore, many breast-feeding women do not have enough iodine in their milk for their newborns. In one study done in Boston, 47 percent of lactating women did not have enough iodine in their milk.[1]

Iodine deficiency may not always be suspected in the United States because of the use of iodized salt. A woman with an enlarged thyroid, low thyroid hormone, and a thyroid scan showing uptake of radioactive iodine is usually deficient in iodine. This can be confirmed by a 24-hour urine iodine level.[7]

Pregnant women not getting enough iodine will have slightly enlarged thyroid glands, with low thyroid hormone and high TSH (thyroid stimulating hormone). If this continues, through breast-feeding and afterward, they can become hyperthyroid and develop multinodular goiters. Without enough iodine women may become obviously hypothyroid and have trouble becoming pregnant and carrying a normal pregnancy to term.[1]

Smoking significantly lowers the amount of iodine in breast milk. This is thought to occur because chemicals in cigarette smoke inhibit the activity of the sodium/iodine symporter. If breast-feeding women do not stop smoking, they should take extra iodine.[8]

Low iodine levels are associated with thyroid cancer. They may also increase the risk of breast, ovarian, uterine, and prostate cancer.[1]

Iodine consumption in Japan can be as high as 10 times what Americans take in. It has been postulated that this may be one of the reasons for a lower rate of breast disease and breast cancer in Japanese women. There is also less autoimmune thyroid disease.[1]

Thyroid status can be checked by measuring thyroglobulin, TSH, T_3 and T_4 (see "Mechanism of Action"). The thyroid gland can also be evaluated by ultrasound, as well as visualized by use of radioactive iodine. While there are other causes of hypothyroidism (low thyroid), inadequate iodine intake does eventually cause hypothyroidism, even if there are periods of hyperthyroidism.

In addition to iodine deficiency, consumption of certain foods, called "goitrogens," can cause problems with thyroid hormone production and lead to goiters.[2]

A naturally occurring chemical that can inhibit iodine uptake is called perchlorate, and it is found in the food and water supply in the United States. This may have an effect on thyroid functioning.[1]

Deficiency of vitamin A, iron, and selenium can also interfere with normal thyroid hormone production. Certain drugs can interfere with the thyroid gland. While these do not alter iodine levels, they can be additive problems.[2]

FOOD SOURCES

The majority of the earth's iodine is in the oceans. There is very little iodine in most foods. The amount varies based on what is in the soil, which is greater in coastal areas.[1]

Fish or other food from the ocean tends to have more iodine because of the iodine in seawater. Seaweed, for example, is very high in iodine. Iodine is found in cow's milk and dairy products.

The amount of iodine in most foods is between 3 to 75 μg a portion. Processed foods may have iodine added.[2]

Most people in the United States get enough dietary iodine in the diet to prevent frank hypothyroidism. Population studies have shown that people who ingest the most iodine are getting near the UL (Upper Limit). Somewhere between 10 and 15 percent of people in the United States take supplementary iodine.

Goitrogens include cassava, millet (especially from polluted water), and crucifera vegetables such as cabbage.[2]

MECHANISM OF ACTION: HOW DOES IT WORK?

Iodine is well absorbed from the gastrointestinal tract in most forms. Much of the iodate form, which is often added to salt, is converted to iodide. It was believed that most of the iodine goes to the thyroid or kidneys. It is concentrated in the thyroid; excess is excreted by the kidneys.[2]

Iodides, as opposed to molecular iodine, are absorbed via the sodium-iodide symporter. The symporter is present in all the parts of the body that concentrate iodine, including the breast, salivary glands, thyroid gland, and cervix of the uterus.[1]

In the thyroid gland, iodide is made into thyroid hormone. Thyroglobulin, a large protein made by thyroid cells, is necessary for the production of thyroid hormone. At the thyroid cells' surfaces, iodide and thyroglobulin meet. Iodide is oxidized and attached to thyroglobulin to produce precursors of thyroid hormone. The precursors are combined into two different forms, tetraiodothyronine (T_4) and triiodothronine (T_3).

There is always thyroglobulin containing iodine in thyroid follicles. This thyroglobulin is about one-third thyroid hormone and the rest precursors. A normal amount of iodine in the thyroid gland is about 15 mg. When thyroid hormone is needed, enzymes digest thyroglobulin to release thyroid hormones. Iodine that is not released as thyroid hormone is recycled within the gland itself.

T_3 and T_4 travel in the bloodstream bound to other proteins, such as thyroxine-binding globulin. When they reach the area needed, T_4 is turned into T_3. This means removing an iodide, which returns to the circulation. T_3 is the active thyroid hormone.

TSH, also called thyrotropin or thyroid stimulating hormone, regulates the release of thyroid hormone. TSH is made in the pituitary gland when thyroid hormone levels drop, and it stimulates the thyroid to make more hormone. When levels rise, TSH goes down. If there is not enough iodine, there will not be enough thyroid hormone made. TSH levels will rise, stimulating the thyroid. This causes the thyroid to enlarge. It can become a diffuse goiter or it can contain nodules. The excess TSH does not usually cause increased hormone with iodine deficiency, but sometimes if there are pockets of iodine, there can be temporary hyperthyroidism with low iodine.[2]

Thyroid hormone is the major regulator of the body's metabolism. Generally speaking, when it is low, everything slows down; when it is high, everything speeds up.

Thyroid hormone is needed for normal development of the central nervous system. It is necessary for myelination, which is the covering of nerves.

Iodine deficiency disorders (IDD), which occur throughout the world wherever iodine intake is low, occur as the result of low thyroid hormone production from inadequate iodine. As noted above, there can be short periods of hyperthyroidism, but usually thyroid hormone levels will be low.

It is now appreciated that iodine goes to other tissues. Whereas there is 15 mg of iodine in the thyroid, there may be 30 to 50 mg in the body. Possibly less than 30 percent of the iodine is in the thyroid.

Iodine goes to the eye, the stomach lining, and as noted, breasts, salivary glands, and uterine cervix. Its primary role in breast tissue has to do with lactation. It is not known what the function of iodine is in the other areas.[1]

There is a sodium/iodide symporter (NIS) in thyroid cancer cells as well as, by some estimates, more than 70 percent of breast cancer cells.[5]

PRIMARY USES

- Iodine is used to prevent and treat iodine deficiency. Where iodized salt is available, that is the most common way to deliver iodine. Iodinated oil is used in countries where there is severe deficiency and medical resources are stretched. The oil contains a large amount of iodine (400 mg) per dose and is enough for a year.

- Supplementation is important in known areas around the world where food is low in iodine. It is especially important during pregnancy and lactation.

- Molecular iodine (I_2) can be used to treat the symptoms of fibrocystic breast disease without affecting the thyroid gland.

- Radioactive iodine is used to treat thyroid cancer.[9]

COMMON DOSAGES

The Food and Nutrition Board of the Institute of Medicine has set dietary requirements for iodine in the United States. According to the FNB, the following are guidelines for iodine intake.

The Average Intake (AI) for iodine is 110 µg a day for infants 0 to 6 months of age. At 7 to 12 months, the AI is 130 µg a day. The Estimated Average Requirement (EAR) for children ages 1 through 8 years is 65 µg a day; the Recommended Dietary Allowance (RDA) is 90 µg. For children ages 9 through 13 years, the EAR is 73 µg a day; the RDA is 120 µg a day. The EAR for both boys and girls ages 14 through 18 years is 95 µg of iodine; the RDA is 150 µg/day.

The EAR for all adults, except pregnant and lactating women, is 95 µg a day and the RDA is 150 µg a day. The EAR for pregnant women is 160 µg a day regardless of the woman's age; the RDA is 220 µg a day. The EAR for lactating women is 209 µg a day; the RDA is 290 µg a day.[2]

In the United States, most people, but not all, get enough iodine in the diet. In many parts of the world, that is not true. It is also not true for some people in certain parts of the United States.

It is important for pregnant women to take enough iodine throughout the entire pregnancy and breast-feeding.[10,11]

The American Thyroid Association recommends that pregnant and breast-feeding women take supplements of 150 µg of iodine a day.[12]

POTENTIAL SIDE EFFECTS

Ingestion of multiple grams of iodine at one time can cause acute poisoning. A very large amount of iodine causes fever; abdominal pain; burning of the mouth, throat, and stomach; nausea; vomiting; diarrhea; heart problems; and coma.[2]

Over the long term, both excessive and inadequate intake of iodine can cause thyroid problems, depending on previous intake of iodine and any underlying problems with the thyroid. People with thyroid autoantibodies, meaning they are making antibodies against their thyroid gland, are more susceptible to problems with both excessive and inadequate intake of iodine.[1]

Excessive iodine ingestion can cause hyperthyroidism, the opposite of low thyroid. It can also cause goiter, thyroid inflammation (thyroiditis), and thyroid cancer. Long-term consumption of excessive amounts of iodine may also cause hypothyroidism. This can happen at any age. The reaction of a person's thyroid to excess iodine may depend on his or her previous levels of iodine and any existing thyroid disease, as noted above. Case reports have shown that high iodine intake can also potentially slow down thyroid function.

There is a serious illness highlighted by a rash specific to high iodine intake called iodermia. The rash can look like acne, hives, or be red and itchy. Iodermia can actually lead to death.[2]

The first measurable change with excess iodine consumption is an elevated TSH. TSH values were used to help set safety limits by the IOM. The No Observed Adverse Effect Level (NOAEL) for adults is 1,000 to 1,200 µg per day. The Lowest Observed Adverse Effect Level (LOAEL) for adults is 1,700 µg a day. The Upper Limit (UL) for adults is 1,100 µg a day. This is the upper limit considered to be completely safe.

Infants should only get iodine from breast milk, food, or formula. The UL for other ages has simply been extrapolated based on size. The UL for children 1 to

3 years of age is 200 µg a day. The UL for children 4 to 8 years of age is 300 µg a day, and for children 9 to 13, the UL is 600 µg a day of iodine.[2]

People who have autoimmune thyroid disease may be more susceptible to problems from increased iodine intake. These are common conditions, especially among older women.[2] One, called Graves' disease, is associated with hyperthyroidism. Another, called Hashimoto's thyroiditis, is associated with hypothyroidism.

In addition to iodine in supplements, iodine is contained in some medications, for example, amiodarone (for irregular heart rhythm). It is also contained in disinfectants like povidine-iodine and in some contrast media used for x-ray studies. Molecular iodine (I_2) does not cause the same problems as iodine (I), and larger amounts may be tolerated.

FACT VERSUS FICTION

Iodine is an essential part of the human diet. In many parts of the world, iodine deficiency is a major public health problem. In places where salt is iodized, most people get enough iodine. However, for people who are restricting their salt intake or electing not to take iodized salt, deficiency is a possibility.

Iodine is especially important during pregnancy. Pregnant and breast-feeding women have an increased need for iodine. If it is not met, there are consequences for both the mother and baby. The normal development of the fetus cannot occur without enough iodine.

Iodine deficiency causes hypothyroidism and goiter. Anyone with low thyroid hormone and an enlarged thyroid should consider whether or not he or she is getting enough iodine. A 24-hour urine test for iodine can be done to check, but this is not common practice. Discussing iodine status with your physician is a good idea if you are not sure.

People with autoimmune thyroid disorders may be less tolerant in the case of iodine excess. Iodine can help lessen the symptoms of fibrocystic breast disease. Molecular iodine (I_2) is the form best used to treat breast symptoms. It is found in seaweed.

Radioactive iodine can be used to treat thyroid cancers and metastases. It is being investigated as treatment for breast cancer and its metastases.

REFERENCES

1. Patrick, L. Iodine: Deficiency and therapeutic considerations. *Altern Med Rev.* 2008;13(2):116–127.
2. Institute of Medicine. Food and Nutrition Board. *Dietary reference intakes for vitamin A, vitamin K, arsenic, boron, chromium, copper, iodine, iron, manganese, molybdenum, nickel, silicon, vanadium, and zinc.* Washington, DC: National Academies Press, 2001.
3. Anguiano, B, Garcia-Solis, Delgado, G, Aceves Velasco, C. Uptake and gene expression with antitumoral doses of iodine in thyroid and mammary gland: Evidence that chronic administration has no harmful effects. *Thyroid.* 2007;17(9):851–859.

4. Aceves, C, Anguiano, B, Delgado, G. Is iodine a gatekeeper of the integrity of the mammary gland? *Journal of Mammary Gland Biology and Neoplasia.* 2005;10(2):189–196.

5. Wapnir, IL, Goris, M, Yudd, A, et al. The Na/I-symporter mediates iodide up-take in breast cancer metastases and can be selectively down-regulated in the thyroid. *Clinical Cancer Research.* 2004;10:4294–4302.

6. Andersson, M, de Benoist, B, Delange, F, Zupan, J. Prevention and control of iodine deficiency in pregnant and lactating women and in children less than 2-years-old: Conclusions and Recommendations of the Technical Consultation. *Public Health Nutrition.* 2007;10(12A):1606–1611.

7. Nyenwe, EA, Dagogo-Jack, S. Iodine deficiency disorders in the iodine-replete environment. *Am J Med Sci.* 2009;337(1):37–40.

8. Laurberg, P, Nøhr, SB, Pedersen, M, Fuglsang, E. Iodine nutrition in breast-fed infants is impaired by maternal smoking. *The Journal of Clinical Endocrinology & Metabolism.* 2004:89(1):181–187.

9. Spitzweg, C, Harrington, KJ, Pinke, LA, et al. Clinical Review 132. The sodium iodide symporter and its potential role in cancer therapy. *The Journal of Clinical Endocrinology & Metabolism.* 2001;86(7):3327–3335.

10. Zeisel, SH. Is maternal diet supplementation beneficial? Optimal development of infant depends on mother's diet. *Am J Clin Nutr.* 2009;89(Suppl): 685S–687S.

11. Moleti, M, Pio lo Presti, V, Mattina, F, et al. Gestational thyroid function abnormalities in conditions of mild iodine deficiency: Early screening versus continuous monitoring of maternal thyroid status. *European Journal of Endocrinology.* 2009;160:611–617.

12. Picciano, MF, McGuire, MK. Use of dietary supplements by pregnant and lactating women in North America. *Am J Clin Nutr.* 2009;89(Suppl):663S–667S.

18

Iron

BRIEF OVERVIEW

Iron is essential for human life. It is at the core of hemoglobin, which transports oxygen to the body via red blood cells. Deficiency of iron eventually leads to anemia, which means a low red blood count. Iron deficiency and anemia can lead to fatigue, exercise intolerance, decreased immunity, adverse outcomes during pregnancy, and a whole host of other problems that are still being studied.

In populations with adequate food intake, menstruating, pregnant, and lactating women are at the highest risk for iron deficiency, along with small children. In populations with inadequate access to food, iron deficiency is common.

On the other hand, excessive amounts of iron are stored in body organs where the iron can cause damage. An example of this is a hereditary disease called hemochromatosis, in which iron is deposited in the liver, the heart, and other organs. Treatment of this disease includes phlebotomy, or removal of blood, to decrease the excess iron. Older people may also accumulate excess iron from the diet and/or supplements, which may increase their risk of certain chronic illnesses.

While there is a control system in the body regulating iron absorption that can delay or mask some of the problems with iron deficiency or excess, a deficiency of iron will eventually produce symptoms, as will a chronic excess.[1]

THE HYPE

Iron Excess

Iron can catalyze oxidation reactions, including those that generate free radicals. Free radical–induced, oxidative reactions may increase the risk of cancer, cardiovascular diseases, and other problems.

Iron often accumulates in older people. The intake of iron can be greater than the loss of iron, and the body has no mechanism for eliminating excess iron. It is not certain whether or not significant iron accumulation can occur simply from

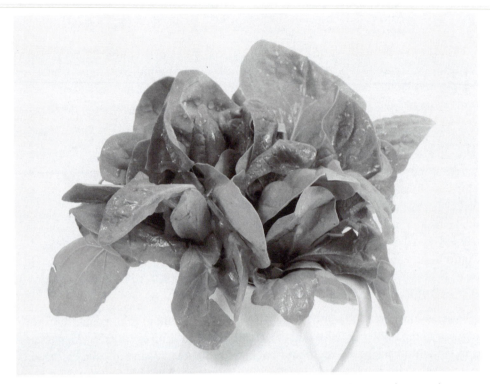

Natural nonheme iron can be found in spinach. (© Ramon Grosso/Dreamstime.com)

dietary intake, or if supplementation has to be involved, such that there is more iron ingested than necessary over a long period of time. One study demonstrated that a diet high in fruit, fruit juices, and red meat, along with iron and vitamin C supplementation can be associated with elevated iron stores in the elderly (ages 68 to 93). If elevated iron stores do in fact cause an increased risk of cancer or cardiovascular disease, this needs to be taken into account. Many people eating a Western diet do not need supplemental iron.[2]

Iron Excess May Increase the Risk of Cardiovascular Disease

The free-radical reactions that ferrous iron can catalyze can cause cell damage. This may contribute to the beginning of coronary artery disease by damaging cell walls, disrupting cholesterol-laden plaques, or causing platelet clumping, among suggested mechanisms. Iron's possible contribution to coronary heart disease risk is called the iron hypothesis.

Many studies have been done examining the risk of coronary heart disease in relation to elevated iron levels. Ferritin, transferrin saturation, serum iron concentration, and total iron-binding capacity, as well as other tests, have been used to assess body iron stores. Types of studies have included prospective studies following groups of people, or prospective epidemiological studies and case control studies. The Institute of Medicine looked at the data in 2000, and came to the conclusion that there was no proof of a causal relationship. However, a possible relationship has not been disproven.[3]

Others have come to similar conclusions, that the data is equivocal at this time, regarding a relationship between high iron levels and coronary artery disease or peripheral arterial disease.[4] It was suggested that the ideal measurement of true iron status has not been found, and that prospective, randomized trials are needed to see if lowering iron content by phlebotomy might improve PAD.

In one such trial, a randomized, controlled, single-blinded trial, called the Iron and Atherosclerosis Study (FeAST), phlebotomy every six months to lower iron stores had no impact on all-cause mortality or death plus nonfatal heart attacks and stroke. This was done in patients with stable peripheral artery disease. There was some evidence that younger patients may have benefited from the reduction in iron.[5]

The discovery of the genetic mutation that causes hemochromatosis (see below) has led to studies of carriers of this gene. They may have elevated iron stores. Could that increase the likelihood of coronary heart disease or other vascular disease? So far there has been no conclusive proof of this.[6]

Iron Excess May Cause an Increased Risk of Cancer

Many studies have shown a possible relationship between iron levels and cancer. In the study group already mentioned that looked at iron excess and peripheral artery disease, cancer occurrence was also monitored. Adult male patients who had periodic blood removal to lower total iron in the FeAST trial had a significantly lower incidence of cancer and mortality over four and a half years.[7] This study included only adult men, and the researchers were careful to say that it did not necessarily apply to other populations. However, their findings, as well as those of other investigators, have led to the theory that there is a level of iron that is toxic over time, which they called "ferrotoxicity." This is discussed further in the section entitled "Potential Side Effects."

Some studies have shown a relationship between higher levels of iron and colon cancer, as well as other cancers. Not all research has found the same correlation. The only definite connection at this time is that patients with hemochromatosis and cirrhosis of the liver have a higher risk of liver cancer.

Further research needs to be done to either confirm or disprove the idea of a link between iron levels and cancer in general.[3]

Iron Deficiency—Possible Effects

There are many known physical effects of iron deficiency, described below in "Deficiency." Other problems are not as clear. This section will deal with problems caused by iron deficiency.

Iron Deficiency Impairs the Immune System; Excess Iron May Benefit the Infecting Organisms

Both humans and infecting organisms need iron. During an illness, absorption and release of iron are decreased, so that iron is not available to the bacteria, viruses.

or parasites. Any increase in iron during infection may actually wind up benefiting the bacteria or other organisms. At the same time, the human immune system, mainly the cellular portion of immunity, is less effective under conditions of iron deficiency.

Supplementing people who are infected with pathogenic organisms can actually cause an increase in the replication of the infecting organism. Iron administration has been shown to reactivate malaria. There is a balance between human host and infectious organisms in terms of where the iron goes.[8] This is a difficult balance to try and maintain.[9] It is more of a problem in countries where iron deficiency, as well as chronic infections, are endemic.

Iron Deficiency Itself May Impair Brain Development

The brain is rich in iron, but the pattern of iron location in the brain varies from infancy to adulthood.[8] Iron is needed in order for the spinal cord and the cerebellar folds in the brain to have normal myelinization—that is, the development of a protective covering of myelin. Iron deficiency may cause a delay in the maturation of motor control in childhood as well as affect behavior.[8] It may also cause cognitive defects.

There is conflicting data on the effect of iron deficiency on the neurotransmitters in the brain. Some research indicates it may affect GABA metabolism and dopamine.[8] Other researchers have found an effect on serotonin and dopamine. Their synthesis is decreased when there is iron deficiency. This can lead to behavioral and cognitive alterations.[10]

There may be a critical time period during which the human brain is susceptible to iron deficiency, and damage occurs that cannot be corrected with iron later on. There are indications that infants between 8 and 15 months old may be susceptible to damage from low iron,[8] which is irreversible.[10] It seems possible that infants and children who are iron deficient up to age 2 years will have permanent damage that can include motor control problems, behavioral problems, and cognitive deficiencies. Older children may have the same type of problems that can be reversed with adequate iron intake.

There is also evidence that deficiency of many other nutrients negatively impacts brain function when it occurs early in development. Since iron deficiency may be accompanied by other deficiencies, it is very difficult to prove that the low iron alone is responsible for abnormalities or deficits.

Even more perplexing to investigators is the fact that anemia itself depresses mental processes and brain functions. Therefore, it is very difficult to say if the anemia of iron deficiency is causing the problem, or if a lesser iron deficiency without anemia would have the same effect.[10]

Athletes May Have Increased Iron Deficiency and Anemia

Highly trained athletes, both male and female, need more iron than those who do not exercise. They may be losing more iron in the stool or urine, or the red cells may be rupturing in the feet of runners.[3]

More athletes have iron-deficiency anemia than occurs in the general population, especially female athletes. This is likely due to a variety of factors, from decreased consumption of iron to increased losses. Anemic athletes perform poorly. Iron status needs to be monitored and appropriate supplements given to athletes.[11]

Iron Deficiency May Cause Restless Legs Syndrome

People with restless legs syndrome have an uncontrollable and distressing urge to move their legs, severe enough to interfere with sleep. Many studies have found a high prevalence of iron deficiency in patients with this problem. Iron testing is recommended, and treatment with iron given if iron is low. It is not clear whether or not the low iron is a cause of the syndrome.[12]

Iron Deficiency with or without Anemia May Contribute to Congestive Heart Failure

Since iron is the key to oxygen transport, even patients without iron-deficiency anemia, but with low iron stores, may have more symptoms from heart failure. A recent study showed that giving intravenous iron to patients with chronic heart failure improved many symptoms, functioning, and quality of life, even in those who were not anemic.[13]

DEFICIENCY

Iron deficiency is a well-known problem. It can occur because of increased loss of iron, in menstrual blood, from bleeding in the intestinal tract, or from major trauma with blood loss. It can also occur because of insufficient iron in the diet or decreased absorption of iron.[14]

Most of the time, iron deficiency occurs slowly. When there is not enough intake of iron to balance losses, it is released from body stores, and hemoglobin and red blood cells remain normal. Anemia is an advanced stage of iron deficiency, when stores have been used up.[14]

A range of symptoms is associated with iron deficiency. Most are likely a direct result of the lack of hemoglobin and the decreased oxygen delivery throughout the body. There may also be effects on the body that are not due to the low hemoglobin but are rather due to an interruption of other iron-related reactions.[8] With iron deficiency, the concentration of myoglobin in muscles drops, which may cause decreased endurance. Myoglobin is similar to hemoglobin but found in skeletal muscle.[3]

Fatigue and lack of energy are prominent, and physical performance is decreased. People with iron deficiency may exhibit pica, which is the desire to eat nonnutritional items such as dirt and ice.[8]

Visible physical changes include a blue tinge to the whites of the eye, spooning of the nails, inflammation of the tongue (glossitis), cracking of the sides of the lips (angular stomatitis), and a measurable anemia.

Iron deficiency leads to an impairment of many of the body's functions, including thermoregulation, mental function, and immune function. It can alter insulin sensitivity, drug metabolism, and absorption of metals like cadmium and lead. It can slow childhood development. While the anemia from iron deficiency is well understood, as are many of the symptoms, some of the other problems, such as the effect iron deficiency has on the development of mental function, are being studied and analyzed.[8,14] (See "The Hype," above.)

Iron deficiency can lead to complications of pregnancy. Moderate to severe anemia increases the risk of maternal death. It also is associated with low birth weight and premature delivery.[3,15] There is evidence associating maternal iron deficiency with cardiovascular disease when the children grow into adulthood.[16] The developing fetus will get iron at the expense of the mother. Full-term babies of normal weight born to iron-deficient mothers may not have obvious iron deficiency. They still may have decreased iron stores. Premature and low birth weight babies may be iron deficient because they did not have enough time or get enough nutrition from their mothers.

People with kidney failure on dialysis often develop iron-deficiency anemia because of iron losses as well as a decrease in erythropoietin, a hormone secreted by the kidney that stimulates red blood cell production.[14] Vitamin A deficiency limits the body's ability to use iron, although it does not cause actual iron deficiency.

Blood can be lost in the intestinal tract because of bleeding from cancer and inflammatory diseases of the intestine like Crohn's disease. Crohn's disease and any others causing general malabsorption can also cause iron deficiency.

Vegetarians can also become iron deficient because the nonheme iron in their diet may not be well-enough absorbed.[14] People who have gastric bypass surgery frequently become iron deficient and need supplements, sometimes intravenously.[17]

Iron deficiency can be detected before anemia occurs. There are a number of blood tests that physicians can perform to measure iron stores. If iron stores are low, supplementation is indicated to prevent anemia and other symptoms.

FOOD SOURCES

Iron is found in food from both plant and animal sources. Animal proteins and some plants contain heme iron. The iron in heme is bound in a ring structure such as hemoglobin. Many plant sources offer nonheme iron. Food enriched with iron contains nonheme iron.

Heme iron is much more easily absorbed in the intestine. Sources include red meats, chicken and other poultry, fish, shellfish, and bivalves like clams. Natural nonheme iron can be found in many kinds of beans, soy and soy derivatives like tofu, as well as spinach, molasses, and raisins. Cereals are often iron-fortified, as are many types of bread.[14]

Iron absorption in the intestine varies depending on the type of iron, the amount of iron in a person's system, the presence of food or medication in the intestinal tract, and other factors. On average, 10 to 15 percent of dietary iron is absorbed.

Iron deficiency causes increased absorption. Between 15 and 35 percent of heme iron is absorbed, as opposed to 2 to 20 percent of nonheme iron. Nonheme iron absorption increases in the presence of vitamin C and meat proteins. The tannins in tea can decrease absorption of nonheme iron, as can calcium, phytates (found in whole grains and legumes), and some proteins in soybeans. For anyone low in iron who wants to get enough iron from a vegetarian diet, care must be taken to try and eat enhancing foods along with nonheme iron.[14]

The diets of people in Western countries usually contain only 10 percent heme iron.[1]

MECHANISM OF ACTION: HOW DOES IT WORK?

Iron is an element than can exist in a number of oxidative states, usually ferric or ferrous, which have different degrees of oxidation. Iron is most commonly bound to oxygen, nitrogen, or sulfur. Its unique chemical properties make it useful in a wide variety of chemical reactions. In the human body, reactions involving iron include oxidation-reduction reactions, oxygen transport and storage, and transfer of electrons.[8]

In humans (and other mammals), iron is contained in proteins. There are the nonenzymatic proteins hemoglobin and myoglobin, enzymes containing iron, enzymes containing heme iron, and a group of enzymes that contain iron in different forms.[8] Hemoglobin and myoglobin transport oxygen. Iron-sulfur enzymes are involved in energy metabolism. Iron-heme enzymes transfer electrons associated with a number of cofactors.

Oxygen transport is the best-known and most important function of iron. Hemoglobin is a protein with two identical subunits, each of which has an iron-containing compound that can bind with oxygen. Hemoglobin transports oxygen from the lungs to the rest of the body. It picks up oxygen from lung capillaries and transports it to capillaries in tissue throughout the body. Iron's primary mechanism of action is its ability to bind oxygen as well as release it. In peripheral tissues, higher concentrations of CO_2 and lower pH favor releasing of oxygen from hemoglobin.

Iron is necessary to make hemoglobin, and hemoglobin is necessary to make red blood cells.[8]

Myoglobin has a single subunit and transports oxygen from red cells to the inside of other cells, especially to mitochondria, the powerhouse of the cell. Myoglobin is found in muscle.

The other chemicals containing iron participate in a variety of reactions in cells all over the body. Most iron in the body is found in one of three places. It is stored in proteins like hemosiderin and ferritin. It is part of proteins or enzymes that are crucial for life, such as hemoglobin. Or iron can be found in the proteins that transport it, like transferrin.[1]

Regulation of Iron Absorption

Because both iron deficiency and iron excess can be damaging, there is a control mechanism in humans to try and maintain correct iron balance. Ingested iron is a "pool" in the intestinal tract. When there is a low amount of iron in the body, more iron in the pool will cross into the cells lining the intestine. A relatively newly discovered peptide called hepcidin regulates the export of iron from the intestinal cells as well as iron stored in liver cells or macrophages.[18] Hepcidin degrades ferroportin, the protein that transports iron out of cells. Hepcidin is also believed to regulate the amount of iron that enters intestinal cells called enterocytes.[19] Ongoing study of hepcidin is increasing the understanding of iron homeostasis in the human body and will lead to better ways to diagnose and treat iron disorders.[20]

Iron is transported out of cells and into the circulation, eventually to the bone marrow where red blood cells are made. Iron can also be retained in the intestinal cells attached to ferritin.[1]

Approximately 80 percent of the iron in the body is inside red blood cells. These cells age and are replaced with new red cells every 120 days. Iron is stored primarily in the liver and spleen as hemosiderin, as well as in individual cells bound to ferritin. Hemosiderin in the liver increases dramatically if there is excess iron.

PRIMARY USES

- The primary use of iron is to treat iron deficiency.
- It can also be used to prevent iron deficiency at predictable times. For example, pregnant women need much more iron, because they have a larger blood volume, need enough iron for the baby, and also will lose blood during delivery. It was estimated by the CDC that in 1999–2000, 12 percent of women ages 12 to 49 years in the United States were iron deficient.[14]

COMMON DOSAGES

The Institute of Medicine of the National Academy of Sciences has developed a number of guidelines for iron consumption. The Recommended Dietary Allowance (RDA) for iron is different between males and females at different ages. The RDA is meant to indicate the amount of a nutrient that will meet the needs of 97 to 98 percent of healthy people. Many people can get the iron they need from food, especially those who do not have increased need for iron.

Healthy infants are born with iron stores to last around 6 months. According to the RDAs, infants ages 7 to 12 months old need 11 mg of iron a day. Children ages 1 to 3 years need 7 mg a day. Children ages 4 to 8 years need 10 mg of iron a day. From 9 to 13 years, both boys and girls need 8 mg of iron a day. From 14 to 18 years and on, there is a difference between girls (and women) and boys (and men). Girls in that age group (or menstruating before age 14) need 15 mg of iron a day, whereas boys only need 11 mg of iron a day. Between ages 19 and 50 years, when women are menstruating, women need 18 mg of iron a day. Pregnant women need 27 mg of iron a day, while breast-feeding women need significantly less, 9 mg a day. After age 51, both men and women need 8 mg of iron a day.[14]

Babies can absorb iron in breast milk very well. They cannot absorb cow's milk iron, which is low. Cow's milk can also cause intestinal bleeding in babies and should not be given to them. Breast milk and then iron-fortified baby foods are recommended.

People with inadequate sources of quality food can develop iron deficiency, particularly in the groups that need more iron. Worldwide, as many as 80 percent of people may be deficient in iron.

Pregnant women are often recommended to take low doses of supplemental iron, in the range of 30 mg/day. If iron-deficiency anemia occurs, higher doses of iron are necessary.[14]

Iron deficiency can be diagnosed by a number of tests, including serum ferritin levels, transferrin saturation, total iron-binding capacity, erythrocyte protoporphyrin, hemoglobin concentration, mean cell volume, and stainable iron in the bone marrow. Ferritin levels may be the most sensitive indicator of how much iron is still in storage. Low serum transferrin saturation indicates that there is not enough iron to continue to make normal amounts of hemoglobin. Doctors can decide which tests need to be done to evaluate a person's iron status. Then iron supplementation can be recommended if necessary. It is very important not to assume that anemia is caused by iron deficiency. If iron is given to individuals without iron deficiency, excess iron can accumulate.

The most easily absorbed type of iron occurs in the form of ferrous iron. Ferrous sulfate has the most available iron, followed by ferrous lactate and ferrous gluconate. A 300-mg tablet of ferrous sulfate has 50 to 60 mg (approximately 20%) of available iron. Ferrous gluconate has only 12 percent iron content.[1]

If all the iron is taken at once, less will be absorbed. Most recommend that when treating iron deficiency, the iron should be split up and taken twice a day. A common dose to treat iron deficiency would be 300 mg of ferrous sulfate two times a day for approximately three months.[14] Iron is absorbed better when taken with vitamin C.

Physicians can monitor the laboratory tests to make sure the iron is absorbed, stores are being replenished, and anemia corrected.

It is very unusual, but sometimes in severe cases of iron deficiency, the iron has to be given by injection, monitored by a health care provider.

The safe upper limit for iron, according to the Institute of Medicine, is 40 mg/day for infants and children up to age 13. Then 45 mg/day is the upper limit for people ages 14 to18 and adults including pregnant and lactating women. The upper limit defines a dose above which most people experience significant adverse effects, with iron, usually gastrointestinal.[3] This upper limit will not prevent overload in patients with hemochromatosis (see the next section).

POTENTIAL SIDE EFFECTS

Iron supplements frequently cause nausea, vomiting, constipation or diarrhea, abdominal discomfort, and dark-colored stools. Dividing up the dose and taking iron with food helps lessen these symptoms. They also usually decrease with time as the body adjusts to the supplements.[14]

High amounts of ingested iron can reduce zinc absorption.[1]

Excessive amounts of iron are very dangerous. If there is too much iron in the intestinal tract, it can overwhelm any feedback mechanism and will be absorbed. High iron can actually kill cells in the intestinal tract. Vomiting and diarrhea will be followed by death if a lethal dose of iron is ingested. A one-time lethal dose is in excess of 180 mg/kg, which would be at least 12,600 mg of iron for an average adult male.[1]

Children can ingest a toxic amount if they eat a lot of iron supplement pills, for example, all of a 100-pill bottle. This is a true emergency. As recently as 1997, the most common cause of poisoning deaths in children less than six years old in the United States was accidental iron ingestion.[3]

Chronic consumption of excess iron can cause intestinal symptoms and constipation. This can occur at doses of 10 to 20 mg/kg, which would be 700 to 1,400 mg of iron daily. As a point of reference, most ferrous sulfate tablets contain 60 mg of iron.[1]

There is also no way for the body to get rid of excess iron. It tends to accumulate in the elderly, especially if they continue to eat a high-iron diet with lots of red meat and similar foods. Ferrotoxic disease may be caused by elevated body stores of iron over time. Ferrotoxicity may occur with ferritin levels about 50 mg/mL.[7] This toxicity may include cancer, cardiovascular disease as well as other chronic illnesses (see "The Hype").

Iron from diet alone does not usually cause iron overload.[3] Supplements are usually involved.

Hemochromatosis is a specific disease related to iron excess. It is an inherited condition that can occur in 1 in 200 to 400 people of northern European ancestry. Hemochromatosis is an autosomal-recessive condition, which means that people who get an abnormal gene from both parents can have the disease. It is possible that people with just one copy of the abnormal gene may have some iron storage problems. In hemochromatosis, iron absorption across the intestinal lining cells is not controlled. Consequently, excess iron is absorbed, and it accumulates in the body. Symptoms do not occur until body stores of iron are quite high. Symptoms start to manifest between 40 and 60 years of age. At this point, a patient with hemochromatosis may have as much as 20 or 30 g of excess iron in his or her body.

The abnormal gene that causes most cases of hemochromatosis has been identified (C282Y). There are other less common genes that can cause hemochromatosis. Also, not everyone with the abnormal genes actually develops the disease. The mechanism by which the disease is manifested is now known to be insufficiency of hepcidin. Hepcidin levels do not increase in these patients with rising iron levels. Iron continues to be absorbed.[21]

Instead of being stored throughout what is called the reticulendothelial system, people with hemochromatosis have excess iron in the cells of critical organs, including the liver and heart. The large amounts of iron stored in the liver can cause cirrhosis and liver cancer. Heart muscle, the pituitary gland, and pancreatic tissue can be damaged. Treatment of this disease includes administration of chemicals that can bind excess iron, and phlebotomy, or removal of blood.[1,3]

FACT VERSUS FICTION

Iron is essential to human life, but there is danger in excess iron as well as deficiency. More thorough understanding of iron regulation in humans has led to greater understanding of both extremes.

While it may be safe for healthy adults, especially women, to take iron supplements at the recommended daily allowance, most people should be evaluated before deciding to take iron on a regular basis. Many patients with anemia are not iron deficient and run the risk of ingesting too much iron. On the other hand, in many parts of the world, the majority of people are iron deficient.

Hemochromatosis is a known disease of iron overload. It is not proven at this time that excess iron causes other disease. However, it may contribute to the risk of cardiovascular disease and cancer as well as other conditions like restless legs syndrome and decreased athletic performance.

Since these are possibilities, it is best for most people to know their iron status and take appropriate action under the care of a physician.

REFERENCES

1. Beard, J. Iron. In: Coates, PM. (Ed). *Encyclopedia of dietary supplements.* New York: Marcel Dekker, 2005, 357–362.
2. Fleming, DJ, Tucker, KL, Jacques, PF, et al. Dietary factors associated with the risk of high iron stores in the elderly Framingham Heart Study cohort. *Am J Clin Nutr.* 2002;76:1375–1384.
3. Institute of Medicine. Food and Nutrition Board. *Dietary reference intakes for vitamin A, vitamin K, arsenic, boron, chromium, copper, iodine, iron, manganese, molybdenum, nickel, silicon, vanadium, and zinc.* Washington, DC: National Academies Press, 2000. http://books.nap.edu/openbook.php?record_id=10026. Accessed January 10, 2010.
4. Ramakrishna, G, Rooke, TW, Cooper, LT. Iron and peripheral arterial disease: Revisiting the iron hypothesis in a different light. *Vasc Med.* 2003;8:203–210.
5. Zacharksi, LR, Chow, BK, Howes, PS, et al. Reduction of iron stores and cardiovascular outcomes in patients with peripheral arterial disease. *JAMA.* 2007;297:603–610.
6. Ma, J, Stampfer, MJ. Body iron stores and coronary heart disease. *Clinical Chemistry.* 2002;48(4):601–603.
7. Zacharksi, LR, Chow, BK, Howes, PS, et al. Decreased cancer risk after iron reduction in patients with peripheral arterial disease: Results from a randomized trial. *Natl Cancer Inst.* 2008;100:996–1002.
8. Beard, JL. Iron biology in immune function, muscle metabolism and neuronal functioning. *J Nutr.* 2001;131:568S–580S.
9. Prentice, AM. Iron metabolism, malaria, and other infections: What is all the fuss about? *J Nutr.* 2008;138:2537–2541.
10. McCann, JC, Ames, BN. An overview of evidence for a causal relation between iron deficiency during development and deficits in cognitive or behavioral function. *Am J Clin Nutr.* 2007;85:931–945.

11. Beard, J, Tobin, B. Iron status and exercise. *Am J Clin Nutr.* 2000;72(Suppl): 594S–597S.

12. Earley, CJ. Restless legs syndrome. *N Engl J Med.* 2003;348:2103–2109.

13. Anker, SD, Comin, CJ, Filippatos, G, et al. Ferric carboxymaltose in patients with heart failure and iron deficiency. *N Engl J Med.* 2009;361:2436–2448.

14. Office of Dietary Supplements. Dietary Supplement Fact Sheet: Iron. National Institutes of Health. http://ods.od.nih.gov/factsheets/iron.asp. Accessed January 12, 2010.

15. Allen, AH. Anemia and iron deficiency: Effects on pregnancy outcome. *Am J Clin Nutr.* 2000;71(Suppl):1280S–1284S.

16. Gambling, L, Danzeisen, R, Fosset, C, et al. Iron and copper interactions in development and the effect on pregnancy outcome. *J Nutr.* 2003;133: 1554S–1556S.

17. Gasteyger, C, Suter, M, Gaillard, RC, Giusti, V. Nutritional deficiencies after Roux-en-Y gastric bypass for morbid obesity often cannot be prevented by standard multivitamin supplementation. *Am J Clin Nutr.* 2008;87:1128–1133.

18. Ganz, T. Hepcidin—a regulator of intestinal iron absorption and iron recycling by macrophages. *Best Pract Res Clin Haematol.* 2005;18:171–182.

19. Pak, M, Lopez, MA, Gabayan, V, et al. Suppression of hepcidin during anemia requires erythropoietic activity. *Blood.* 2006;108:3730–3735.

20. Collins, JF, Wessling-Resnick, M, Knutson, MD. Hepcidin regulation of iron transport. *J Nutr.* 2008;138:2284–2288.

21. Piperno, A, Girelli, D, Nemeth, E, et al. Blunted hepcidin response to oral iron challenge in HFE-related hemochromatosis. *Blood.* 2007;110:4096–4100.

19

L-Glutamine

BRIEF OVERVIEW

L-glutamine is a conditionally indispensable amino acid. This means that there are conditions under which it must be ingested. L-glutamine can be synthesized by the body by glutamine synthetase, which converts ammonia and glutamate into glutamine. Excess glutamine can be broken down into glutamate and ammonia by the enzyme glutaminase. Glutamine can also be converted into other amino acids, used in other reactions, and become part of the body's protein.

However, when there are not enough precursors for the body to make glutamine, and the demand for it is high, it must be taken in, or the body will become glutamine deficient.

Amino acids are the building blocks of proteins. Proteins make up the structure of cells. They also work as enzymes, carriers for other substances, in cell membranes, and as hormones. Amino acids are precursors for the nucleic acids that make up RNA and DNA, the genetic blueprints. Glutamine fulfills all of these functions as an amino acid.

However, glutamine has many other biological functions in addition to being an essential part of human proteins. It is important for energy metabolism as well as nitrogen metabolism. It stimulates the immune system. It is important for cell growth and proliferation, helping provide the materials as well as the energy. This is critical for rapidly growing, dividing cells like the lining of the intestine and those of the bone marrow.

At the current time, there is much research focused on these other roles of glutamine.

(In this chapter, L-glutamine and glutamine will be used interchangeably.)

THE HYPE

Much of the initial research on glutamine was in the laboratory, using cell cultures or animals. There have also been studies on humans, which seem to prove some hypotheses and disprove others. At the current time, there are larger trials in progress that may provide answers to some of the questions about the best uses of glutamine.

For patients that are critically ill with sepsis or injury, adding glutamine to the intravenous fluid they are getting has been tested and proven beneficial. This is crucial for anyone who is getting all nutrition by vein (total parenteral nutrition, TPN). While glutamine had been considered dispensable and not necessarily given to people in these conditions, it seems probable that glutamine may be more important than some other nutrients and should be used in large doses.[1,2]

Of the many trials looking at glutamine's effect on critically ill patients, intravenous, high-dose glutamine trials have usually showed a positive effect. The trials of oral or enteral (into the intestine) glutamine, especially at lower doses, have often not shown any effect.

While it had been thought that replacing low glutamine levels during stress might be helpful as a fuel, it is now believed that, among other things, glutamine helps the immune system and signals cells in order to trigger genes needed to help the body.

Glutamine and the Immune System

Lymphocytes, one type of white blood cells, are dependent upon glutamine from skeletal muscle for much of their functioning. Monocytes and macrophages are other types of cells critical to the immune system that need glutamine to function normally.

The behavior of both lymphocytes and monocytes in response to various levels of glutamine has been studied in laboratory settings. Glutamine has many actions in these cells that allow them to function properly.

Glutamine probably also affects other parts of the immune system.

There are many chemical changes that have been measured in these cells in vitro, in the laboratory, as the result of changes in the amount of available glutamine.[3] What is visible in the laboratory correlates with what has, at least in part, been observed in patients and in human studies.

HIV/AIDS

In HIV/AIDS there is usually glutamine deficiency. This may be because of rapid cell turnover. During later phases of AIDS, muscle wasting further depletes glutamine. At this stage there are often infections as well as poor absorption of nutrients. In a double-blind, placebo-controlled study of AIDS patients who had lost weight, half received standard treatment, the other half also took 40 g of glutamine a day as well as antioxidants. After three months, the patients taking glutamine gained significantly more lean body mass.[4] Studies have shown improvements in immune function as well as maintenance of lean body mass in patients with HIV/AIDS.[1]

Glutamine and Sepsis, Severe Burns, and Injuries

Under extreme stress, cells make certain necessary proteins, called the HSPs (heat shock proteins). These proteins protect cells under this kind of severe stress; in animals, they lessen organ damage and death. In situations when glutamine is extremely low, such as severe bloodstream and body infection (sepsis) or multiple traumatic injuries, white blood cells cannot make normal amounts of the heat shock proteins.

Studies indicate that the protective effect of glutamine in these conditions of severe stress may be related to HSP production.[3] Studies in lab animals indicate that a single dose of glutamine administered one hour after induction of sepsis can increase production of a number of heat shock proteins in the lungs. This increases survival.[5]

A similar experiment showed that glutamine not only protected the lungs, but also the small intestinal cells, liver, and kidney. Both studies emphasized the use of glutamine early.[6]

Glutamine is required for the synthesis of glutathione (see "Mechanism of Action"), which is another reason it helps in conditions of stress. Glutathione protects cells against free radical damage. Glutathione is necessary for lymphocytes to grow. Glutathione can protect the liver after injury.

Trials in humans undergoing surgery and needing total peripheral hyperalimentation have also shown improvement in outcome with glutamine supplementation. In one study, adding glutamine to the solution resulted in less pneumonia and less metabolic problems such as hyperglycemia, leading to less adverse events in total for the glutamine-treated patients.[7]

In another study, critically ill patients in the intensive care unit receiving TPN with or without glutamine had better outcomes with glutamine. The incidence of pneumonia, urinary tract infections, and organ failure was decreased in patients given glutamine.[8]

A review of a number of the recent trials summarized the successes in using parenteral glutamine. Some studies have shown reduced infectious rates, especially pneumonia, as well as lowered mortality and lowered gastrointestinal bleeding in at least one study. Others have shown that intravenous glutamine improves glucose control in critically ill patients.[2] There is ongoing data collection from multiple sites, and as of 2009, it was recommended by many experts that all TPN have added glutamine. The reasons people get total peripheral hyperalimentation are all reasons to replace glutamine. Glutamine supplementation is associated with reduced mortality, infections, and length of hospital stay in critically ill patients.[9]

The same case cannot be made for glutamine given through the intestinal tract, although it seems to be beneficial in burn and trauma patients.[2]

It is possible that glutamine is not absorbed fully or quickly enough to be as helpful in the intestine as by vein. It has been noted that in one study it took five days for the target glutamine level to be achieved with intestinal administration.[10]

Another review of studies conducted in 2009 found that there was sufficient evidence to add glutamine to TPN solutions for all critically ill patients not receiving any nutrition via the gastrointestinal tract. There are less infectious complications, shorter hospital stays, and decreased mortality in surgical as well as medical patients. This review recommended the use of glutamine in patients with catabolic stress, including burns, trauma, surgery, and chemotherapy, in which glutamine deficiency is known to occur. These reviewers stated that there were insufficient data to recommended glutamine for patients with pancreatitis, after bone marrow transplantation, or for newborns.[11]

Glutamine in Intestinal Illnesses Such as Inflammatory Bowel Disease

Intestinal cells do not make glutamine but must get it from elsewhere; usually skeletal muscle makes glutamine that is taken up by cells in the small intestine. In catabolic states like those above, there is often damage to the small intestine, as there is with many types of chemotherapy for cancer. Glutamine can protect the intestinal cells from this type of damage. There is evidence that glutamine can protect the bowel during critical illness (see above). Most of the successful trials have used intravenous glutamine in TPN. There has been some limited success with oral glutamine.[1]

A number of studies using oral glutamine for patients with Crohn's disease, an inflammatory bowel disease, did not have positive results, however. Intestinal permeability was not decreased, and no markers of disease improved.[12]

In developing countries, lack of growth is not just caused by malnutrition, but also by inflammation in the intestinal tract that limits digestion of nutrients. However, oral glutamine supplements do not necessarily improve weight gain along with increased nutrients. A study of Gambian infants failed to show any benefit for glutamine.[13]

Glutamine for Cancer Patients, to Prevent Complications like Inflammation of the Mucous Membranes during Chemotherapy, Peripheral Neuropathy from Chemotherapy, and Complications from Radiation Therapy or Bone Marrow Transplant

Glutamine has been suggested and/or used for all of the above reasons.[1]

Glutamine has been given to patients with cancer on chemotherapy to prevent inflammation of the mucosal membranes. At doses of 7.5 g a day for three weeks, it reduced stomatitis without side effects. In another study, patients were given 30 g a day for 15 days; reduction of mucositis was also found without side effects.[3]

In a pilot study, glutamine given to cancer patients receiving oxaliplatin reduced the incidence and severity of peripheral neuropathy (damage to nerves going to the arms and legs) without reducing the effectiveness of cancer treatment. The dose was 30 g a day. There were no side effects.[14] It is believed that cancer uses so much glutamine that it depletes body stores. Nerve tissue is sensitive to a lack of glutamine. Replenishing glutamine protects the nerve cells.

In a double-blind, placebo-controlled trial of oral glutamine given to patients getting chemotherapy for colorectal cancer, there were less changes in intestinal absorption and permeability in the patients given glucosamine. There was also less diarrhea.[15]

Patients undergoing bone marrow transplants as well as stem cell transplants after their own bone marrow has been ablated have been given glutamine in their TPN in a number of studies with mixed results. In one recent study, randomly assigned, and placebo-controlled, patients with leukemia had their bone marrow nullified and then were given stem cell transplants from siblings. In addition to all other therapy, half of the patients got glutamine in their TPN. The group that got glutamine had increased length of survival. However, the glutamine did not decrease intestinal permeability. It must work in some other way, possibly by stimulating immunity.[16]

Will Glutamine Be Used by the Body or Cancer Cells?

Cancer cells are rapidly growing and have a high demand for glutamine. They can quickly use up the body stores. Cancers have been called "glutamine traps." There was a concern that giving patients with cancer glutamine might strengthen the cancer, but that has not been the case in clinical trials.[1]

Glutamine and Glucose

It has been suggested that glutamine might help prediabetic and diabetic patients from getting worse or gaining weight. This was confirmed in at least one trial.[3]

Patients undergoing surgery who are on TPN or very sick often develop high blood sugars. Intravenous glutamine improves glucose metabolism in this situation.[7]

Glutamine and Athletes

The body's supply of glutamine is principally made and stored in skeletal muscle. Athletes in training and competition use much of the glutamine and do show a less active immune system (see above).

While testing has shown that taking glutamine can in fact help normalize the levels of glutamine, it does not necessarily improve the immune function in athletes. Multiple studies have failed to show a benefit from glutamine supplementation.[17] Studies of the immune cells of exercising athletes who were given supplemental glutamine or placebo have shown that while the glutamine levels can be normal, various measures of immune function including activated white blood cells and immunoglobulins do not normalize.

One randomized, double-blinded, placebo-controlled study followed the clinical course of athletes given glutamine immediately before and after marathon running. Athletes filled out questionnaires about their health during the seven days after the marathon. Of those who got glutamine, 81 percent had no upper respiratory tract infections during that week. Of those who got placebo, only 49 percent had no respiratory infections during the week.[18] The doses in this study were not large enough to maintain glutamine levels. More research into the way glutamine may help immune function in marathon runners is necessary.

Other claims for glutamine's benefits include increased absorption of water and maintenance of a normal acid-base balance, as well as preventing the breakdown of muscle protein. There are no good studies to support these claims. Glutamine does not cause as much of an increase in growth hormone as exercise does. Glutamine may help improve the synthesis of glycogen immediately after exercise. However, this is not a clear benefit beyond what an athlete would get by eating the proper diet after exercise, which is high in carbohydrate and also contains protein.[18]

The area in which glutamine may be useful concerns anabolic processes, meaning improving protein synthesis and glycogen synthesis. More good quality studies are needed. Until there is more evidence, many experts cannot recommend glutamine supplements for athletes.[18] However, there are those who believe glutamine will help preserve muscle mass and increase growth hormone release, in athletes as well as older people and those on calorie-restricted diets.[19]

DEFICIENCY

Glutamine is a conditionally indispensible amino acid. There is no recommended daily amount of glutamine, because the body can make it.

However, under conditions of stress, glutamine levels become low. Glutamine deficiency occurs only under stresses as described elsewhere in this chapter. In these cases, glutamine is necessary for recovery. Glutamine is necessary for so many chemical reactions in the body and so many processes that health is not possible without sufficient glutamine.[3]

FOOD SOURCES

Glutamine can be found in most protein. Some of the best sources are fish, poultry, beef, dairy products, cabbage, and beets.[19]

MECHANISM OF ACTION: HOW DOES IT WORK?

L-glutamine is important as an amino acid and therefore part of protein. It is also a necessary part of the balancing of energy and nitrogen in the body. Glutamine stimulates the immune system, as well as being a cell regulator.[3]

Another crucial activity of glutamine is that it is one component of glutathione. Glutathione is made from glutamic acid (from glutamine), cysteine, and glycine. Glutathione is an extremely important antioxidant in the body. It also helps detoxify the waste products and potential injurious chemicals in the liver.[3,20]

L-glutamine is considered a conditionally indispensible amino acid. Glutamine can be made from the amino acids glutamic acid plus ammonia. This synthesis may not be possible under certain conditions, when the body is under stress, for example, trying to heal from a severe injury. This can also be true if enough precursors are not taken in through the intestine or are not available. Recommended dietary intakes of "conditionally indispensible" amino acids like glutamine have not been definitively set.[21]

Glutamine is synthesized principally in muscle by the enzyme glutamine synthetase, and it is broken down mainly in the liver, by glutaminase. It can be metabolized in other parts of the body.[3]

There is a small pool of free amino acids in the human body. The amount of glutamine in this pool is significant, containing 10 to 15 g of nitrogen. There are also free amino acids inside cells that have not yet been made into protein. Amino acids inside the cell and outside can be made into protein, and protein can be broken down into amino acids. Amino acids can be ingested or synthesized, and they can be recycled or excreted.

In muscle, amino acids are parts of the reactions that provide energy for the cells. One of the byproducts of these reactions is ammonium ion, which becomes part of glutamine. Glutamine goes to the kidneys. Glutaminase removes the ammonium, which is excreted, with glutamate remaining. The glutamate can be used to make glucose inside the kidneys. Ammonium helps maintain the acid-base balance in the body.

Nitrogen is one of the end products of protein digestion, usually in the form of urea and ammonia. Because glutamine has two nitrogen-containing ammonia groups, it is critical to the metabolism of nitrogen. It can both accept and release ammonia.[20] High ammonia levels can cause many problems, from alterations in mental functions, to coma and death.

Glutamine has been called a "nitrogen shuttle," moving nitrogen around to make sure that blood ammonia levels do not get too high. It can accept nitrogen as well as giving it to other compounds, allowing the formation of some of the other amino acids, as well as amino sugars, nucleotides (the building blocks of DNA and RNA), and urea for excretion.[1] Glutamine contributes nucleotide precursors, as well as being involved in glucose production.

As the most abundant amino acid, glutamine is part of all the protein in the human body. Approximately 5–6 percent of the amino acids in body protein are glutamine. Amino acids including glutamine are necessary for making the many types of protein in the human body, from keratin and collagen, to the structure and function of most cells, to carrier molecules, hair, fingernails, hormones, and more. Health and reproduction are not possible without adequate protein.[21]

Proteins make up a large part of the human body. A 70 kg adult man will have the largest single type of protein, that found in skeletal muscle (43%). There is also protein wherever there is a need for structural support; approximately 15 percent of the protein is in blood and another 15 percent is in the skin. Organs do not contain as much protein. Liver and kidney contain about 10 percent of the protein, together. The rest is in other organs and bone.

There is only a very small reserve of protein that can be used during conditions of insufficient dietary intake for whatever reason. The reserve is small, made up of structural proteins that are probably stored in the liver and visceral tissues. It is perhaps 1 percent of the body's protein. It will be used by the body when enough protein is not being consumed. It is still necessary for the body.

Normally the body can adapt to a wide range of protein intake. But there are certain pathological states, such as severe disease or injury, in which protein will be used for energy. Muscle protein is lost in these cases.

The body needs both sufficient protein and the correct balances of amino acids to grow and survive. The body loses protein every day through the intestinal tract, urine, and from skin and hair to a lesser extent.

While it is not the primary source of energy for the body, protein can be used to produce energy and will be used when there is no other source.

Catabolism means the breaking down of body tissues. It occurs when molecules are needed from the tissues, such as amino acids and glucose. It happens during serious injury or illness, starvation, or with extreme exercise. Under conditions of extreme catabolic stress, the level of glutamine inside cells can drop 50 percent or more. Glutamine will be released from skeletal muscle in large amounts. Glutamine will be continuously released from muscle even if essential amino acids are used for its synthesis.

PRIMARY USES

Oral Supplements

Supplements can be taken:

- To reduce symptoms from the gastrointestinal tract during chemotherapy such as diarrhea and mouth ulcers.
- To treat peripheral neuropathy from chemotherapy.
- During dieting to try and maintain muscle mass.
- To improve performance and maintain muscle strength during marathons and other similar athletic activities.
- To enhance immune function in patients with immune deficits or after strenuous exercise.
- As an antioxidant (because it is a precursor of glutathione).

Glutamine can be given by mouth or into the intestine for hospitalized patients but the benefits are not clear. Hospitalized patients need glutamine supplementation by vein.

Intravenous Supplementation in Parenteral Nutrition

- Glucosamine added to TPN improves outcomes for most critically ill patients, with trauma, burns, sepsis, and after surgery.

COMMON DOSAGES

There are general protein requirements. The RDA for men and women is 0.8 g of good-quality protein a day/kg. In certain situations, glutamine may be necessary in the diet, but there is no general dietary requirement.[21]

Children ages 2 to 12 should take in 23 mg/kg/day of protein or 10 mg/pound. Adults should take 12 mg/kg/day.

A normal diet contains approximately 5 to 10 g of glutamine a day. The body makes 60 to 100 g a day of glutamine. When more glutamine is necessary, the body can usually synthesize it. When there is great metabolic stress, this may not be enough. Levels of glutamine inside cells can drop 50 percent or more, and the concentration in blood plasma can drop 30 percent. This is when glutamine supplements are necessary.[20]

Glutamine can be taken by mouth, injected intravenously, or put into the intestinal tract by tube. A dipeptide is added to glutamine to make it stable in solution.

For athletes in training, 1,000 mg/day are recommended as supplements.[18]

For very sick adults, such as those with cancer or AIDS, as much as 10 to 40 g a day may be taken in divided doses.[1]

POTENTIAL SIDE EFFECTS

If too much glutamine is ingested, and it is converted to ammonia and glutamic acid, both ammonia and glutamic acid can be toxic to the nervous system, at least in theory.

This can be a problem for patients with liver failure. Glutamine can cause their blood ammonia level to increase enough to affect their mental state, and in fact, precipitate liver-failure–induced brain dysfunction and coma.[3]

However, glutamine has generally proved safe in most situations. There was one report of an increase in liver enzymes in patients receiving all their nutrition by vein. Glutamine was added to the solution. There were some increases in liver enzymes that resolved after treatment stopped.

Higher doses than used in the above study have not been associated with any side effects or toxicity. Therefore the IOM has not established an UL for glutamine. Doses as high as 0.3 g/kg/day have been given to low birth weight babies, and 0.57 g/kg/day to adults with no problems reported. A number of studies have investigated glutamine given orally, by vein, and as part of a total peripheral alimentation (all calories by vein) in healthy volunteers, with no toxicity.

However, many cancer cells need glutamine. It is possible that glutamine may help cancers grow. Cancers can take in the body's entire glutamine pool. Glutamine is used by the tumors that are growing the fastest. While this effect is known, there is no data to show that giving glutamine to patients with cancer has actually promoted the growth of the cancer.[21]

Even critically ill patients can tolerate doses of glutamine 30 to 40 g a day for an approximately 70 kg patient.

Healthy athletes have taken 20 to 30 g during a few hours without problems; 0.65 g/kg have been given to pediatric cancer patients without problems.[18]

There is no definitive evidence either way about long-term safety of glutamine administration. However, it appears to be extremely safe.

FACT VERSUS FICTION

Glutamine is a conditionally essential amino acid that can become depleted when the body is under significant stress. It functions in many ways beyond that of being a protein building block.

Critically ill, hospitalized patients need glutamine added to their TPN solutions or intravenous solutions.

Oral supplements are not as helpful for people with serious illnesses but can be tried.

Oral supplements can be taken to bolster the immune system, to try and add lean muscle mass during dieting or with aging. Athletes like marathon runners can take glutamine to improve their immunity. Patients with cancer getting chemotherapy can take it to prevent intestinal symptoms like diarrhea, ulcers in the mouth, and symptoms from nerve irritation.

It may be helpful in patients with inflammatory bowel disease, but this is far from certain.

Since glutamine is very safe, trying it for any of these reasons is reasonable.

More information will be forthcoming about L-glutamine since there are a number of large-scale trials in progress. A search of clinical trials listed at the NIH under "glutamine" yielded 83 studies in various phases.

REFERENCES

1. L-Glutamine. *Altern Med Rev.* 2001;6(4):406–410.
2. Wischmeyer, PE. Glutamine: Role in critical illness and ongoing clinical trials. *Current Opinion in Gastroenterology.* 2008;24:190–197.
3. Roth, E. Nonnutritive effects of glutamine. *J Nutr.* 2008;138:2025S–2031S.
4. Patrick, L. Nutrients and HIV: Part Three—N-acetylcysteine, alpha-lipoic acid, L-Glutamine, and L-Carnitine. *Altern Med Rev.* 2000;5(4):290–305.
5. Singleton, KD, Serkova, N, Beckey, VE, Wischmeyer, PE. Glutamine attenuates lung injury and improves survival after sepsis: Role of enhanced heat shock protein expression. *Crit Care Med.* 2005;33:1206–1213.
6. Oliveira, GP, Oliveira, MBG, Santos, RS, et al. Intravenous glutamine decreases lung and distal organ injury in an experimental model of abdominal sepsis. *Critical Care.* 2009;13:R74.
7. Aboelmagd, R, Moez, K, Salem, W. Role of parenteral glutamine supplementation on patient outcome in the surgical ICU. *Critical Care.* 2009;13 (Suppl 1):P136.
8. Grau, TG, Bonet, A, Miñambres, E, et al. Efficacy of glutamine dipeptide-supplemented total parenteral nutrition in critically ill patients: A prospective, double-blind randomized trial. *Critical Care.* 2008;12(Suppl 2):P146.
9. Critical Care Nutrition. Composition of parenteral nutrition: Glutamine supplementation. January 31, 2009. http://www.criticalcarenutrition.com/index.php?option=com_content&task=view&id=17&Itemid=40. Accessed April 1, 2010.
10. Andrews, FJ, Griffiths, RD. Glutamine: Essential for immune nutrition in the critically ill. *British Journal of Nutrition.* 2002;87(Suppl 1):S3–S8.
11. Stein, J, Boehles, HJ, Blumenstein, I, et al. Amino acids—Guidelines on parenteral nutrition. Chapter 4. *GMS German Medical Science.* 2009;7:1–8.
12. Wild, GE, Drozdowski, L, Tartaglia, C, Clandinin, MT, Thomson, ABR. Nutritional modulation of the inflammatory response in inflammatory bowel disease: From the molecular to the integrative to the clinical. *World J Gastroenterol* 2007;3(1):1–7.
13. Williams, EA, Elia, M, Lunn, PG. A double-blind, placebo-controlled, glutamine-supplementation trial in growth-faltering Gambian infants. *Am J Clin Nutr.* 2007;86:421–427.

14. Wang, W-S, Lin, J-K, Lin, T-C. Oral glutamine is effective for preventing oxaliplatin-induced neuropathy in colorectal cancer patients. *The Oncologist.* 2007;12:312–319.
15. Daniele, B, Perrone, F, Gallo, C, et al. Oral glutamine in the prevention of fluorouracil induced intestinal toxicity: A double blind, placebo controlled, randomised trial. *Gut.* 2001;48:28–33.
16. da Gama Torres, HO, Vilela, EG, da Cunha, AS, et al. Efficacy of glutamine-supplemented parenteral nutrition on short-term survival following allo-SCT: A randomized study. *Bone Marrow Transplantation.* 2008;41:1021–1027.
17. Gleeson, M, Bishop, NC. Modification of immune responses to exercise by carbohydrate, glutamine and anti-oxidant supplements. *Immunology and Cell Biology.* 2000;78:554–561.
18. Gleeson, M. Dosing and efficacy of glutamine supplementation in human exercise and sport training. *J Nutr.* 2008;138:2045S–2049S.
19. Scipione, A. Glutamine. This amino acid helps to preserve muscle mass while bolstering immune and gastrointestinal health. *Life Extension Magazine.* January 2006. http://search.lef.org/cgi-src-bin/MsmGo.exe?grab_id=0&page_id=1300&query=glutamine&hiword=GLUTAMIN%20GLUTAMINES%20GLUTAMINIC%20glutamine%20. Accessed April 2, 2010.
20. Miller, AL. Therapeutic considerations of L-glutamine: A review of the literature. *Altern Med Rev.* 1999;4:239–248.
21. Institute of Medicine. Food and Nutrition Board. *Dietary reference intakes for energy, carbohydrate, fiber, fat, fatty acids, cholesterol, protein, and amino acids (macronutrients).* Washington, DC: National Academies Press, 2005.

20

L-Lysine

BRIEF OVERVIEW

L-lysine is an essential amino acid in humans. Amino acids are the building blocks of proteins. Some can be synthesized in the human body. Others, like L-lysine, cannot. The only way to have enough lysine for protein synthesis is to ingest it in food or take supplements.

Proteins make up the structure of cells. They also work as enzymes, carriers for other substances, in cell membranes, and as hormones. Amino acids are precursors for the nucleic acids that make up RNA and DNA, the genetic blueprints. Proteins can also be used as sources of energy, when necessary. Lysine is the rate-limiting step in the creation of new protein in humans.

Most people get plenty of lysine in their diet. Vegetarians, however, may not, because they eat a limited amount of protein, and what they do eat is often low in lysine. Since it is essential, there are definite symptoms when the body does not have enough lysine.

Lysine may have other uses, including preventing reoccurrence of herpes simplex lesions, as well as having a role in the metabolism of other substances.

(In this chapter L-lysine and lysine will mean the same thing.)

THE HYPE

Lysine Is Involved in the Absorption of Calcium; Perhaps Lysine can Help Treat or Prevent Osteoporosis

Lysine decreases the amount of calcium that is excreted in the urine and also increases the amount of calcium absorbed by the body.[1]

Lab studies have indicated that a combination of lysine and arginine, which is another amino acid, activates osteoblasts (cells that make bone) and increases collagen synthesis.[2]

These properties might mean that lysine could be used to help treat or prevent osteoporosis.

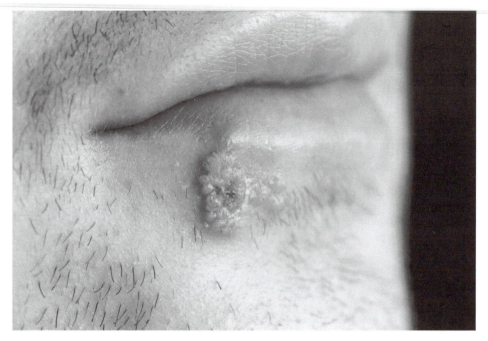

L-lysine may help prevent cold sores. (© Kuhar/Dreamstime.com)

L-Lysine Is Advertised as a Dietary Supplement for Bodybuilders

Bodybuilders want to increase their muscle mass, so they are interested in amino acids and protein, because muscle is made of protein. There is a substance called growth hormone (GH) that the body releases in response to exercise. There is a question of whether or not lysine, with or without arginine, can cause the release of extra GH. In one study, the ingestion of soy protein, either intact or hydrolyzed, as well as a mix of all amino acids caused a larger amount of GH release than just arginine and lysine.[3]

A review of the research indicated that it is probably true that specific amino acids, including lysine, arginine, and ornithine, can cause GH release when taken by mouth or intravenously. However, the oral doses necessary to increase the release of GH above what already happens with exercise would cause gastrointestinal distress, like nausea and vomiting.[4]

No studies have shown that oral amino acid supplements taken before exercise cause a greater release in GH than would happen as a result of exercise alone. The authors of this paper stated that there have been no good studies to determine if there is a greater increase in strength or muscle mass after the use of amino acids than with just strength training.[4]

There is continuing research in this area.

Treatment of Angina Pectoris or Coronary Heart Disease

In the early 1990s, Dr. Linus Pauling reported on several cases of angina pectoris (heart pain from low blood supply, or coronary artery disease) improved by lysine given with high doses of ascorbic acid.[1]

In coronary artery disease, fatty plaques are attached to the inside of the arteries. They are filled with cholesterol. There are many factors that influence how much gets deposited in the arteries, the most obvious being elevated cholesterol. However, there are other things that have to take place, including microscopic damage to the arteries. Dr. Pauling thought that the lysine and vitamin C might protect the vessel walls.

Others have taken Dr. Pauling's work further. Investigators have used multinutrient therapy to try and reverse damaging changes in the coronary arteries. The nutrients include vitamins C, E, A, D, and multiple B vitamins as well as many minerals, including calcium, magnesium, and others, coenzymes like biotin and folic acid, as well as amino acids lysine and arginine and others. In one study, a multinutrient supplement was given to 55 patients with documented coronary artery disease (CAD) for a year. The supplements seemed to slow the progression of CAD or even reverse early disease, as measured by ultrafast computed tomography. There is no way to ascertain how important lysine is within the group of nutrients.[5]

One laboratory study used a mixture of ascorbic acid, lysine, proline, arginine, cysteine, and green tea phenolics, which were applied to smooth muscle cells from the human aorta. There was a demonstrable change in the behavior of the cells away from actions that can cause damage and growth of fatty plaques in arterial walls. Again, there is no way to tell how important the lysine was in this mixture.[6]

There is no evidence that lysine alone can improve or prevent CAD, and even with the multinutrient mix, the research is extremely preliminary.

Lysine Is Needed for the Production of Carnitine, Which Is Very Important in the Metabolism of Cholesterol and Fatty Acids

Lysine, in particular, along with methionine is made in the liver and kidney into carnitine. Carnitine is needed to transport long-chain fatty acids.[7] This is undoubtedly true. That does not mean that taking extra lysine will lower cholesterol.

L-Lysine Is Advertised as a Way to Prevent and/or Treat Recurrent Herpes Simplex Infections

While it is apparently very useful in some animals for herpes simplex infection, it has not always proven effective in humans.[2]

The herpes simplex virus uses less lysine and more arginine in its proteins than humans. Lysine may decrease available arginine for the virus in a variety of ways. Lysine and arginine share a transport system, so supplements of lysine can reduce the absorption of arginine.

There have been a number of studies, some of which indicate lysine may help prevent herpes outbreaks, and some that have shown that it does not help. It may depend on the dose, and the patient, as well as how much arginine is in the diet.[8,9]

One reported study involved 45 patients followed between two months and three years. Lysine 312 mg to 1,200 mg was given daily, and foods rich in arginine were restricted. There was a dramatic reduction in recurrence; after discontinuation of lysine, lesions reappeared quickly.[10]

At least one double-blind, placebo-controlled, crossover trial has been performed with 500 mg and 1,000 mg of lysine, which showed a decrease in herpes lesions with the lysine. This, along with all of the trials with good results, included a reduction in arginine-rich foods and an increase in lysine-rich foods.[8] It may be that lysine cannot prevent herpes recurrences if there is too much arginine in the diet.

Lysine May Be Useful to Treat Anxiety

There have been a number of early studies that indicate lysine plus or minus arginine may improve symptoms of stress and anxiety.[11]

A double-blind, randomized, placebo-controlled study used the combination of L-lysine and L-arginine taken for 1 week to evaluate baseline anxiety as well as stress-induced anxiety in a group of 180 healthy Japanese men and women. They found that trait (baseline) anxiety decreased at the end of a week of treatment, as did anxiety in response to stress. In men but not women, the values of chemical markers of stress in saliva were reduced. These investigators concluded that the amino acids were decreasing anxiety, and that there must be additional ways beyond the hormone changes, because the women were equally less anxious.[12]

The reason why it could lessen anxiety may be twofold: it has been shown to elevate serotonin levels, a neurotransmitter that helps us deal with stress, and it may decrease cortisol levels, the stress hormone.

DEFICIENCY

Deficiency of lysine is uncommon in most people eating a regular diet in developed countries.

Vegetarians can become lysine deficient, especially if they are not careful enough to balance their proteins. Beans (legumes) are the best choice to increase lysine in the diet of a vegan or vegetarian.

People with severe burns can become lysine deficient. So can athletes.

Symptoms of lysine deficiency include anemia, fatigue and slow growth, as well as dizziness, loss of appetite, nausea, reproductive disorders, agitation, and bloodshot eyes.[2]

FOOD SOURCES

Lysine is found in protein-rich foods. This would include animal proteins such as meat, cheese, and some other dairy products, certain fish, nuts, eggs, soybeans. Beans, some other legumes, Brewer's yeast, and certain herbs also contain lysine.[2] Grain proteins are for the most part low in lysine, except for wheat germ, which is a good source.

While grains and bread for human consumption have not been fortified with lysine, animal feed has been fortified.

The lysine in some foods can be rendered impossible to absorb because of the reaction known as carmelization, the browning of foods with sugar in desserts and pastries. In this reaction, lysine links with a sugar.[1]

MECHANISM OF ACTION: HOW DOES IT WORK?

Lysine is an essential amino acid necessary for making the many types of protein in the human body, proteins like keratin, elastin, and collagen. Other proteins are key to the structure and function of most cells. Carrier molecules, like the ones that transport iron, are proteins. There is protein in hair, fingernails, hormones, and more. The amino acids can also be converted to coenzymes, nucleic acids, and other essential molecules. Health, including a vigorous immune system, growth, development, and reproduction, is not possible without adequate protein. Adequate protein is not possible without the essential amino acid lysine, which the human body cannot make.

Once lysine is ingested, it goes to the liver and undergoes a variety of metabolic steps. Lysine can aid in the formation of glucose, glycogen, and lipids. This means that lysine contributes to energy production. Other amino acids cannot do this.[1]

Lysine is very well absorbed and transported throughout the body and to muscle quickly. The pool of free lysine in the body may mainly be inside muscle cells.[1]

Lysine in particular, along with methionine, is metabolized in the liver and kidney into carnitine. Carnitine is needed to transport long-chain fatty acids.

Proteins are made from strings of amino acids. All the amino acids are at least slightly different from one another and perform slightly different tasks in combining to make proteins. Some amino acids are modified after joining others to make a protein. Lysine, for example, is converted into hydroxylysine once it is in collagen. This helps collagen cross-link and be stable. Lysine is important in the structure of bone.

Proteins make up a large part of the human body. The largest single type of protein is that found in skeletal muscle (43%). There is also protein wherever there is a need for structural support; approximately 15 percent of the protein is in blood and another 15 percent is in the skin. Organs do not contain as much protein. Liver and kidney contain about 10 percent of the protein, together. The rest is in other organs and bone.

The proportion of muscle in the body increases with age, from newborn to adult.

There are four proteins that constitute almost 50 percent of the body's protein. They are myosin and actin (in muscle), collagen (in connective tissue), and hemoglobin (in red blood cells).

There is only a very small reserve of protein that can be used during conditions of insufficient dietary intake for whatever reason. This small reserve is made up of structural proteins that are probably stored in the liver and visceral tissues. It is perhaps 1 percent of the body's protein. It will be used by the body when enough protein is not being consumed.

Normally the body can adapt to a wide range of protein intake. But there are certain pathological states, such as severe disease or injury, in which body protein will be used for energy. Muscle protein is lost in these cases.

PRIMARY USES

- The primary use for lysine is as a supplement to individuals who do not get enough in their diet. This can be true for vegetarians. It can also occur as the result of an increased need for lysine, when the body is extremely stressed due severe burns or other injury. Athletes performing at high levels can also need more lysine.

- Lysine supplements may prevent recurrences of herpes simplex in some people. It is also used to treat active outbreaks.

- Bodybuilders take lysine along with other amino acids in an attempt to get more growth hormone released and thereby increase muscle mass and strength.

- It may be used in a cocktail with other amino acids, vitamins, and minerals for heart health.

COMMON DOSAGES

There are general protein requirements as well as specifics for lysine. The RDA for men and women is 0.8 g of good-quality protein per kilogram per day. The protein needs to contain lysine in a certain proportion, 51 mg of lysine per gram of protein.[7]

Protein in General

The recommended amounts of protein at various ages have been calculated by the Institute of Medicine Food and Nutrition Board using a variety of methods. The higher quality the protein, the more will be absorbed and the more specific requirements for amino acids will be met.[7]

The AI (Adequate Intake) for infants 0 to 6 months is 1.52 g/kg/day. The EAR (Estimated Average Requirement) for older infants ages 7 to 12 months is 1.0 g/kg/day. The RDA (Recommended Dietary Allowance) for this group is 1.2 g/kg/day or 11.0 g/day of protein.

The EAR for boys and girls 1 to 3 years of age is 0.87 g/kg/day of protein. From 4 up to 13 years it is 0.76 g/kg/day. The RDA for children 1 to 3 years old is 1.05 g/kg/day or 13 g/day. For children ages 4 to 13 years, it is 0.95 g/kg/day or 34 g/day of protein.

The EAR for boys ages 14 to 18 is 0.73 g/kg/day; for girls of that age it is 0.71 g/kg/day of protein.

The RDA for boys 14–18 years of age is 0.85 g/kg/day of protein or 52 g/day of protein. The RDA for girls 14–18 years of age is 0.85 g/kg/day of protein or 46 g/day of protein.

The EAR for men and women ages 31o 50 is 0.66 g/kg/day of protein. The same is true for older adults.

The RDA for men 19 through 50 is 0.80 g/kg/day or 56 g/day of protein. For women it is 0.80 g/kg/day or 46 g/day. The same is true for older men and women.

The EAR for pregnancy in any age group is 0.88 g/kg/day of protein or plus an additional 21 g/day of protein. The RDA for pregnancy is 1.1 g/kg/day of protein or plus an additional 25 g/day.

The EAR for lactation is 1.05 g/kg/day of protein or plus an additional 21 g/day. The RDA for lactation is 1.3 g/kg/day of protein or plus an additional 25 g per day.

Lysine Specifically

The IOM/FNB used many different methods to estimates lysine requirements, which were published in 2005. Values from earlier reports, as well as values used by the World Health Organization, had been criticized by many investigators.[13,14]

There seems to be some agreement that these recommendations are reasonable. This was noted by experts like Kurpad and Young, who saw the IOM report before publication.[15]

The lysine AI for infants 0 to 6 months is 640 mg/day or 107 mg/kg/day. At 7 to 12 months, the EAR is 62 mg/kg/day and the RDA is 89 mg/kg/day. For boys and girls ages 1 to 3 years, the EAR for lysine is 45 mg/kg/day, and the RDA is 58 mg/kg/day. For boys 4 to 13 years of age, and girls ages 4 to 8 years of age, the EAR is 37 mg/kg/day and the RDA is 46 mg/kg/day. For girls 9 to 13 and boys ages 14 to 18, the EAR is 35 mg/kg/day and the RDA is 43 mg/kg/day. For girls ages 14 to 18, the EAR is 32 mg/kg/day and the RDA is 40 mg/kg/day.

For all adults 19 years of age and older, the EAR is 31 mg/kg/day, and the RDA is 38 mg/kg/day. A 70 kg man would need to take in 2,660 mg of lysine a day, or 2.66 g. As noted above, he would need 56 g of protein in total.

For pregnancy, the EAR is 41 mg/kg/day, and the RDA is 51 mg/kg/day. For breast-feeding women, the EAR is 42 mg/kg/day and the RDA is 52 mg/kg/day.[7]

While the IOM/FNB used much data and analysis to determine AI, EAR, and RDA values for amino acids, they have not been able to establish a UL (Tolerable Upper Intake Limit) for any amino acid. For lysine, the highest 99 percent of intake estimated in this country is 12.6 g per day. The median (average) intake is 7.5 grams a day. That can give some idea of what amounts can be taken safely. There are also investigators trying to define a UL for lysine as well as other amino acids.[11] Some have suggested 300 to 400 mg/kg/day should be the NOAEL, the No Observed Adverse Effect Level, based in part on animal data.[16,17]

Between 312 and 1,500 mg of lysine daily has been recommended generally as a dietary supplement.[18]

Humans do absorb some lysine synthesized by bacteria in the intestine. It is not clear how much, but it is measurable.[19]

For Herpes

The optimal dose is not clear. To prevent breakouts, a dose between 500 mg and 3,000 mg a day has been given. For prophylaxis, 500 mg to 1,000 mg is a reasonable dose; 3,000 mg a day can be taken for active herpes lesions.[1]

POTENTIAL SIDE EFFECTS

Lysine in the diet is safe.[7] However, large amounts of supplemental lysine can interfere with the metabolism of protein in the diet and also with arginine transport. Lysine and arginine share a transport mechanism in the intestines. They also compete with each other in the kidney for reabsorption, as well as transport into cells.[1]

Supplementary lysine has caused gallstones and increased cholesterol in animals. Very high doses have caused renal failure in dogs.[17]

There have only been limited studies in humans taking high doses of lysine, without any real evidence of serious side effects. In one small study, levels of carnitine rose in healthy adults given high doses of lysine. In another study, 3 out of 27 people had slight gastrointestinal upset.[7] This upset can include diarrhea, cramps, and nausea.[1]

People with liver or kidney damage or failure should discuss supplementation with a health care provider.[1]

There are rare genetic disorders involving lysine metabolism, and in those cases lysine should not be given. The principal condition is called lysinuric protein intolerance. With this disease, the body cannot absorb or use lysine, arginine, and ornithine, which is very serious. There is a genetic defect in a transport protein, leading to a shortage of these amino acids in the body and an excess in the urine. The lack of ornithine and arginine cause problems related to the way nitrogen is handled in the body, and ammonia accumulates. The lack of lysine leads to weakness in collagen and therefore skin, tendons, ligaments, and bones. People with this condition are short in stature and have osteoporosis. They also have protein deposits in the lungs, enlarged liver and spleen, and protein deposition in the kidneys. The lung and kidney problems, as well as the excess of ammonia, can be causes of death. Treatment includes protein restriction and administration of citrulline; sometimes kidney transplants are done.[20]

Lysinuric protein intolerance is a very rare congenital disorder affecting approximately 1 in 60,000 people of Finnish descent, and 1 in 57,000 of Japanese descent. It is much less frequent in other populations.[21]

FACT VERSUS FICTION

Lysine is clearly a necessary nutrient. Those people who may not be getting enough dietary lysine because they are vegetarians, or have increased needs with athletic training, can consider supplements.

Supplements of lysine are safe over a wide range of doses.

Lysine and arginine share a transport mechanism in the intestine. They are related in many ways. In many studies, both arginine and lysine are used together, while at other times, they need to be separated.

Lysine may prevent recurrences of herpes simplex, especially if used along with a diet low in arginine. This is a case where lysine is needed to be increased and arginine lowered.

Lysine may be useful in other situations that are still being studied. One is reducing anxiety. Preliminary research indicates that it might be useful for this, along with arginine. Similarly, lysine and arginine ingestion may help bodybuilders, but there is not enough research to make definite conclusions.

Multinutrient therapy for the heart may actually be beneficial, but there is not enough research to support its use at this time. There is also no way to separate the contribution of the various components that have been used. Lysine may or may not help prevent coronary artery disease.

Lysine's ability to raise calcium levels and stimulate osteoblasts may mean that it could be used to help prevent or treat osteoporosis. Further research needs to be conducted.

Because lysine is safe, people may take it for any of these reasons and see if they find it beneficial. Further, clear indications of lysine's uses will be learned in the future.

REFERENCES

1. L-Lysine. *Altern Med Rev*. 2007;12(2):169–172.
2. University of Maryland Medical Center. Medical Reference. Complementary Medicine. Lysine. 2009. http://www.umm.edu/altmed/articles/lysine-000312. htm. Accessed March 15, 2010.
3. Van Vught, AJAH, Nieuwenhuizen, AG, Brummer, RJM, Westerterp-Plantenga, MS. Effects of oral ingestion of amino acids and proteins on the somatotropic axis. *J Clin Endocrinol Metab*. 2008;93:584–590.
4. Chromiak, JA, Antonio, J. Use of amino acids as growth hormone-releasing agents by athletes. *Nutrition*. 2002;18(7–8):657–661.
5. Rath, M, Niedzwieck, A. Nutritional supplement program halts progression of early coronary atherosclerosis documented by ultrafast computed tomography. *Journal of Applied Nutrition*. 1996;48(3):67–78.
6. Ivanov, V, Roomi, MW, Kalinovsky, T, et al. Anti-atherogenic effects of a mixture of ascorbic acid, lysine, proline, arginine, cysteine, and green tea phenolics in human aortic smooth muscle cells. *Journal Cardiovasc Pharmacol*. 2007;49:140–145.
7. Institute of Medicine. Food and Nutrition Board. *Dietary reference intakes for energy, carbohydrate, fiber, fat, fatty acids, cholesterol, protein, and amino acids (macronutrients)*. Washington, DC: National Academies Press, 2005.
8. Gaby, AR. Natural remedies for Herpes simplex. *Altern Med Rev*. 2006; 11(2):93–101.
9. Beauman, JG. Genital Herpes: A review. *American Family Physician*. 2005;72(8):1527–1534.
10. Griffith, RS, Norins, AL. Kagan, C. "A multicentered study of lysine therapy in Herpes simplex infection." *Dermatologica*. 1978;156(5):257–267.
11. Pencharz, PB, Elango, R, Ball, RO. An approach to defining the upper safe limits of amino acid intake. *J Nutr*. 2008;138:1996S–2002S.
12. Smriga, M, Ando, T, Akutsu, M, et al. Oral treatment with L-lysine and L-arginine reduces anxiety and basal cortisol levels in healthy humans. *Biomedical Research*. 2007;28(2):85–90.
13. Kurpad, AV, El-Khoury, AE, Beaumier, L, et al. An initial assessment, using 24-h [13C] leucine kinetics, of the lysine requirement of healthy adult Indian subjects. *Am J Clin Nutr*. 1998;67:58–66.
14. Millward, DJ, Fereday, A, Gibson, NR, et al. Efficiency of utilization of wheat and milk protein in healthy adults and apparent lysine requirements determined by a single-meal [1–13C] leucine balance protocol. *Am J Clin Nutr*. 2002;76:1326–1334.

15. Kurpad, AV, Young, VR. What is apparent is not always real: Lessons from lysine requirement studies in adult humans. *J Nutr.* 2003;133:1227–1230.

16. Tsubuku, S, Mochizuki, M, Mawatari, K, Smriga, M, Kimura, T. Thirteen week oral toxicity study of L-lysine hydrochloride in rats. *Int J Toxicol.* 2004;23:113–118.

17. Tomé, D, Bos, C. Lysine requirement through the human life cycle. *J Nutr.* 2007;137:1642S–1645S.

18. Merck Medicus Facts and Comparisons. L-lysine. http://www.merckmedi cus.com/pp/us/hcp/frame_textbooks.jsp?pg=http://online.factsandcompari sons.com/MonoDisp.aspx?monoID=fandc-hcp11242. Accessed February 16, 2010.

19. Metges, CC. Contribution of microbial amino acids to amino acid homeostasis of the host. *J Nutr.* 2000;130:1857S–1864S.

20. Tanner, LM, Nanto-Salonen, K, Ninkoski, H, et al. Nephropathy advancing to end-stage renal disease: A novel complication of lysinuric protein intolerance. *J Pediatr.* 2007;150:631–634.

21. U.S. National Library of Medicines. Genetics home reference. Lysinuric protein intolerance. March 2008. http://ghr.nlm.nih.gov/condition=lysinuricprote inintolerance#treatment. Accessed March 18, 2010.

21

L-Tyrosine

BRIEF OVERVIEW

Amino acids are the building blocks of proteins. Some, like L-tyrosine, can be synthesized in the human body. L-tyrosine can be made from phenylalanine, another amino acid. Either enough phenylalanine or tyrosine must be ingested for the human body to synthesize proteins.

Proteins make up the structure of cells. They also work as enzymes, carriers for other substances, in cell membranes, and as hormones. Amino acids are precursors for the nucleic acids that make up RNA and DNA, the genetic blueprints. Proteins can also be used as sources of energy, when necessary.

Additionally, tyrosine specifically can be metabolized into other very active molecules, such as neurotransmitters, including catecholamines, as well as thyroid hormone and melanin.

(L-tyrosine is the form of tyrosine used in the human body. Tyrosine will be used interchangeably with L-tyrosine.)

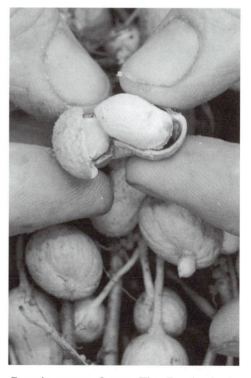

Georgia peanut farmer Tim Burch checks peanuts in a Baker County, Georgia, field. Peanuts are a good food source of L-tyrosine. (AP Photo/Ric Feld)

THE HYPE

Tyrosine is involved in so many important biochemical processes that dietary supplements are popular. The supplement industry is looking at ways to make more tyrosine safely and efficiently.[1]

Much research has been done to see how supplemental tyrosine could help with a variety of diseases and problems, some with positive results. However, it has also been discovered that trying to lower tyrosine might actually be more helpful in some situations, where it would be best not to take any supplemental tyrosine.

Depression

The catecholamine theory of depression postulates that lowered amounts of certain brain chemicals, called catecholamines, cause depression. The most likely are norepinephrine and serotonin, and probably to a lesser extent, dopamine. Conversely, too much norepinephrine in the brain can cause mania. Tyrosine is a precursor of a number of catecholamines. It can be converted in the brain via a number of steps to dopamine. In nerve cells transmitting impulses with dopamine, no further metabolism is necessary. For other nerve cells, dopamine can be converted to norepinephrine, and finally, for other cells, epinephrine.

Because depressed patients respond to medications that raise these neurotransmitters, it has long been thought that tyrosine might be helpful in treating depression. In 1980, one depressed patient was treated successfully with tyrosine.[2] There was another very small study in the 1980s that found that tyrosine had some effect on depression.[3] However, most of the subsequent research has not found it effective as a treatment for depression.[4,5]

For example, 65 patients were enrolled in a randomized, double-blind trial and given 100 mg/kg/day of tyrosine, the antidepressant imipramine, or placebo for four weeks. No effect on depression by tyrosine was seen in this study.[6]

In 2007, a review of alternate and complementary medical treatment of depression said that results with tyrosine are "unequivocally negative."[7]

One of the problems is that the rate-limiting step in synthesis of these chemicals is the enzyme tyrosine hydroxylase. It can only handle so much tyrosine, so that taking in more does not necessarily lead to higher levels of the catecholamines.

Researchers have found ways to decrease the amount of tyrosine in the brain, with resulting lowered catecholamines. They give research subjects a mixture of amino acids missing phenylalanine and tyrosine. The body, using the ingested amino acids to make new protein, has to take free phenylalanine and/or tyrosine out of the system to make complete proteins, thus lowering the tyrosine level in the brain. This has been done in lab animals and in people. The reverse has also been done, raising brain levels of tyrosine.

The effects on the body of either lowering or raising tyrosine are unclear. Some have postulated that the catecholamine progression serves as a trigger to increase protein ingestion if levels are low and decrease it when levels are high. This seems to be the case in animals.[8]

Investigators have studied the short-term effects of lowering levels of tyrosine and phenylalanine on mood. Normal subjects in small studies whose levels have been lowered reported a depressed mood, which was worsened by stress.[9]

A subsequent study of 15 women who had recovered from major depression who had their tyrosine lowered did not show any return of symptoms, although there were chemical indications that their dopamine levels were lower.[10]

Similar research has been done with other patients who have recovered from a major depression. In one study, tyrosine and phenylalanine were lowered in an attempt to lower dopamine. Lowering tyrosine levels, in one study, did not cause any depressive symptoms to reoccur. However, there was one parameter changed in this study, "lowered sensitivity to reward in a gambling game." This was considered a marker of anhedonia in depression, the lack of ability to enjoy various things. This particular study was designed to lower dopamine, but the manner in which it was done would have also lowered other catecholamines.[11]

Mania

Mania is the other side of depression in patients with bipolar illness. Perhaps lowering tyrosine might help patients with mania. This has been tested using the method of lowering brain aromatic amino acids by giving BCAAs. The aromatic amino acids tyrosine, phenylalanine, and tryptophan use the same transport mechanism to get into the brain, past the blood-brain barrier, as do the branched-chain amino acids (BCAAs) leucine, isoleucine, and valine. Giving subjects a lot of BCAAs will lower levels of aromatic amino acids, including tyrosine, in the brain. In at least one randomized, blinded, placebo-controlled trial, this was effective. BCAAs were given to 25 patients with mania. The patients given the BCAAs had symptoms of mania resolve more quickly than those given placebo. More research is needed in this area.[12]

Another study showed that pretreating healthy volunteers with tyrosine and phenylalanine-free amino acid mixtures, which lower brain tyrosine and dopamine, blunt the response to amphetamines. This may serve as a model for mania, in which dopamine is implicated.[13]

Hypertension

There have been a few small studies, none showing a consistent lowering of blood pressure in response to tyrosine. An early, randomized, placebo-controlled, double-blind trial in 1985 found that in 13 people with mild hypertension who were given tyrosine for two weeks, blood pressure remained the same. While the level of blood tyrosine rose, nothing else changed, including blood levels of norepinephrine.[14]

Stress

Tyrosine is the precursor to neurotransmitters released during stress, epinephrine and norepinephrine. There is some evidence that the body may not be able to make enough tyrosine from phenylalanine during psychological stress. Tyrosine may improve performance during stress, as well as during sleep deprivation.[4]

Tests done by the U.S. military to simulate battle conditions or sleep deprivation as well as cold have shown that people taking up to 100 mg/kg of tyrosine perform better under stressful conditions.[15,16]

For example, the performance of 10 men and women on multiple task battery and simple task battery tests was measured, one hour after receiving either placebo or 150 mg/kg of tyrosine. The subjects given tyrosine showed improvement in only the memory retrieval part of the tests. This suggested to the military investigators that tyrosine might be useful in situations involving multitasking.[17]

Cognitive Function and Memory

Cognitive function and memory have been tested in healthy adults under stress, to see if tyrosine would help improve performance. Some of the tests have been done by the military, such as the one above.

In another study, 16 healthy young adults were given either tyrosine (100 mg/kg) or a placebo. They were then tested, doing stress-sensitive tasks while being stressed with high levels of noise. The subjects given tyrosine showed improved performance doing cognitive tasks while stressed.[18]

Parkinson's Disease

As explained previously, tyrosine can be metabolized into dopamine, which should help patients with Parkinson's disease who have low amounts of dopamine. Treatment with L-dopa helps patients with Parkinson's. However, studies have not found tyrosine useful in this condition.[5]

Migraine Headaches

There has been some evidence that products of tyrosine metabolism, which can include dopamine and other amines, might be part of what precipitates migraine as well as cluster headaches.[19] If this is true, tyrosine-lowering techniques might prove helpful.

ADHD

There have been a number of small studies indicating that tyrosine could help the symptoms of ADHD. However, any improvement wears off quickly; there seems to be a tolerance built up to tyrosine in this situation.[20]

Athletic Performance Enhancer

While there are athletes that use tyrosine to enhance their performance, there is no clear evidence of its effectiveness.[4]

Some studies have shown minimal or conflicting results. For example, in one study, 10 male athletes were given a variety of substances to try and enhance performance. They were given placebo, tyrosine (20 g), 21 g of branched-chain amino acids (BCAA), or paroxetine (Paxil, an antidepressant) and then exercised. There was little difference of significance between any measure of function or fatigue between the groups given amino acids.[21] This study did indicate that subjects perceived exhaustion earlier when treated with paroxetine, which increases brain serotonin.

This relates to a theory that exercise fatigue is mediated by serotonin. If tyrosine is given in high enough levels to compete with and reduce uptake of tryptophan, the serotonin precursor, there will be less serotonin in the central nervous system and less fatigue. Other studies have not confirmed this hypothesis.[22]

Cirrhosis

People with cirrhosis can develop what is called encephalopathy, a dysfunction of the brain that progresses to coma. Many of the symptoms are from elevated levels of aromatic amino acids, which may be metabolized into other amines that affect the brain. Giving patients with cirrhosis branched-chain amino acids (BCAAs) has been found to decrease neurologic symptoms.[23] This would be another situation where less tyrosine is needed, not more.

DEFICIENCY

Patients with phenylketonuria (PKU) cannot make tyrosine from phenylalanine. Eating a normal diet will lead to a buildup of phenylalanine in the system in patients with PKU, and it is the phenylalanine that causes brain damage. Babies are tested for PKU at birth. Treatment with a phenylalanine-free diet is extremely effective. They do not usually need supplements with tyrosine unless there is not enough tyrosine in their diet.

There are other, rare genetic defects in which tyrosine or other neurotransmitter precursors cannot be metabolized. None of these is treated with tyrosine.[24]

There is no specific, described deficiency state due to low tyrosine.

FOOD SOURCES

Tyrosine exists in all protein sources, vegetable and animal. Some good sources of tyrosine include poultry, eggs and dairy products, fish, soy products, lima beans, avocados, bananas, almonds, peanuts, sesame and pumpkin seeds, wheat germ and oats.[20]

Ingested tyrosine goes to the liver. Any tyrosine not taken up by the liver will then be shuttled into one of three metabolic pathways. One pathway involves tyrosine in tissues all over the body, being used in protein synthesis, as well as the synthesis of peptides. A second pathway is the conversion of a small amount of tyrosine into thyroxin (thyroid hormone), melanin (skin pigment), and neurotransmitters (see above). Finally tyrosine can also be metabolized to an intermediate substance used for the production of glucose, called gluconeogenesis.[20]

As stated previously, the aromatic amino acids including tyrosine use the same transport mechanism to get into the brain, past the blood-brain barrier, as do branched-chain amino acids. Since there are a lot of BCAAs in most protein, and large amounts get into the circulation, they regularly compete for transport into the brain with the aromatic amino acids. This direct competition has been well documented in animals.[23] It also occurs in humans.

MECHANISM OF ACTION

L-tyrosine is considered a conditionally indispensable amino acid. Tyrosine can be made from other amino acids under normal conditions. Tyrosine can be made from phenylalanine in the liver, and probably other places in the body, like the kidneys.

However, people with phenylketonuria (PKU) cannot make tyrosine from phenylalanine; they must ingest tyrosine itself. Usually people with PKU need to eat proteins rich in tyrosine but do not need to take supplements. The most important thing is that people with PKU cannot ingest phenylalanine because they cannot metabolize it. Excess phenylalanine causes the brain damage that is seen in people with untreated PKU.[4] Babies are tested for PKU at birth.

Tyrosine itself is the precursor of a number of important substances, which include certain neurotransmitters (catecholamines), hormones and skin pigments.

Tyrosine does cross the blood-brain barrier, which does not allow everything in the blood to reach the brain. As explained previously, under some conditions, there is competition over this transport mechanism between the aromatic amino acids and branched-chain amino acids. Once in the brain, tyrosine can be metabolized to the catecholamines norepinephrine, epinephrine, and dopamine. This is why tyrosine has been considered as a possible antidepressant.[20]

Melanin, the skin pigment, is derived from tyrosine, as is thyroxin (thyroid hormone). Tyrosine influences adrenal and pituitary function and stimulates growth hormone. Many substances with biologic activity contain tyrosine, including enkephalins, which are natural opioid-like pain killers made in the body. It is also an antioxidant, capable of stopping free radical damage.[20]

While tyrosine plays an essential role in maintaining neurotransmitters as well as the other hormones and chemicals mentioned, it is also an amino acid that the body uses to make protein. As an amino acid, tyrosine is distributed in tissues and incorporated into protein. Amino acids are necessary for making the many types of protein in the human body, proteins like keratin, elastin, and collagen. Proteins are keys to the structure and function of most cells. Carrier molecules, like the ones that transport iron, are proteins. There is protein in hair, fingernails, hormones, and more. Amino acids can also be converted to coenzymes, nucleic acids, and other essential molecules. Health, including a vigorous immune system, growth, development, and reproduction is not possible without adequate protein.

Proteins are made from strings of amino acids. All the amino acids are at least slightly different from one another and perform slightly different tasks in combining to make proteins. Some amino acids are modified after joining others to make a protein.[25]

Proteins make up a large part of the human body. The largest single type of protein is that found in skeletal muscle (43%). There is also protein wherever there is a need for structural support; approximately 15 percent of the protein is in blood and another 15 percent is in the skin. Organs do not contain as much protein. Liver and kidney contain about 10 percent of the protein, together. The rest is in other organs and bone.

The proportion of muscle in the body increases with age, from newborn to adult.

There are four proteins that constitute almost 50 percent of the body's protein. They are myosin and actin (in muscle), collagen (connective tissue), and hemoglobin (in red blood cells).

There is only a very small reserve of protein that can be used during conditions of insufficient dietary intake for whatever reason. This small reserve is made up of structural proteins that are probably stored in the liver and visceral tissues. It is perhaps 1 percent of the body's protein. It will be used by the body when enough protein is not being consumed.

Normally the body can adapt to a wide range of protein intake. But there are certain pathological states, such as severe disease or injury, in which protein will be used for energy. Muscle protein is lost in these cases.

The body needs both sufficient protein and the correct balances of amino acids to grow and survive. The body loses protein every day through the intestinal tract, urine, and from skin and hair to a lesser extent.

While it is not the primary source of energy for the body, protein can be used to produce energy and will be when there is no other source.

PRIMARY USES

- Tyrosine and phenylalanine are parts of a normal diet.
- Tyrosine may be taken for depression.
- Athletes take it to try and improve performance.
- Others may take it to try and reduce symptoms of fatigue.
- It may be used in the military to improve performance under conditions of stress.

COMMON DOSAGES

For use as a supplement, tyrosine can be taken in doses of 500 to 1,000 mg three times a day, usually before each meal.[4]

Every person needs protein, which will include phenylalanine with or without tyrosine, depending on the source of the protein. The RDA for men and women is 0.8 g of good-quality protein per kilogram per day. The protein needs to contain tyrosine and/or phenylalanine in a certain proportion, which is 47 mg/g of protein.[25]

Protein in General[25]

The recommended amounts of protein at various ages have been calculated by the Institute of Medicine (IOM), Food and Nutrition Board using a variety of methods. The higher quality the protein, the more will be absorbed and the more specific requirements for amino acids will be met. It is recommended in general that phenylalanine and tyrosine together make up 47 mg per gram of protein.

The AI (Adequate Intake) for infants 0 to 6 months is 1.52 g/kg/day. The EAR (Estimated Average Requirement) for older infants ages 7 to 12 months is 1.0 g/kg/day. The RDA (Recommended Dietary Allowance) for this group is 1.2 g/kg/day or 11.0 g/day of protein.

The EAR for boys and girls 1 to 3 years of age is 0.87 g/kg/day of protein. From 4 up to 13 years it is 0.76 g/kg/day. The RDA for children 1 to 3 years old is 1.05 g/kg/day or 13 g/day. For children ages 4 to 13 years, it is 0.95 g/kg/day or 34 g/day of protein.

The EAR for boys ages 14 to 18 is 0.73 g/kg/day; for girls of that age it is 0.71 g/kg/day of protein.

The RDA for boys 14–18 years of age is 0.85 g/kg/day of protein or 52 g/day of protein. The RDA for girls 14–18 years of age is 0.85 g/kg/day of protein or 46 g/day of protein.

The EAR for men and women ages 18 to 50 is 0.66 g/kg/day of protein. The same is true for older adults.

The RDA for men ages 19 through 50 is 0.80 g/kg/day or 56 g/day of protein. For women it is 0.80 g/kg/day or 46 g/day. The same is true for older men and women.

The EAR for pregnancy in any age group is 0.88 g/kg/day of protein or plus an additional 21 g/day of protein. The RDA for pregnancy is 1.1 g/kg/day of protein or plus an additional 25 g/day.

The EAR for lactation is 1.05 g/kg/day of protein or plus an additional 21 g/day. The RDA for lactation is 1.3 g/kg/day of protein or plus an additional 25 g per day.

Tyrosine Plus Phenylalanine[25]

Tyrosine can be made from phenylalanine. These recommendations are for the total of one plus the other.

The AI for infants 0 to 6 months is 807 mg/day or 135 mg/kg/day of phenylalanine plus tyrosine. At 7 to 12 months, the EAR is 58 mg/kg/day and the RDA is 84 mg/kg/day. For boys and girls ages 1 to 3 years, the EAR for lysine is 41 mg/kg/day, and the RDA is 54 mg/kg/day. For boys ages 4 to 13, and girls ages 4 to 8, the EAR for the two amino acids is 33 mg/kg/day, and the RDA is 41 mg/kg/day. The EAR for girls ages 9 to 13 is 31 mg/kg/day, and the RDA is 38 mg/kg/day.

The EAR for adults is 27 mg/kg/day of tyrosine and phenylalanine. The RDA is 33 mg/kg/day.

The EAR for pregnant women is 36 mg/kg/day, and the RDA is 44 mg/kg/day. The EAR for breast-feeding women of all ages is 41 mg/kg/day, while the RDA is 51 mg/kg/day.

POTENTIAL SIDE EFFECTS

There have been no adverse effects noted with any amino acids in the diet. Taken as a supplement, tyrosine has not been associated with any adverse effects even at very high doses of 500 mg/kg/day. Large amounts of tyrosine do raise the level of the amino acid in the blood, and of some of the brain neurotransmitters, but there have not been any clinical problems as a result in normal individuals.

However, in the autosomal-recessive genetic disease, tyrosinemia II, high levels of tyrosine can lead to skin problems and lesions on the cornea of the eye.

The IOM has not been able to set a UL (Tolerable Upper Intake Level) for tyrosine or any other amino acid. It is not known what level might cause the eye and skin lesions or what the changes in the neurotransmitters might mean.[25]

Tyrosine can cause migraine headaches in some people, as well as stomach upset. Tyrosine can elevate the levels of thyroid hormone. It should not be taken by people who already have a condition associated with elevated thyroid hormone, like Grave's disease,[4] or who are taking replacement thyroid hormone.

As stated previously, tyrosine may exacerbate mania. It should not be taken by anyone with liver cirrhosis or failure from any cause.

Interactions

Tyrosine must not be taken by people on monoamine oxidase inhibitors for depression. These include Marplan (isocarboxazid), Nardil (phenelzine), Parnate (tranylcypromine), and selegiline. Anyone taking one of these medications who ingests tyrosine can have a "hypertensive crisis" with elevated blood pressure and risk of heart attack and stroke.

FACT VERSUS FICTION

Research is ongoing in every area mentioned. So far there is little proof that supplemental tyrosine is helpful for most conditions related to the central nervous system. It may be, as stated previously, that since the rate-limiting step in the synthesis of catecholamines from tyrosine is tyrosine hydroxylase, it may be difficult to actually raise brain levels by simply taking supplements of tyrosine.

While it is clearly vital to all brain functions, tyrosine may not be helpful as a supplement in many conditions. In fact, in some cases, lowering tyrosine is advisable. More research needs to be done to clarify the benefits of tyrosine.

Tyrosine is possibly useful in the following cases:

- Depression: results are mixed and definitive conclusions cannot be made.
- Stress: there is some evidence tyrosine may help the reaction to stress.
- Cognitive function and memory: tyrosine may help strengthen these, especially under stress.
- Athletic performance: although there is no solid evidence for performance enhancement, tyrosine may lessen fatigue.

Tyrosine does not seem to have any long-term benefit for the following conditions:

- Hypertension: tyrosine does not lower blood pressure.
- Parkinson's disease: tyrosine does not improve Parkinson's disease.
- ADHD: Although tyrosine may temporarily improve symptoms of ADHD, the improvement is short-lived.

Tyrosine should not be taken in the following cases:

- Cirrhosis: symptoms such as brain dysfunction (encephalopathy) can worsen with tyrosine. Tyrosine may need to be lowered.
- Mania: Lowering tyrosine may improve mania.
- Migraines: Tyrosine can worsen migraine and cluster headaches.

REFERENCES

1. Kim, DY, Rha, E, Choi, S-L, et al. Development of bioreactor system for l-tyrosine synthesis using thermostable tyrosine phenol-lyase. *J. Microbiol Biotechnol*. 2007;17(1):116–122.
2. Gelenberg, AJ, Wojcik, JD, Growdon, JH, et al. Tyrosine for the treatment of depression. *Am J Psychiatry*. 1980;137(5):622–623.
3. Meyers, S. Use of neurotransmitter precursors for treatment of depression. *Altern Med Rev*. 2000;5(1):64–71.
4. University of Maryland Health Center. Complementary Medicine. Tyrosine. Last reviewed May 6, 2009. http://www.umm.edu/altmed/articles/tyrosine-000329.htm. Accessed March 23, 2010.
5. Fernstrom, JD. Can nutrient supplements modify brain function? *Am J Clin Nutr*. 2000;71(Suppl):1669S–1673S.
6. Gelenberg, AJ, Wojcik, JD, Falk, WE, Baldessarini, RJ. Tyrosine for depression: A double-blind trial. *J Affect Disord*. 1990;19(2):125–132.
7. Tachil, AF, Mohan, R, Bhugra, D. The evidence base of complementary and alternative therapies in depression. *J Affect Disord*. 2007;97(1–3):23–35.
8. Fernstrom, JD, Fernstrom, MH. Tyrosine, phenylalanine, and catecholamine synthesis and function in the brain. *J Nutr*. 2007;137:1539S–1547S.
9. Leyton, M, Young, SN, Pihl, RO, et al. Effects on mood of acute phenylalanine/tyrosine depletion in healthy women. *Neuropsychopharmacology*. 2000;22:52–63.
10. McTavish, SFB, Mannie, ZN, Harmer, CJ, Cowen, PJ. Lack of effect of tyrosine depletion on mood in recovered depressed women. *Neuropsychopharmacology*. 2005;30(4):786–791.
11. Roiser, JP, McLean, A, Ogilvie, AD, et al. The subjective and cognitive effects of acute phenylalanine and tyrosine depletion in patients recovered from depression. *Neuropsychopharmacology*. 2005;30(4):775–785.

12. Scarna, A, Gijsman, HJ, McTavish, SF, Harmer, CJ, Cowen, PJ, Goodwin, GM. Effects of a branched-chain amino acid drink in mania. *Br J Psychiatry.* 2003;182:210–213.

13. McTavish, SFB, McPherson, MH, Sharp, T, Cowen, PJ. Attenuation of some subjective effects of amphetamine following tyrosine depletion. *Journal of Psychopharmacology.* 1999;23(2):144–147.

14. Sole, MJ, Benedict, CR, Myers, MG, Leenen, FH, Anderson, GH. Chronic dietary tyrosine supplements do not affect mild essential hypertension. *Hypertension.* 1985;7:593–596.

15. Life Extension Magazine. Report: Don't fall victim to frailty. March 2010. http://search.lef.org/cgi-src bin/MsmGo.exe?grab_id=0&page_id=1459&query=tyrosine&hiword=tyrosine%20. Accessed March 23, 2010.

16. Lieberman, HR. Nutrition, brain function and cognitive performance. *Appetite.* 2003;40(3):245–254.

17. Thomas, JR, Lockwood, PA, Singh, A, Deuster, PA. Tyrosine improves working memory in a multitasking environment. *Pharmacol Biochem Behav.* 1999;64(3):495–500.

18. Deijen, JB, Orlebeke, JF. Effect of tyrosine on cognitive function and blood pressure under stress. *Brain Research Bulletin.* 1994;33(3):319–323.

19. D'Andrea, G, Nordera, GP, Perini, F, Allais, G, Granella, F. Biochemistry of neuromodulation in primary headaches: Focus on anomalies of tyrosine metabolism. *Neurol Sci.* 2007;28(Suppl 2):S94–S96.

20. L-tyrosine. *Altern Med Rev.* 2007;12(4):364–368.

21. Struder, HK, Hollmann, W, Platen, P, Donike, M, Gotzmann, A, Weber, K. Influence of paroxetine, branched-chain amino acids and tyrosine on neuroendocrine system responses and fatigue in humans. *Horm Metab Res.* 1998;30(4):188–194.

22. Chinevere, TD, Sawyer, RD, Creer, AR, et al. Effects of L-tyrosine and carbohydrate ingestion on endurance exercise performance. *J Appl Physiol.* 2002;93:1590–1597.

23. Fernstrom, JD. Branched-chain amino acids and brain function. *J Nutr.* 2005;135:1539S–1546S.

24. Hyland, K. Inherited disorders affecting dopamine and serotonin: Critical neurotransmitters derived from aromatic amino acids. *J Nutr.* 2007; 137:1568S–1572S.

25. Institute of Medicine. Food and Nutrition Board. *Dietary reference intakes for energy, carbohydrate, fiber, fat, fatty acids, cholesterol, protein, and amino acids (macronutrients).* Washington, DC: National Academies Press, 2005.

22

Melatonin

BRIEF OVERVIEW

Melatonin is a hormone produced in a part of the brain called the pineal gland. It is most commonly known for its role in maintaining the circadian rhythm of humans. Also called "The Dark Hormone," it is secreted mainly during the night. Melatonin secretion markedly decreases during the day.

Melatonin is one of the regulators of sleep, which it affects in a number of different ways. It is part of the biological clock of every person. When the rhythm of melatonin secretion is disrupted, for example, by night-time light exposure, there are adverse consequences. Sleep problems often occur, but there are other less obvious effects.[1] In addition to melatonin's key role in chronobiology, it is now known to be a powerful antioxidant with other functions.

THE HYPE

Sleep

The suprachiasmatic nucleus (SCN) is a part of the brain that is called the circadian pacemaker. It receives information about conditions of light and dark, and in dark, sends signals to the pineal gland to secrete melatonin. Melatonin acts on other parts of the brain to induce sleep.

Since melatonin affects the sleep-wake cycle, it has been used to treat insomnia. As a natural substance, it should be a safe insomnia treatment. Since so many people suffer from difficulty sleeping at one time or another, there is much interest in melatonin for this purpose. There are many ongoing trials looking at the best ways to use melatonin to help people who cannot sleep. As a consequence, there have been many studies, as well as reviews, trying to analyze the data from the different studies.

There are different kinds of sleep disturbances. In one called delayed sleep phase syndrome, people have difficulty going to sleep at the appropriate time, as well as waking up at the desired time. Studies have shown that melatonin may be effective in treating this condition; people fall asleep more quickly when they take it.[2,3] Melatonin does seem to shorten sleep onset latency, which may help people with other disorders of sleep onset as well as delayed sleep phase syndrome.[5]

Melatonin seems to work best when used to help initiate sleep, but not to maintain it. In primary insomnia, there is difficulty falling asleep as well as staying asleep. Therefore, melatonin has not proven to be helpful in primary insomnia.[2,4] Melatonin is metabolized very quickly, which may prevent it from maintaining sleep. Melatonin does not cause sleep directly. It interacts in a complex way with many areas of the brain. The SCN as well as other parts of the brain are all involved in the sleep-wake cycle.

It is possible that melatonin does not help maintain sleep because of its short half-life. To test that theory and try and find a way to help people with primary insomnia, prolonged-release formulations of melatonin have been developed, as have synthetic drugs with melatonin-like actions.[6]

Prolonged-release melatonin has been studied, and in Europe, studied and approved under the trade name Circadan. In one of the larger studies, Circadan decreased sleep onset latency in elderly patients with primary insomnia. It did not necessarily improve measured sleep maintenance. However, many patients felt that they slept better and were more alert the next day.[7] Multiple studies of prolonged-release melatonin demonstrated that it may be useful in reducing the length of time it takes to fall asleep for elderly individuals with insomnia.[6]

More studies are being done with Circadan and other extended-release formulations of melatonin. Immediate-release melatonin, as well as prolonged release, may also improve the sleep of children with neuropsychiatric disorders.[3] Other populations that may benefit include schizophrenics and patients with Alzheimer's disease.[6]

Melatonin definitely helps reduce symptoms of jet lag. There are conflicting reports about how melatonin helps. Does it actually improve sleep, or does it just reduce symptoms? In the case of jet lag, it probably helps reset the sleep-wake cycle.[2,3,8]

Melatonin agonists—drugs that are similar to melatonin in structure and function—have been made, studied, and at least one (Rozerem—ramelteon) has been FDA approved for insomnia. This is a prescription drug and not a supplement.

Depression

There is evidence of phase shifting of melatonin in depression.[9] When depression is treated by any one of a number of antidepressants, there is usually a normalizing of melatonin secretion. There is also a melatonin agonist called agomelatine that has been used successfully to treat depression.[10]

It is not clear that melatonin itself can help people with depression. There are ongoing investigations into the antidepressant properties of melatonin.

General

As people age, the circadian rhythm is disrupted. Melatonin production declines and is shifted to later in the evening. Cortisol secretion is increased and occurs earlier in the night. In addition to causing delayed sleep onset, this imbalance may influence blood pressure, metabolism, and mood. Giving melatonin to elderly patients with insomnia can readjust the excessive and early cortisol secretion. This may have many other benefits.[11]

The list of illnesses and conditions thought by some to be influenced by melatonin secretion is a long one.[10] In some cases, increased or altered melatonin secretion may actually cause or worsen certain illnesses, including autoimmune diseases like rheumatoid arthritis. Melatonin may help increase bone mass. It may have an effect on body mass and composition, as well as sexual maturation.[10] Low melatonin levels may contribute to idiopathic scoliosis.[10,12] Some of these associations are based on observations made about melatonin in animals and may not be significant in humans.

Cancer

As an antioxidant, melatonin might be useful in treating diseases due to oxidative stress and the damage it causes, like cancer. A review article in 2005 came to the conclusion that, when used as either a treatment itself, or as an adjunct to other treatment of solid-tumor cancers, melatonin reduced the risk of death at one year across all the trials reviewed. There were few adverse effects.[13] The authors pointed out that the trials they reviewed were not blinded (doctors and patients knew what they were getting), and all took place in the same institution. More studies are needed and are being done.

One study in 2002 randomly assigned patients with metastatic non–small cell lung cancer to receive chemotherapy with or without melatonin. The two-year survival rate was zero in the patients who received only chemotherapy, while 6 percent of the patients who also received melatonin were alive after five years. The patients receiving melatonin also tolerated the chemotherapy better.[14]

Melatonin may be an inhibitory factor to cancer cells, both in culture, and in actual patients. In 2006, the International Agency for Research on Cancer (IARC) stated that shift work disrupting the circadian rhythm is probably carcinogenic to humans. There is a higher incidence of breast cancer and colorectal cancer in shift workers, for example.[10] Ongoing research is investigating this phenomenon, which may very well be related to melatonin levels.[1]

Whether or not changes in melatonin levels contribute to the development of cancer is a separate issue from whether or not melatonin can help treat cancer.

Degenerative Neurologic Diseases

As an antioxidant, melatonin may be able to play a role in degenerative diseases thought to be caused by oxidative stress in the nervous system. These could include Alzheimer's disease, amyotrophic lateral sclerosis, and others. There is a model of Alzheimer's disease in mice; melatonin is effective therapy for the disease in mice. Obviously humans are not mice. There is continued investigation of this treatment. Melatonin has been shown to help patients with Alzheimer's disease sleep better and possibly slow the progression of the disease.[10]

However, in 2006, a (systematic) Cochrane Review of studies using melatonin for patients with cognitive decline and dementia showed insufficient evidence to conclude that it is of any benefit.[15]

DEFICIENCY

There is no known melatonin deficiency state. There can be alterations in melatonin secretion, which happens in the elderly.

Melatonin is not just synthesized by the pineal gland, but also in multiple other places in the human body.

FOOD SOURCES

Although melatonin is found in just about all sources of food, both plant and animal, there are some experts who note that it has not been proved that consuming melatonin in food raises levels of melatonin in humans.[16]

However, melatonin in chicken feed has been proven to raise plasma levels of melatonin in chickens. Plant melatonin fed to rabbits inhibits binding of tagged melatonin to the brain. While this does not prove that melatonin in food raises levels in humans, it is certainly likely that it does.[17]

Others assume that dietary melatonin can be absorbed. It has been noted that many Chinese herbal medicines are rich in melatonin. They are considered to have medicinal effects on multiple diseases.[10,18] Melatonin found in herbs is absorbed.

Assuming people can absorb melatonin from food, they can get it from any animal or plant source. However, since it is a hormone produced by the human body, it is not something that people need to take as a supplement.

MECHANISM OF ACTION: HOW DOES IT WORK?

While the pineal gland is part of the brain, it is outside what is called the blood-brain barrier. This means that the melatonin it produces gets into both the bloodstream, into the cerebrospinal fluid around the brain and spinal cord, and directly into cells in the nervous system and elsewhere.

Melatonin is made by the body from the amino acid tryptophan via a number of steps. Tryptophan is converted to serotonin, which is in turn converted to melatonin. Serotonin is stored in the pineal gland. When signals come in from the suprachiasmatic nucleus of the brain, this information is transmitted to the pineal gland and triggers the conversion of serotonin to melatonin. Melatonin is very lipid soluble and can get into cells and fluids anywhere in the body.

There are melatonin receptors located throughout the body. The best known are MT_1, which is found in the brain and blood vessels in the heart, MT_2, which is found in other areas of the brain, and MT_3, which is found in many organs including kidney and brain. Both MT_1 and MT_2 can be found in the suprachiasmic nucleus, so that melatonin acts on the very area that causes it to be secreted.[16] Melatonin supplements do not just go to the brain, but also to these other receptors. Most of melatonin's actions occur via its effects on the melatonin receptors. All of its functions are not yet completely understood.[10]

Light intensity is not the only signal that affects melatonin synthesis. When people are placed in darkened rooms around the clock, it takes a number of days for their melatonin secretion patterns to change. If the secretion was simply light dependant, it should change more quickly.

Melatonin influences the circadian rhythm in humans, and thus the phasing (timing) of sleep. It also directly promotes sleep.

Some of melatonin's actions may occur because of its antioxidant properties.

PRIMARY USES

- Melatonin is used for jet lag, which is especially problematic for people traveling east and across two to five time zones.[19] It works less well for travelers going west and across fewer time zones.[8]

- It is also used to treat patients with circadian rhythm sleep disorders. People with prolonged sleep onset latency from whatever cause may benefit from taking melatonin. This can include people with delayed sleep phase syndrome, shift workers, and others. It is also effective in treating the elderly with insomnia.

- Some blind people lose the synchronicity of their circadian rhythms, and melatonin can help to return them to a 24-hour cycle.[20]

- Melatonin has not proved effective in patients with chronic primary insomnia.[6] However, many people chose to try it.

COMMON DOSAGES

Melatonin can be synthesized or isolated from the pineal glands of beef cattle. It can be obtained in a short-acting form or in a prolonged-release form.

Many authorities believe that melatonin should not be sold as a supplement and should be regulated by the FDA. Instead of being available over-the-counter, it should be given to patients by prescription, since it is a hormone like estrogen or thyroid hormone.[16] At the current time it is sold as a supplement in a wide variety of doses.

For jet lag, doses from 0.5 mg to 5 mg of melatonin can be taken at about the destination bedtime starting the day of travel and continuing for two to four nights.[8,19] The dose of 5 mg works best; larger doses do not seem to work any better. It appears to be safe and effective for this short-term use.

As much as 50 mg of melatonin has been taken for sleep, although 5 to 10 mg are more commonly used. Both quick-release and prolonged-release forms are available. Research is being done on transdermal preparations that may allow for longer daytime sleep for night-shift workers who have to sleep during the day.[21]

POTENTIAL SIDE EFFECTS

Melatonin is generally safe when used for a short term.[5] Long-term safety has not been documented.

A number of side effects have been reported, including headache, drowsiness, and depression, nausea, and dizziness.[2,19] Melatonin must be taken at the appropriate time so as to avoid daytime sleepiness.[5]

Melatonin has so many effects on the body, involving multiple systems, that there are certain groups of people that should not take melatonin. Melatonin affects other hormones, as well as the immune system, the gastrointestinal tract, and blood vessels, among other things. It should probably not be taken by men or women actively trying to conceive a baby. It is also not recommended for patients with Parkinson's disease.[6]

Since melatonin can stimulate the immune system, it is not a good choice for people with autoimmune diseases. There are studies that show melatonin can worsen rheumatoid arthritis.[22]

Melatonin may increase the risk of seizures in patients with epilepsy and may interfere with the actions of the anticoagulant warfarin[3] and possibly other blood thinners. There have been reports of elevated cholesterol and elevated blood sugar. Melatonin can alter mood and should be used with caution by people with psychiatric disorders. Anyone contemplating taking large doses of melatonin, or taking any dose for a prolonged period of time, should consult a health care professional.[3]

FACT VERSUS FICTION

There is no doubt that melatonin is an active hormone involved in many processes. It is an important component in the regulation of the human biologic clock and circadian rhythm. It can be used to help restore normal sleep to people whose sleep cycle has been disrupted by a wide variety of causes. In a long-acting formulation, it may also be useful to help treat primary insomnia, but that has not yet been proved.

There may be other uses for melatonin, in treating depression, cancer, and possibly other illnesses. These uses for melatonin are being studied. It may turn out that a melatonin agonist—a drug with some of melatonin's features—will actually be useful, when plain melatonin is not. These agonists are already arriving on the market, as prescription medications.

There is no need to take melatonin as a supplement because there is no evidence of a deficiency state. Taking it as suggested for jet lag or other sleep phase disruptions seems very reasonable.

REFERENCES

1. Erren, TC, Reiter, RJ. Defining chronodisruption. *J Pineal Res.* 2009;46(3): 245–247.
2. Buscemi, N, Vandermeer, B, Pandya, R, Hooton, N, Tjosvold, L, Hartling, L, Baker, G, Vohra, S, Klassen, T. *Melatonin for treatment of sleep disorders.* Evidence Report/Technology Assessment: Number 108. Agency for Healthcare Research and Quality, Rockville, MD. http://www.ahrq.gov/clinic/epcsums/ melatsum.htm. Accessed December 1, 2009.
3. Natural Standard Research Collaboration. Melatonin. Medline Plus. Last update August 26, 2009. http://www.nlm.nih.gov/medlineplus/druginfo/natural/ patient-melatonin.html. Accessed December 1, 2009.
4. Silber, MH. Chronic insomnia. *N Engl J Med.* 2005;353:803–810.

5. Buscemi, N, Vandermeer, B, Hooton, N, et al. The efficacy and safety of exogenous melatonin for primary sleep disorders: A meta-analysis. *J Gen Int Med.* 2005;20:1151–1158.

6. Hardeland, R. New approaches in the management of insomnia: Weighing the advantages of prolonged-release melatonin and synthetic melatoninergic agonists. *Neuropsychiatric Disease and Treatment.* 2009;5:341–354.

7. Lemoine, P, Nir, T, Laudon, M, Zisapel, N. Prolonged-release melatonin improves sleep quality and morning alertness in insomnia patients aged 55 years and older and has no withdrawal effects. *J Sleep Res.* 2007;16:372–380.

8. Herxheimer, A, Petrie, KJ. Melatonin for the prevention and treatment of jet lag. *Cochrane Database of Systematic Reviews.* 2009:4 (first published 2002, no change). 2002;(2):CD001520.

9. Crasson, M, Kjiri, S, Colin, A, Kjiri, K, L'Hermite-Baleriaux, M, Ansseau, M, Legros, JJ. Serum melatoninand urinary 6-sulfatoxymelatonin in major depression. *Psychoneuroendocrinology.* 2004;29:1–12.

10. Pandi-Perumal, SR, Srinivasan, V, Maestroni, GJ, et al. Melatonin: Nature's most versatile biological signal? *FEBS Journal.* 2006;273:2813–2838.

11. Zisapel, N, Tarrasch, R, Laudon, M. The relationship between melatonin and cortisol rhythms: Clinical implications of melatonin therapy. *Drug Development Research.* 2005;65(3):119–125.

12. Grivas, TB, Savvidou, OD. Melatonin the "light of night" in human biology and adolescent idiopathic scoliosis. *Scoliosis.* 2007;2(6). doi:10.1186/1748-7161-2-6.

13. Mills, E, Wu, P, Seely, D, Guyatt, G. Melatonin in the treatment of cancer: A systematic review of randomized controlled trials and meta-analysis. *J Pineal Res.* 2005;39(4):360–366.

14. Lissoni, P, Chilelli, M, Villa, S, Cerizza, L, Tancini, G. Five years survival in metastatic non-small cell lung cancer patients treated with chemotherapy alone or chemotherapy and melatonin: A randomized trial. *J Pineal Res.* 2003;35:12–15.

15. Jansen, SL, Forbes, D, Duncan, F, Morgan, DG. Melatonin for cognitive impairment. *Cochrane Database of Systematic Reviews.* 2009:4 (first published 2006, no change).

16. Wurtman, RJ. Melatonin. In: Coates, PM., (Ed.). *Encyclopedia of dietary supplements.* New York: Marcel Dekker, 2005;457–466.

17. Hattori, A, Migitaka, H, Iigo, M, Itoh, M, Yamamoto, K, Ohtani-Kaneko, R, Hara, M, Suzuki, T, Reiter, RJ. Identification of melatonin in plants and its effects on plasma melatonin levels and binding to melatonin receptors in vertebrates. *Biochem Mol Biol Int.* 1995;35(3):627–634.

18. Chen, G, Huo, Y, Tan, D, et al. Melatonin in Chinese medicinal herbs. *Life Sciences.* 2003;73(1):19–26.

19. The Merck Manuals Online Medical Library for Healthcare Professionals. Melatonin. Last full review/revision May 2009 by Ara DerMarderosian, PhD. http://www.merck.com/mmpe/sec22/ch331/ch331v.html?qt=melatonin&alt=sh#sec22-ch331-ch331t-340. Accessed December 1, 2009.

20. Sack, RL, Brandes, RW, Kendall, AR, Lewy, AJ. Entrainment of free-running circadian rhythms by melatonin in blind people. *N Engl J Med.* 2000;343: 1070–1077.

21. Aeschbach, D, Lockyer, BJ, Dijk, DJ, Lockley, SW, Nuwayser, ES, Nichols, LD, Czeisler, CA. Use of transdermal melatonin delivery to improve sleep maintenance during daytime. *Clin Pharmacol Ther.* 2009;86(4):378–382.

22. Cutolo, M, Straub, RH. Insights into endocrine-immunological disturbances in autoimmunity and their impact on treatment. *Arthritis Research & Therapy.* 2009;11:218–215.

23

MSM

MSM stands for methylsulfonylmethane, which is also known as dimethyl sulfone. It occurs naturally in plants and animals.

It is a close chemical relative, a metabolite (a metabolic product), of DMSO, dimethylsulfoxide. DMSO has been used for decades to treat horses with painful, inflammatory conditions, in a topical form as well as orally. While effective in horses, DMSO has side effects including skin irritation and a garlic odor imparted to the user.

Some DMSO is converted to MSM in the body. MSM appears to have the same effects, but not the same side effects as DMSO. Like DMSO, it has been used for painful and/or inflammatory conditions such as arthritis. Other uses are being investigated.

MSM is sold as a dietary supplement, not a drug. Sales have made the supplement its own industry. Long before any real evidence was accumulated for its efficacy, MSM was being sold in large quantities online, in vitamin and supplement stores, and in bulk for consumers at places like Costco. Many books were published, such as *The Definitive Guide. A Comprehensive Review of the Science and Therapeutics of Methylsulfonylmethane*[1] and *The Miracle of MSM: The Natural Solution for Pain*, claiming it was a cure for just about everything, especially pain.[2]

THE HYPE

Arthritis and Other Pain

MSM is a very popular supplement for people with osteoarthritis (OA), for a reason. There is a real need for safe and effective treatment for arthritis. People with serious osteoarthritis of large joints like the knees do not have good choices. They can take nonsteroidal anti-inflammatory medicines (NSAIDs) but not over long periods of time. The older the person, the more likely a bad reaction, such as gastrointestinal bleeding, can occur. Acetaminophen does not give the same kind of pain relief. People with very bad osteoarthritis in the knees or hips can have their joint or joints replaced but often put surgery off for as long as they can. The hip surgery is very successful but the replacement joints don't last forever. The knee surgery is still very difficult.

In addition to osteoarthritis, there are other forms of arthritis like rheumatoid arthritis that can be very difficult to treat. Patients with pain from most forms of arthritis, as well as other painful conditions like fibromyalgia rheumatica, are all looking for safe alternative treatments.

MSM appears to be very safe, according to researchers in the field.[3] It has been said, "Methylsulfonylmethane is one of the least toxic substances in biology, similar in toxicity to water."[4]

The question is, is it effective? Early trials were small, unpublished, and lacking a lot of relevant data. One unpublished study, said to be double-blind, using 750 mg of MSM a day for six weeks, found improvement in 80 percent of those treated for osteoarthritis, compared to 20 percent improvement in the placebo group.[3]

Two trials were sponsored by a manufacturer of MSM, Lignisul MSM, which is sold on the Web site www.msm.com. Lignisul's first sponsored study, called "MSM (methylsulfonylmethane): A Double-Blind Study of Its Use in Degenerative Arthritis," was on the Lignisul Web site in 2002,[4] although it was apparently not there in 2009. It can be found at http://www.vitaflex.com/res_msmdjdstudy.php. It describes a small trial involving 16 patients with x-ray evidence of degenerative arthritis as well as pain. In total, 10 were randomly chosen to receive 2,250 mg of MSM per day, while the other 6 received placebo. There was an average of an 82 percent decrease in pain for the subjects given MSM, versus 18 percent with placebo.[5] There was no raw data presented, and the study was never published in a medical journal.

The second report, called "MSM in the Treatment of Acute Athletic Injuries," was also on the Lignisul Web site in 2002, although it was apparently not there in 2009 (it can be found on the Web site http://www.vitaflex.com/res_lignisulmsm.php). Twenty-four patients with athletic injuries requiring chiropractic treatment were randomly split into two groups. Both got the same other care, but one group received an unspecified dose of MSM, the other, placebo. The report says that the patients and chiropractors did not know who got MSM. The injuries in one group called "A" included nine sprain/strain injuries, one case of knee pain from the kneecaps, one case of tennis elbow, and one person with back pain with radiation of pain. The other group, B, comprised patients with similar diagnoses, with one more strain/sprain and no patient with kneecap pain. Pain was assessed by the patients and the chiropractor.

The MSM-treated group (A) reported a 58.3 percent reduction of symptoms as opposed to a 33.3 percent reduction for patients given placebo. The MSM-treated patients needed two less visits to the chiropractor. This was a double-blind, randomly controlled trial, but the assessments were all subjective. The diagnoses varied. The report used the patients' assessments, for example, stating that their symptoms resolved in two weeks less than with treatment they had received at a previous time.[6] This report was never published in a medical journal and again was sponsored by an MSM manufacturer.

In 2004, a review article was published documenting how many people were already taking MSM, often in addition to other supplements for their OA or other pain. Researchers gave a questionnaire to approximately 600 people seen in a primary care, university-based setting, including Spanish speakers. The patients had OA, rheumatoid arthritis, or fibromyalgia. Of these patients, 90 percent had at least tried alternative therapy; 4.6% of the patients with OA were using MSM, as were 4.2% of the patients with rheumatoid arthritis, and 9.9% of the patients with fibromyalgia.[7]

Researchers have looked at some of the combination supplements for arthritis that contain MSM. There is a specific formula used for OA called AR7 Joint Complex that has been on the market for many years. It includes sternum collagen, methylsulfonylmethane, cetyl myristoleate (CMO), lipase, vitamin C, and bromelain. A randomized, blinded, placebo-controlled trial of 89 subjects was done, using this formula for osteoarthritis. After three months, the patients treated with AR7 reported significantly less pain and stiffness and improved quality of life. It is not possible to separate out the effects of MSM.[8]

Larger and more rigorous trials were eventually undertaken. In 2004, 118 patients with "mild to moderate" osteoarthritis of the knee were randomized to take MSM, glucosamine (also an alternative treatment for arthritis), the two together, or placebo. Patients were evaluated for 12 weeks, with a number of relatively objective scales, such as 15-minute walking time, the Lequesne Index, and the need to take rescue medication—meaning pain was bad enough to take something else, like an NSAID or stronger pain medicine. MSM alone significantly decreased pain and swelling, and the combination of MSM and glucosamine improved symptoms more than either alone.[9]

In 2006, another randomized, double-blind, placebo-controlled trial of MSM was done, with 50 men and women who had knee osteoarthritis. They received MSM 3 g or placebo twice a day. Using the WOMAC scale (Western Ontario MacMaster Osteoarthritis Index pain subscale) to assess pain and function, the researchers found that MSM produced significant decreases in both pain and functional impairment. There were no major adverse events. The authors of this study stated that more investigation is needed.[10]

Reviewers in 2006, writing for *Arthritis Research & Therapy,* thought that there was moderate evidence of efficacy of MSM for osteoarthritis based on the previous two trials.[11] In an article in the *American Family Physician,* other writers concluded that, as of 2008, there was not enough evidence of long-term effectiveness or safety of MSM to recommend its use.[12] Yet another analysis of the various trials in 2009 concluded that neither MSM nor DMSO have been proved effective in reducing joint pain.[13]

Since there has been some success in the small trials using MSM, further research would be very useful in determining if MSM can be used safely over a prolonged period, and how much relief it might provide to people with arthritis. Many reviewers note that MSM has promise,[14] calling it at the current time, "possibly effective."[15]

MSM Is Also Proposed as a Treatment for Allergic Rhinitis (Hay Fever)

In one open-label trial 50 patients were give 2,600 mg of MSM for 30 days. Patients reported decreased upper and lower respiratory symptoms as well as more energy.[3] There were no changes in laboratory tests such as IgE levels.[16] There was a letter criticizing the study published in the *Journal of Alternative and Complementary Medicine,* the same journal that first published the study. Requests were made for pollen counts and other data that might make the study more persuasive. Pollen counts were later supplied. However, there have not been further controlled studies of this treatment.

MSM Is Proposed as Treatment for Interstitial Cystitis

Both MSM and DMSO have been used to treat interstitial cystitis, a painful inflammation of the urinary bladder without a clear cause, with some success.[3,4] A researcher reported on one small group of six patients with interstitial cystitis who were given 30 to 50 cc of MSM, instilled into the bladder. Four patients derived benefit from this treatment.[17]

MSM Is Proposed as a Cancer Preventative

Tests in animals and in labs have suggested that MSM might prevent tumor growth.[3]

There has been little actual study of MSM and cancer in humans. One large study called the VITamins and Lifestyle study found an inverse association between the use of MSM and incidence of colorectal cancer.[18]

Other Indications

MSM has been suggested as treatment for autoimmune disorders and stress injuries.[3] There was also a small trial using MSM topically to the throat for snoring. The patients and their bed partners indicated snoring decreased during the four nights of the trial.[19]

DEFICIENCY

There is no deficiency disease related to MSM. It is a source of sulfur (see below), but there are many other sources of sulfur in the diet.

FOOD SOURCES

MSM can be found in many foods of plant or animal origin. Cow's milk is possibly the best source, with probably the highest concentration of MSM. It can also be found in tomatoes, Swiss chard, corn, fruit, and alfalfa. MSM is also in beer, coffee, and tea. In terms of herbal sources, MSM has been isolated from horsetail.[3]

However, supplements of MSM are manufactured rather than extracted, because the concentration of MSM in food sources is very low. Dimethyl sulfoxide

(DMSO) and hydrogen peroxide are combined to make MSM, which can also be called dimethyl sulfone. After it is synthesized, it is purified, usually by distillation, using heat to separate out any other substances. Manufacturers who are making MSM properly and safeguarding its purity have ways to check for contamination.

MECHANISM OF ACTION: HOW DOES IT WORK?

In laboratory testing, MSM shows anti-inflammatory and antioxidant properties.[3] MSM may stabilize the membranes of damaged cells to prevent leakage and may also stop the injury that can be caused by free radicals.[13]

However, it is possible that MSM helps with pain and inflammation not necessarily because of these properties, but because it is a source of sulfur.[4,13] Sulfur is found in all connective tissue and is needed for repair of cartilage. MSM is one of the sources of sulfur in the diet. It had been thought that the main dietary sources of sulfur for humans were the sulfur-containing amino acids methionine, cysteine, and taurine. It is now believed that MSM may also be an important source of sulfur.[4] Approximately one-third of MSM is sulfur.[20] There is sulfur in chondroitin sulfate and glucosamine sulfate, which are also promoted as good for joint health, and often combined with MSM in supplements.[4]

Sulfur is a critical element of the diet. Sulfur is found both in colostrum and breast milk. Of the minerals in the adult body, sulfur is the third most prominent. Sulfur is involved in the human clotting system, since some of the elements contain sulfur. It is also critical in a number of metabolic reactions.[4]

Forms of sulfur have been used to treat many skin problems including dandruff and acne. Sulfur is a folk remedy for many other skin conditions. Sulfur-containing baths were used for centuries to treat patients with rheumatism and other ailments. "Taking the waters" in Europe usually meant water containing sulfur.

PRIMARY USES

- Most people who take MSM take it for pain, usually arthritis pain, or muscular pain. Some people take it for joint health, based on the idea that it might prevent joint problems in the future.

COMMON DOSAGES

For osteoarthritis, some suggest 1 to 3 g of MSM a day.[3] Others suggest 2 to 5 g.[20] Up to 18 g a day have been given.[3] For allergic rhinitis, 2,600 mg a day have been given in two divided doses. For snoring, one spray containing 150 mg of MSM was used.

MSM is often packaged with other supplements for 'joint health," which can include glucosamine and chondroitin sulfate, among other ingredients.

For interstitial cystitis, 30 to 50 cc are instilled into the urinary bladder.

POTENTIAL SIDE EFFECTS

Large doses of MSM have caused gastrointestinal symptoms like diarrhea.[15] There has been one report of bladder spasm caused by MSM, when used for interstitial cystitis, but this could have been a symptom of the disease. One person in the hay fever trial developed hives. It is unclear if MSM provoked this reaction.[15]

It has been written that MSM is believed to be nontoxic because of animal testing.[3] The lethal dose of DMSO in mice is more than 20 g per kg of body weight. Since MSM is a metabolite of DMSO, it is thought to have a similar safety protocol.[4]

When given to pregnant rats, doses as high as 1,000 mg/kg/day caused no damage to the female rates or the fetuses.[21] In another study, the rats tolerated acute doses of 2 g/kg and subacute chronic doses of 1.5 g/kg.[22]

FACT VERSUS FICTION

There appears to be some evidence, however limited, that MSM may help with the pain of osteoarthritis and possibly other arthritis. This may be because MSM is a source of sulfur or because of its anti-inflammatory or antioxidant properties. Many more studies are needed to confirm long-term safety and efficacy.

Other claims for MSM are not substantiated at this time.

REFERENCES

1. Jacob, SW, Appleton, J. *MSM: The definitive guide. A comprehensive review of the science and therapeutics of methylsulfonylmethane.* Topanga, CA: Freedom Press, 2003.
2. Jacob, S, Lawrence, RM, Zucker, M. *The miracle of MSM: The natural solution for pain.* New York: Penguin-Putnam, 1999.
3. Anonymous. Methylsulfonylmethane. *Altern Med Rev.* 2003;8(4):438–440.
4. Parcell, S. Sulfur in human nutrition and applications in medicine. *Altern Med Rev.* 2002;7(1):22–44.
5. Lawrence, RM. Methyl-sulfonyl-methane (M.S.M.): A double blind study of its use in degenerative arthritis (a preliminary correspondence). http://www.vitaflex.com/res_msmdjdstudy.php. Accessed December 11, 2009.
6. Lawrence, RM, Sanchez, D, Grosman, M. LIGNISUL MSM in the treatment of acute athletic injuries. http://www.vitaflex.com/res_lignisulmsm.php. Accessed December 11, 2009.
7. Herman, CJ, Allen, P, Hunt, WC, Prasad, A, Brady, TJ. Use of complementary therapies among primary care clinic patients with arthritis. *Prev Chronic Dis.* 2004;4(1):1–15. http://www.cdc.gov/pcd/issues/2004/oct/03_0036.htm. Accessed December 11, 2009.
8. Xie, Q, Shi, R, Xu, G, et al. Effects of AR7 Joint Complex on arthralgia for patients with osteoarthritis: Results of a three-month study in Shanghai, China. *Nutrition Journal.* 2008;7(31):1–6.

9. Usha, PR, Naidu, MUR. Randomised, double-blind, parallel, placebo-controlled study of oral glucosamine, methylsulfonylmethane and their combination in osteoarthritis. *Clinical Drug Investigation.* 2004;24:353–363.

10. Kim, LS, Axelrod, LJ, Howard, P, Buratovich, N, Waters, RF. Efficacy of methylsulfonylmethane (MSM) in osteoarthritis pain of the knee: A pilot clinical trial. *Osteoarthritis Cartilage.* 2006;14:286–294.

11. Ameye, LG, Chee, WSS. Osteoarthritis and nutrition. From nutraceuticals to functional foods: A systematic review of the scientific evidence. *Arthritis Research & Therapy.* 2006;8:R127. doi:10.1186/ar2016.

12. Gregory, PJ, Sperry, M, Wilson, AF. Dietary supplements for osteoarthritis. *American Family Physician.* 2008;77(22):177–184.

13. Brien, S, Prescott, P, Lewith, G. Meta-analysis of the related nutritional supplements dimethyl sulfoxide and methylsulfonylmethane in the treatment of osteoarthritis of the knee. *Evidence-based Complimentary and Alternative Medicine.* eCam Advance Access published online on May 27, 2009. http://ecam.oxfordjournals.org/cgi/content/full/nep045. Accessed December 4, 2009.

14. Ramsbottom, H, Lockwood, G. Nutraceuticals for healthy joints. *Pharmaceutical Journal.* 2006;277(7431):740–746.

15. Chen, L, Boon, H. Professional review: Herb & supplements: MSM. *CAMline.* 2007. http://www.camline.ca/professionalreview/pr.php?NHPID=65. Accessed December 18, 2009.

16. Barrager, E, Velmann, JR, Schauss, AG, Schiller, RN. A multicentered, open-label trial on the safety and efficacy of methylsulfonylmethane in the treatment of seasonal allergic rhinitis. *The Journal of Alternative and Complementary Medicine.* 2002;8(2):167–173.

17. Childs, SJ. Dimethyl sulfone (DMSO$_2$) in the treatment of interstitial cystitis. *Urologic Clinics of North America.* 1994;21(1):85–88.

18. Satia, JA, Littman, A, Slatore, CG, Galanko, JA, White, E. Associations of herbal and specialty supplements with lung and colorectal cancer risk in the VITamins and Lifestyle study. *Cancer Epidemiol Biomarkers Prev.* 2009;18(5):1419–1428.

19. Blum, JM, Blum, RI. The effect of methylsulfonylmethane (MSM) in the control of snoring. *Integrative Medicine: A Clinician's Journal.* 2005; 3(6):24–30.

20. Talbott, SM. *A guide to understanding dietary supplements.* Binghamton, NY: Haworth Press, 2003.

21. Magnuson, BA, Appleton, J, Ryan, B, Matulka, RA. Oral developmental toxicity study of methylsulfonylmethane in rats. *Food Chem Toxicol.* 2007;45(6):977–984.

22. Horváth, K, Noker, PE, Somfai-Relle, S, Glávits, R, Financsek, I, Schauss, AG. Toxicity of methylsulfonylmethane in rats. *Food Chem Toxicol.* 2002;40(10):1459–1462.

24

N-Acetylcysteine

BRIEF OVERVIEW

N-acetylcysteine has been in medical use for more than 50 years as a mucolytic agent—a chemical that helps make sputum (phlegm) more liquid and easier to cough up and out of the lungs. It is also well known as a treatment for acetaminophen overdose, which can cause liver failure.

However, N-acetylcysteine (NAC) is a much more versatile supplement. By providing the body with a precursor to glutathione, it increases glutathione and all its antioxidant and other mechanisms of detoxifying foreign substances; see Chapter 13, "Glutathione (GSH)." NAC may also act as a vasodilator as well as an antioxidant in its own right.

NAC is now being studied as treatment for a wide variety of diseases and problems.

THE HYPE

NAC is proven to raise levels of glutathione,[1] which means that it should have all the effects of glutathione, including its protective effects on cells. This is because of glutathione's antioxidant capabilities, as well as other cellular protective mechanisms. In addition, NAC is also a vasodilator, increasing the action of nitric oxide.[2]

NAC is being used or studied for use as a treatment for chronic obstructive pulmonary disease (COPD), influenza, idiopathic pulmonary fibrosis, and as a preventative of contrast dye-induced kidney damage. It is being used to treat polycystic ovary disease and has been tested as a chemoprotective agent in cancer treatment, a substance that can help get rid of Helicobacter pylori in the stomach (associated with ulcers), and a preventative of hearing loss in certain toxic situations.[2]

COPD

Chronic obstructive pulmonary disease is a progressive deterioration of lung function most often due to cigarette smoking. Multiple studies have found NAC useful for treatment of COPD symptoms, as well as prevention of worsening lung function. Laboratory research has focused on showing how much oxidative stress does to cause COPD. Many experts believe that oxidative stress is a major component of COPD.

In COPD patients, NAC provides some of its own antioxidant capacity, as well as delivering an important precursor so that glutathione can be synthesized. Many studies have shown that NAC use can cause a measurable decrease in various measures of oxidative stress in the lungs.

In one large, open-label trial, COPD patients taking NAC showed less deterioration in lung function over a period of five years than patients not taking it.[3] In another open-label study, patients given NAC had clinical improvement in symptoms.[2]

Multiple studies have looked at whether or not NAC can reduce the normal deterioration that occurs in COPD and prevent the exacerbations that are the natural course of the disease. More than one analysis of a large number of available trials showed a definite decrease in the number of exacerbations in patients treated with NAC. There was also a small improvement seen in measures of lung function.[2,3] One study demonstrated a lower rate of hospitalization in patients taking NAC.[4] Doses in various studies have ranged from 600 mg three times a week to 1,200 mg a day.

However, a large, prominent trial called BRONCUS that followed patients for three years did not show any benefit to the use of NAC in terms of number of exacerbations or deterioration of lung function. There may have been some improvements in subgroups of the BRONCUS trial, such as patients not taking inhaled steroids, who had fewer exacerbations.[2,3] It is also possible that the 600-mg dose used was not high enough. More controlled studies are needed.

Other Lung Diseases and Upper Respiratory Illnesses

Idiopathic pulmonary fibrosis is a scarring lung disease of unknown cause. In at least one study, patients taking NAC 600 mg three times a day showed less deterioration in lung function than those not taking NAC. Both groups were already on a standard regimen of azathioprine, and patients taking NAC had less damage to their bone marrow from the azathioprine than those who did not take it.[2]

NAC might be useful in cystic fibrosis, acute respiratory distress syndrome in adults, and bronchopulmonary dysplasia in premature infants, but studies to date have not demonstrated any definite benefit.[4]

Some have used NAC for the upper respiratory symptoms of rhinosinusitis, due to allergy and/or infection, attributing its success in these cases to its ability to thin mucous.[5]

Viral Illnesses

One study reported a decrease in influenza and influenza-like diseases when NAC was given during winter, especially in elderly people.[2,4]

People with AIDS have significant glutathione deficiency, which NAC can help reverse. However, there are excellent antiviral treatments available, and NAC has not been tested for use along with these medications.[4]

Liver Disease—Acetaminophen Overdose and More

NAC is the established treatment for acetaminophen overdose, either accidental or purposeful, to prevent severe liver damage. A small amount of any ingested acetaminophen (called paracetamol in other countries, brand name Tylenol) is metabolized into a toxic metabolite. In overdose situations there can be enough of this metabolite to cause severe liver injury and death. The metabolite is detoxified via interaction with glutathione. NAC replenishes glutathione in acetaminophen overdose situations. It also has separate actions that limit the liver injury, improving blood flow and oxygen use. There are protocols for when and how much NAC to use in the case of acetaminophen overdose, in the emergency room or other hospital setting.[6]

What about NAC and other liver insults or diseases? There have been conflicting results from small studies, for example, in patients with chronic hepatitis C.[4]

One retrospective study done in England, looking at the outcomes for children with acute liver failure (not associated with acetaminophen) with and without NAC treatment, showed a beneficial effect of NAC on a number of parameters. Children with acute liver failure of unknown origin treated with NAC had shorter hospital stays, greater survival with their own liver and not a transplant, better survival after liver transplant if it was done, and longer overall survival. This study also looked at side effects and found that NAC was well tolerated by children. As of 2008, these investigators were participating in a prospective, randomized controlled trial.[7]

There have also been case studies of NAC helping to treat poisoning by other xenobiotics (chemicals not natural to the body), from carbon tetrachloride to heavy metals. These are preliminary reports.[8] NAC been suggested as a treatment for mushroom poisoning by Amanita phalloides.[4]

Protection against Kidney Damage from Intravenous Contrast Media Used in X-Ray Studies

There is a risk of kidney damage from the agents given intravenously to enhance images in many different kinds of x-ray studies. People with preexisting reduced kidney function are at higher risk, as are diabetics. But it can happen in approximately 2 percent of people with apparently normal kidney function. It can cause increased mortality, the need for dialysis, and other problems.

When an article in the *New England Journal of Medicine* reported success using NAC to protect against contrast-induced nephropathy (kidney damage) in 2000, many randomized clinical trials were started. There have been at least 20 trials and 13 meta-analyses looking at all the data. Of the analyses, seven found benefit from the use of NAC, five said the data was inconclusive, and one concluded that NAC was ineffective for this purpose. It has been noted that the clinical studies were very different from one to the other.[2] One analysis in 2008 noted that NAC is more protective of renal function than any other medication tested. Since it is safe and inexpensive, it seems reasonable to use it, especially in high-risk patients.[9]

In one trial of patients set to undergo angioplasty (opening of the coronary arteries) who needed contrast media–enhanced radiography to visualize the arteries before the procedure, those who took NAC before and after had a lower incidence of kidney damage, a lower mortality rate in the hospital, lower rates of acute renal failure, and less need for mechanical ventilation. This group of patients was being treated because of coronary artery disease and had evidence of cardiac damage, so they were at higher risk of complications. This was a prospective, randomly assigned, placebo-controlled study. The investigators also concluded that NAC may have been protective of the heart during these procedures.[10]

The protocol used in this study is the only one that has shown reduced mortality. While NAC is not the standard of care during the use of intravenous contrast material, when it is used, the protocol from the above study is often followed.[2]

Protection against Acute Kidney Failure during Surgery

N-acetylcysteine may help prevent some of the complications that occur during major surgery, such as kidney failure.[2]

There have been small studies that show benefit under specific circumstances.[4]

It has been tried for patients undergoing cardiothoracic surgery, including surgeries during which the heart is bypassed temporarily. An analysis of a number of these trials failed to show any benefit to NAC, except for a lowered risk of atrial fibrillation, an abnormal heart rhythm. This particular analysis noted a trend toward lower risk of acute kidney failure, stroke, heart attack and death, but these trends were not statistically significant. More studies need to be done.[11]

A very recent analysis concluded that there have not been enough good-quality trials to know if NAC or any other tested medication can actually prevent acute kidney injury during cardiac surgery.[12]

Polycystic Ovary Syndrome (PCO)

Women with PCO have cystic ovaries, obesity, infertility, and insulin resistance, which contributes to their infertility. NAC may be able to increase insulin sensitivity. In two double-blind, placebo-controlled studies, adding NAC to the treatment resulted in increased ovulation and pregnancy.[2]

Cancer

There has been interest in using NAC to help prevent reoccurrence of cancer, and also to minimize side effects of chemotherapy. EUROSCAN, a large randomized trial, looked at whether or not NAC and vitamin A could prevent tumor recurrence, or prevent new primary cancers in patients with head and neck cancer as well as lung cancer. During the two years of the trial, neither NAC nor vitamin A was of any benefit.[4]

There has been some success in reducing markers of inflammation and stress in some patients with cancer, and NAC has also been able to reduce liver damage from the anticancer agent busulfan.[4]

Raynaud's Phenomenon

Raynaud's phenomenon is a problem with circulation to the hands that can occur by itself or in association with other diseases such as scleroderma. In at least one small study, NAC treatment improved Raynaud's phenomenon in 20 patients with scleroderma.[13]

DEFICIENCY

There is no deficiency syndrome associated with lack of NAC as it is not an essential nutrient. It is synthesized from cysteine, an amino acid that is also not essential. Cysteine can be synthesized in the body from other sulfur-containing molecules such as methionine. NAC is made outside the body.[14]

N-acetylcysteine may be used to treat glutathione deficiency; see Chapter 13, "Glutathione (GSH)."

FOOD SOURCES

N-acetylcysteine is not found in food. It is synthesized from the amino acid cysteine, which is found in protein-rich foods.[14]

MECHANISM OF ACTION: HOW DOES IT WORK?

NAC works in a number of different ways. As a mucolytic, it breaks bonds between parts of the glycoproteins contained in mucus.

One of NAC's functions is its contribution to protection from damage done by reactive oxygen species and other toxic substances. NAC has direct antioxidant effects of its own.[3]

Additionally, NAC supplementation is one of the best ways to provide the cysteine group for glutathione synthesis, which must occur in the body. It is the body's main antioxidant. A rate-limiting step in glutathione synthesis is the amount of cysteine available. Increased levels of GSH can be measured after oral administration of NAC.[1]

Glutathione can detoxify many drugs and poisons, and giving NAC to increase glutathione is an effective way to achieve detoxification. A key example is the treatment of acetaminophen's toxicity to the liver.[4]

NAC also has other actions. For example, it can inhibit the activation of certain white blood cells, and also cause vasodilation.[4]

PRIMARY USES

- N-acetylcysteine is used to help reduce symptoms and slow deterioration of lung function in patients with COPD. It may be useful for treating other lung diseases.
- It can be given to patients with coughs or respiratory illness to help thin mucous.

- It is the cornerstone treatment for acetaminophen poisoning, where it can save lives. It is proving to be useful in other cases of ingestion of poisons that can damage the liver.
- It can protect the kidney during administration of intravenous contrast material and possibly during a variety of surgeries.
- It can help replenish glutathione anytime the body is under stress.

COMMON DOSAGES

NAC is sold as capsules containing from 500 mg to 1,000 mg. The 600-mg dose is the most commonly used. It is sold as a solution for intravenous administration and also as a solution to administer with a nebulizer into the lungs.

As a mucolytic agent, the oral dose is 400 to 1,200 mg daily.[4]

For COPD, many of the clinical studies used 600 mg a day. However, laboratory studies indicate that 1,200 mg a day cause a bigger measurable drop in markers of inflammation.

To treat or prevent influenza, 600 mg twice a day is used, before and throughout influenza season.

For idiopathic pulmonary fibrosis, doses of 1,800 mg a day have been used.

The FDA-approved protocol for an acute acetaminophen overdose is 140 mg/kg of body weight, followed by repeated doses of 70 mg/kg every 4 hours until 17 doses are given. This is only for use in medical facilities. The intravenous dose is 150 mg/kg of body weight infused over 15 to 60 minutes, followed by 12.5 mg/kg per hour over 4 hours, then 6.25 mg/kg per hour over a 16-hour period. These are extremely high doses relative to what is suggested for COPD and other diseases.

POTENTIAL SIDE EFFECTS

At 1,200 mg a day, there are few side effects. These include nausea, vomiting, diarrhea, rash, flushing, stomach pain, and constipation.[2]

NAC can enhance the effect of nitroglycerin, taken for angina (heart pain). People who take nitroglycerin or related nitrates should not take NAC; together they can cause very low blood pressure.[2]

NAC does not smell or taste good; vomiting is common especially with oral doses for acetaminophen toxicity. Even at those high doses, 95 percent of patients are able to take the treatment by mouth. There is very little serious toxicity even at high doses.[6]

There is an allergic-like reaction to intravenous NAC, with swelling, rash, itching, trouble breathing, rapid pulse, and low blood pressure. This may happen in as many as 14 percent of patients treat with intravenous NAC. Vomiting is common, as noted, as is flushing.

The allergic-like reactions occur because the large doses of NAC are causing the release of histamine. They can be treated with antihistamines, corticosteroids, and medicines to stop wheezing. NAC can be stopped and restarted when symptoms are controlled.[6]

FACT VERSUS FICTION

At the current time there are at least 126 trials in various stages registered with the U.S. government using N-acetylcysteine on humans. There are countless studies in progress and being published on NAC effects in the lab. For example, a recent research showed that NAC could reduce noise-induced hearing loss in guinea pigs.[15] There will undoubtedly be more uses found for NAC.

It is safe, inexpensive, and has been found to be effective in treating the conditions mentioned above. It is important as a way to replenish glutathione but also has a lot to offer in and of itself.

REFERENCES

1. Zembron-Lacny, A, Slowinksa-Lisowska, M, Szugula, Z, et al. The comparison of antioxidant and hematological properties of N-acetylcysteine and α-lipoic acid in physically active males. *Physiol Res.* 2009;58:855–861.
2. Millea, PJ. N-acetylcysteine: Multiple clinical applications. *American Family Physician.* 2009;80(3):265–269.
3. Dekhuijzen, PNR, van Beurden, WJC. The role for N-acetylcysteine in the management of COPD. *International Journal of COPD.* 2006;1(2):99–106.
4. Aitio, M-L. N-acetylcysteine—passe-partout or much ado about nothing? *Br J Clin Pharmacol.* 2005;61(1):5–15.
5. Helms, S, Miller, AL. Natural treatment of chronic rhinosinusitis. *Altern Med Rev.* 2006;11(3):196–207.
6. Heard, KJ. Acetylcysteine for acetaminophen poisoning. *N Engl J Med.* 2008;359:285–292.
7. Kortsalioudaki, C, Taylor, RM, Cheeseman, P, et al. Safety and efficacy of N-acetylcysteine in children with non-acetaminophen-induced acute liver failure. *Liver Transplantation.* 2008;14:25–30.
8. N-acetylcysteine. *Altern Med Rev.* 2000;5(5):467–471.
9. Kelly, AM, Dwamena, B, Cronin, P, et al. Meta-analysis: Effectiveness of drugs for preventing contrast-induced nephropathy. *Ann Intern Med.* 2008; 148:284–294.
10. Marenzi, G, Assanelli, E, Marana, I, et al. N-acetylcysteine and contrast-induced nephropathy in primary angioplasty. *N Engl J Med.* 2006;354:2773–2782.
11. Baker, WL, Anglade, MW, Baker, EL, et al. Use of N-acetylcysteine to reduce post-cardiothoracic surgery complications: A meta-analysis. *Eur J Cardiothorac Surg.* 2009;35:521–527.
12. Park, M, Coca, SG, Nigwekar, SU, et al. Kidney injury in patients undergoing cardiac surgery: A systematic review. *Am J Nephrol.* 2010;31:408–418.
13. Gaby, AR. Natural remedies for scleroderma. *Altern Med Rev.* 2006;11(3): 188–195.

14. Laifer, S. N-acetylcysteine, a potent antioxidant that protects against harmful toxins. *Life Extension Magazine.* August 2004. http://www.lef.org/magazine/mag2004/aug2004_aas_01.htm. Accessed May 24, 2010.
15. Fetoni, AR, Ralli, M, Sergi, B, et al. Protective effects of N-acetylcysteine on noise induced hearing loss in guinea pigs. *Acta Otorhinolaryngologica Italica.* 2009;29:70–75.

25

Niacin (Vitamin B3)

Niacin has been well known for its positive effects on HDL. Its effects on LDL have been more modest. Such modesty, however, deserves special attention in that it is indeed associated with an increase in LDL particle size and a shift from small LDL to the less atherogenic, large LDL subclasses. Therefore, we are looking at niacin from a standpoint of quality of LDL that it promotes, not just the quantity that it would reduce it by. This is a crucial point.

Note that a 2006 study in the *American Journal of Cardiology* showed that three months of ER niacin use in subjects w/CAD increased large-particle LDL by 82 percent and decreased small-particle LDL by 12 percent.[1]

BRIEF OVERVIEW

Niacin (nicotinic acid) is a vitamin, a substance that is necessary to prevent a deficiency disease. The deficiency disease associated with a lack of niacin (vitamin B3) is called pellagra, first described in the 1700s. Pellagra is known by the four Ds, which are dermatitis (skin rash), diarrhea, dementia (altered mental function), and death. This disease usually occurs in people eating a diet that is severely deficient in niacin.

In the body nicotinic acid and its derivative nicotinamide are converted to NAD and NADP. These chemicals are coenzymes necessary for hundreds of reactions in which oxidation-reduction occurs. These energy-producing reactions are essential for many cellular functions in the human body. Among many other things, NAD is also critical to many processes in which components are added to proteins inside cells.

In addition to being an essential nutrient, niacin has been shown raise HDL (high density lipoprotein), sometimes called "good" cholesterol. Niacin is one of the many drugs used to lower the risk of coronary heart disease as well as other vascular disease caused by elevated cholesterol and plaque formation. Because of this and many other properties, niacin is both an essential nutrient and a disease-modifying drug.

THE HYPE

It is known that niacin prevents and treats pellagra.[2]

Its effectiveness in treating coronary and other vascular disease has been tested and proven. However, it does more than raise HDL. It has an effect on the blood vessels themselves, as well as on other lipids. There is much research being done, trying to discover all of the ways niacin affects abnormal lipid levels and vascular disease.[2]

Since niacin has anti-inflammatory properties, and is important in so many cell processes, there are research projects underway looking at many different possible uses. It is possible that niacin and nicotinamide may have many therapeutic uses that have not yet been fully understood.

It was thought niacin might protect the cells in the pancreas that make insulin and help prevent diabetes. There have been a number of trials with inconclusive results when nicotinamide is given to people at risk for diabetes.[3,4] In diabetics, niacin can actually cause a small but manageable increase in blood sugar.[5,6]

Can niacin help treat or prevent cancer? Can it help halt the progression of HIV/AIDS?[3]

One researcher titled an article "Pellagra: A Clue as to Why Energy Failure Causes Diseases?" in which it was noted that the symptoms of pellagra are similar to aging, cancer, inflammatory diseases, and metabolic syndromes.[7] Perhaps niacin can help treat this wide array of conditions.

Other researchers have observed that a complete understanding of all the specific reactions of nicotinamide (or niacin) in the body must occur before specific treatments can be fashioned.[8]

DEFICIENCY

Deficiency of niacin causes the symptoms of pellagra. The dermatitis or rash from niacin deficiency is symmetrical and pigmented and occurs in areas exposed to sunlight. In addition to diarrhea, there can also be vomiting and even constipation. The neurologic symptoms include headache and fatigue, as well as apathy, depression, and loss of memory. A clue to the diagnosis of pellagra is the bright red tongue people with the disease manifest.

Pellagra was common in the United States in the early 1900s, especially in the southern states. In 1937, it was discovered that niacin cured pellagra. During the 1940s, the federal government as well as individual states began to require enrichment of grains with vitamins. In addition, more nutritious food was available to more people as the decades passed.[9] Pellagra because of dietary deficiency of vitamin B3 has essentially disappeared from the United States and Canada and anywhere that the food quality is high and/or grains are enriched. It can still be seen in India, China, and Africa.[2] The treatment for pellagra is niacin, although tryptophan can also help.

Whereas it was originally believed that pellagra was due to vitamin B3 deficiency, it is now known that it can be due to a combination of niacin and riboflavin deficiencies in differing amounts.[2] Since the amino acid tryptophan can be converted into niacin, if there is adequate meat intake, even without enough niacin, tryptophan will be converted to niacin and pellagra will be prevented. However, riboflavin deficiency can impair this conversion, as can deficiency of vitamin B6 and iron.

Pellagra still can occur in chronic alcoholics with cirrhosis. Medications can disrupt the conversion of tryptophan to niacin, such as isoniazid, which is used to treat tuberculosis. People with carcinoid syndrome need more niacin because tryptophan is not available to be converted into niacin; in cases of carcinoid syndrome, tryptophan is converted to other substances. Hartnup's disease, a genetic disorder, causes decreased absorption of tryptophan from the intestine and kidney; therefore more niacin needs to be ingested.[2] Patients with Crohn's disease can also become niacin deficient.[10]

FOOD SOURCES

Niacin is present in foods derived from plants and animals. However, it is bound in cereal grains and is not easily absorbed. In areas dependant on corn or maize, such as the United States and Europe in the early 20th century, pellagra was common.

Animal protein is the best source of niacin, including poultry, lean meat, dairy products, eggs, and fish. Cereals and breads that have been fortified with niacin are also good sources, as are nuts. Milk and eggs are actually good sources because they are rich in tryptophan.[11]

Treating grain with alkali makes niacin easier to absorb. Niacin occurs as NAD/NADP in meats and is much more fully absorbed. Added niacin (for enrichment) is also more available for absorption.

Both niacin (nicotinic acid) and nicotinamide are absorbed from the stomach and intestines. Niacin is converted to NAD and NADP in just about any bodily tissue, wherever it is needed.[2]

The body can convert tryptophan, from dietary protein, into niacin. There are other nutrients needed for this to take place. There are also diseases that prevent the tryptophan conversion, as well as medications that can interfere (see above).

MECHANISM OF ACTION: HOW DOES IT WORK?

Niacin has many mechanisms of action. Nicotinic acid can be converted inside the body to nicotinamide, or nicotinamide can be ingested. Nicotinamide is made into NAD or NADP. These are coenzymes, necessary for what are called "redox reactions." This means that either of them can accept or donate electrons, necessary for many cellular functions, from cellular respiration, to fuel utilization and synthesis of fatty acid and steroids. Many of niacin's key mechanisms of action involve these redox reactions.

NAD is needed for DNA synthesis. It is also involved in transferring chemical components to proteins. These transfers can be catalyzed by substances called PARPs (poly-ADP-ribose-polymerases), which regulate the transfer of many ADP-ribose units from NAD to proteins. These reactions are part of DNA repair, cell-to-cell signaling, cell differentiation, cell death, and much more. Much research is ongoing, exploring all the functions and actions of niacin, PARPs, and their relationship to health and disease.[2,3]

Niacin has a number of effects on cholesterol and lipoproteins. There is a constantly evolving level of knowledge about how niacin improves lipid profiles and reduces vascular disease. The Coronary Drug Project, from 1966 to 1975, followed more than 8,000 men who had already experienced a heart attack. Five drugs were tested. Only niacin showed a benefit. It slightly decreased repeat heart attacks but not total mortality during the treatment period. However, during the period after the trial, a total of about 15 years, the patients treated with niacin had 11 percent lower mortality.[12] This was the first clear evidence of niacin's protective effect against vascular disease.

Studies investigating niacin's mechanism of action have shown that, among other things, it lowers LDL (low density lipoproteins, one of the "bad" cholesterols), raises HDL, and has effects on plaque and thickness of arterial walls. The ways niacin does this are very complicated. Much of the changes take place in the liver and affect the way the liver handles cholesterol, triglycerides, and lipoproteins. For example, niacin inhibits a specific liver enzyme that is involved in the synthesis of triglycerides; this leads to lower levels of triglycerides. Niacin lowers the expression of another liver chemical (beta-chain adenosine triphosphate synthase), which has the effect of increasing HDL by decreasing its breakdown.[13,14]

By increasing the redox state of vascular endothelial cells lining the inside of blood vessels, niacin lowers the expression of cytokines, which are involved in the building up of cholesterol-filled plaque in arterial walls.[15]

PRIMARY USES

- Niacin or nicotinamide is the treatment for pellagra, which still occurs in some places and circumstances.

- Niacin is used to treat Hartnup's disease.[11]

- Niacin is used to treat abnormal lipids, in order to prevent coronary heart disease and other vascular disease; it is also used to prevent existing disease from causing further problems.

- Niacin is able to significantly lower the likelihood of repeat myocardial infarction (heart attack) or death after a myocardial infarction.

- Niacin is the most effective medication available to raise HDL cholesterol levels. Increases of 20 to 35 percent can be expected.[12,14] Niacin improves lipid profiles and also has an anti-inflammatory effect on blood vessels. Niacin is probably the drug that should be added if a statin does not significantly improve target lipids.[16]

COMMON DOSAGES

As a Vitamin

Niacin requirements are often given in terms of niacin equivalents, because niacin may also be made from tryptophan. Approximately 60 mg of tryptophan are equivalent to 1 mg of niacin.

The RDA for niacin is 16 mg of niacin equivalents (NEs) per day for men and 14 mg of NEs per day for women. Most people in the United States and Canada get enough niacin in their diets, as do people in countries with high-quality food or that enrich grains and cereals.[2]

The AI (adequate intake) level for infants 0 to 6 months old is around 2 mg. For infants 7 to 12 months old, the adequate intake is estimated at 4 mg.[2]

For older children, an estimate of the average requirement, or EAR, has been determined by the Institute of Medicine. The EARs are the same for boys and girls in early childhood. From 1 to 3 years of age, children need 5 mg of niacin equivalents a day, and 6 mg a day is needed by children 4 to 8 years of age. Children between the ages of 9 and 13 require 9 mg of NEs a day. Boys ages 14 to 18 years of age need 12 mg of niacin equivalents a day, whereas girls 14 to 18 years old need 11 mg of NEs a day. After 18, the adult RDAs are appropriate. Pregnant women need more niacin; the RDA during pregnancy is 18 mg of niacin equivalents a day; the RDA while breast-feeding is 17 mg of NEs a day.[2]

The tolerable upper limit for niacin has been set at the amount that causes flushing, which is 35 mg a day. People take 50 times that much for dyslipidemia; the upper limit is meant to signify the most that needs to be taken as a vitamin, not a medication. Niacin is available without a prescription at up to 400 mg.

The National Health Interview Survey in 1986 found that approximately 26 percent of people were taking supplemental niacin at that time.[2] Many physicians believe that it is reasonable for people to take multivitamins that contain water-soluble vitamins such as niacin in average doses.[17]

To Treat Actual Pellagra

When pellagra is advanced, it needs to be treated with injectable and oral niacin. Nicotinamide can be injected into muscle at doses of 50 to 100 mg three times a day for three or four days. The same amount should then be taken by mouth, in addition to a protein-rich diet (100 g of protein a day). It must also be remembered that other vitamin deficiencies can contribute to pellagra, and any other deficiencies should be corrected.[11]

For Dyslipidemia

Treatment for low HDL, high LDL, and high triglycerides usually starts with 500 mg a day at bedtime. In order to minimize flushing, the dose should be gradually increased (see below). The total daily dose can be up to 2,000 mg. The newer extended-release preparations may be tolerated the best.

Niacin can be given with other medications, such as statins, to improve lipid profiles. A niacin/statin combination is very effective.[18] There are fixed combination pills available that include niacin and a statin.

POTENTIAL SIDE EFFECTS

There are few side effects when niacin is taken as a vitamin. The tolerable upper limit has been set at the amount that causes flushing, so doses less than that cause little or no side effects.

The best-known side effect of niacin is the flush, which usually happens when niacin is given in high doses to lower lipids. Flushing is redness of the face, sometimes with warmth, itching, or tingling. It is not an allergic reaction. The flush is mediated by specific prostaglandins.[14,15] The facial flushing can be controlled by raising the dose slowly, as tolerance to niacin develops quickly and the flushing decreases. If it is absorbed more slowly, there is less flushing. If the prostaglandins or their targets are blocked, that can also decrease the flushing.

Quickly released crystalline niacin causes flushing essentially 100 percent of the time. Sustained-release niacin used in the past did cause less flushing but also caused liver toxicity and worked less well to improve lipid profiles. Newer extended-release niacin products cause less flushing while still improving lipids and cause essentially no liver damage. Taking 325 mg of aspirin 30 minutes before taking the niacin decreases flushing, as does taking it before bedtime. Eating a low-fat snack also helps, as does avoiding hot and spicy foods. It is also important to start with a low dose and slowly increase it. There are other drugs in trials to see if they can reduce the flush without compromising the effectiveness of the niacin. However, it may be impossible to separate the flush from the positive clinical effects. People taking niacin should try and be patient as their dosage is titrated, knowing that it will not be long before the side effect stops.[14]

Very high doses of niacin can cause liver damage, which may also be more likely with older slow-release formulations that are no longer in use. Newer extended-release preparations are able to cause less flushing with less toxicity.[13,14,19] However, there are still reports of liver damage with long-term use of very high doses of niacin, in the range of 3 to 9 g a day.[2]

Niacin can cause an upset stomach (dyspepsia), nausea, and vomiting. It may be related to development of ulcers.[20]

An increase in blood glucose levels as well as uric acid levels can occur in people taking niacin as a medication.[5] The increase in blood sugar needs to be kept in mind, because many patients with cardiovascular disease and undesirable lipid profiles are also diabetic. However, the amount of glucose increase is usually small and easily managed with adjustments in oral medications for people with type 2 diabetes, when niacin doses are less than or equal to 2,500 mg. New diabetes as a result of niacin therapy is infrequent. Significant lowering of cardiovascular risk is still achieved in individuals on niacin who are diabetic, if the niacin improves their lipid profiles.[6]

Niacin can cause visual side effects including blurred vision and double vision because of damage to the retina. This is very rare and seems to be reversible.[2]

FACT VERSUS FICTION

There is no question that niacin cures pellagra. There is also no question that in high doses it helps abnormal lipid profiles and lowers cardiovascular risk in people with abnormal lipids.

Individuals without abnormal lipids can take 15 to 20 mg of niacin equivalents a day in a multivitamin with little risk. Using high doses to treat dyslipidemia should be done under the supervision of a health care practitioner.

Because of the myriad of reactions involving niacin and related chemicals, it seems very likely that there will be other therapeutic uses discovered for niacin. At the current time, it is not clear what those specific uses will be.

REFERENCES

1. Kuvin, JT, Dave, DM, Sliney, KA, et al. Effects of extended-release niacin on lipoprotein particle size, distribution, and inflammatory markers in patients with coronary artery disease. *Am J Cardiol.* 2006 Sep 15;98(6): 743–745.
2. Institute of Medicine. Food and Nutrition Board. Niacin. Chapter 6 in: *Dietary reference intakes for thiamin, riboflavin, niacin, vitamin B6, folate, vitamin B12, pantothenic acid, biotin, and choline.* Washington, DC: National Academies Press, 1998, 123–149.
3. Higdon, J. Niacin. Linus Pauling Institute, Micronutrient Information Center. 2002, updated in 2007. http://lpi.oregonstate.edu/infocenter/vitamins/niacin/. Accessed December 22, 2009.
4. Bingley, PJ, Mahon, JL, Gale, EAM. Insulin resistance and progression to type 1 diabetes in the European Nicotinamide Diabetes Intervention Trial (ENDIT). *Diabetes Care.* 2008;31(1):146–150.
5. Ashen, MD, Blumenthal, RS. Low HDL cholesterol levels. *N Engl J Med.* 2005;353:1252–1260.
6. Goldberg, RB, Jacobson, TA. Effects of niacin on glucose control in patients with dyslipidemia. *Mayo Clin Proc.* 2008;83(4):470–478.
7. Williams, AC, Ramsden, DB. Pellagra: A clue as to why energy failure causes diseases? *Med Hypotheses.* 2007;69(3):618–628.
8. Maiese, K, Chong, ZZ, Hou, J, Shang, YC. The vitamin nicotinamide: Translating nutrition into clinical care. *Molecules.* 2009;14(9):3446–3485.
9. Park, YK, Sempos, CT, Barton, CN, et al. Effectiveness of food fortification in the United States: The case of pellagra. *American Journal of Public Health.* 2000;90(5):727–738.
10. World Health Organization, Food and Agriculture Organization of the United Nations. *Vitamin and mineral requirements in human nutrition.* 2nd edition. Geneva: World Health Organization, 2004, 173–175.
11. Bourgeois, C, Cervantes-Laurean, D, Moss, J. Niacin. Chapter 25 in Shils, ME, Shike, M, Ross, CA, Caballero, B, Cousins, RJ (Eds.): *Modern nutrition in health and disease.* 10th edition. Philadelphia: Lippincott Williams & Wilkins, 2006, 442–451.
12. Canner, PL, Berge, KG, Wenger, NK, et al. Fifteen year mortality in Coronary Drug Project patients: Long-term benefit with niacin. *J Am Coll Cardiol.* 1986;8:1245–1255.
13. Kamanna, VS, Ganji, SH, Kashyap, ML. Niacin: An old drug rejuvenated. *Curr Atheroscler Rep.* 2009;11(1):45–51.
14. Kamanna, VS, Ganji, SH, Kashyap, ML. The mechanism and mitigation of niacin-induced flushing. *Int J Clin Pract.* 2009;63(9):1369–1377.

15. Kamanna, VS, Kashyap, ML. Mechanism of action of niacin. *Am J Cardiol.* 2008;101(8A):20B–26B.

16. Taylor, AJ, Villines, TC, Stanek, EJ, et al. Extended-release niacin or ezetimibe and carotid intima-media thickness. *N Engl J Med.* 2009;361:2113–2122.

17. Willett, WC, Stampfer, MJ. What vitamin should I be taking, doctor? *N Engl J Med.* 2001;345(25):1819–1824.

18. Brown, BG, Xue-Qiao, Z, Chait, A, et al. Simvastatin and niacin, antioxidant vitamins, or the combination for the prevention of coronary disease. *N Engl J Med.* 2001;345(22):1583–1592.

19. Kamanna, VS, Ganji, SH, Kashyap, ML. Nicotinic acid: Recent developments. *Curr Opin Cardiol.* 2008;23(4):393–398.

20. Medline Plus. Niacin. Medline Plus: U.S. National Library of Medicine and NIH. http://www.nlm.nih.gov/medlineplus/ency/article/002409.htm. Accessed December 22, 2009.

26

Omega-3 Fatty Acids

BRIEF OVERVIEW

While it is easy to think of fats and fatty acids as bad for your health, in the case of omega-3 fatty acids, the reverse is true. They are polyunsaturated fatty acids (PUFAs). Most people get PUFAs in their diet from vegetable oils. While there are two groups of PUFAs, omega-3 and omega-6 fatty acids, omega-3 fatty acids are more important for good health. Most vegetable oils have more omega-6 than omega-3 fatty acids. Omega-3s come from different sources, with fish being the best-known food rich in omega-3s.

The omega-3s include three fatty acids called alpha-linolenic acid (ALA), eicosapentaenoic acid (EPA), and docosahexaenoic acid (DHA). These have slightly different pathways and functions in the body. ALA is converted in small amounts to EPA and DHA. EPA may be more important for heart health, while DHA may be more critical to brain function, although both EPA and DHA contribute to good health.

ALA can be found in green leafy vegetables, as well as vegetable oil. EPA and DHA are found in fatty fish and fish oil. The omega-3s found in fish oil have probably received the most public attention, and they are found in a myriad of supplements. They are the only oils made as a pharmaceutical product that requires prescription.

Most of the studies and most of the data about omega-3 fatty acids refer to fish oil and not other sources. This means a mixture of mainly EPA and DHA. Some studies have used separate components, such as DHA alone, or EPA alone, but most have not.

Many groups, including the American Heart Association, have endorsed and encouraged the consumption of omega-3 fatty acids for heart health. Other uses are being discovered and investigated.

The North American diet contains more omega-6 fatty acids than omega-3. It may be that more omega-3 fatty acids than omega-6 fatty acids need to be consumed to gain the full benefit from omega-3s.

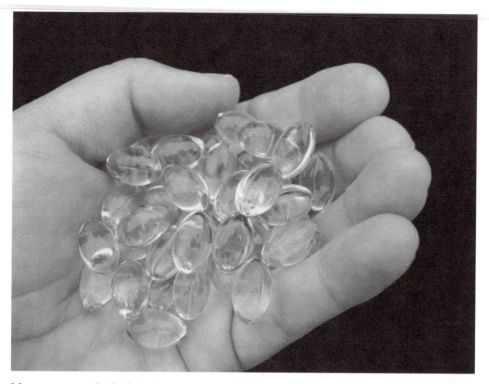

Many groups, including the American Heart Association, have endorsed and encouraged the consumption of omega-3 fatty acids for heart health. (© Inger Anne Hulbækdal/Dreamstime.com)

THE HYPE

There is a plethora of evidence about the benefits of omega-3 PUFAs on health, particularly cardiovascular health. To review this type of data, as they do when evaluating any medical treatment, investigators look at three levels of evidence. With supplements, this information is often incomplete, but in regard to omega-3s, there are all three levels of evidence. The first is epidemiological data that links increased intake of omega-3 PUFAs to various positive outcomes. Second, experimental studies (in the lab, on animals or tissue cultures) show many types of positive effects. Most important, there are a number of good prospective clinical trials that show the effects of omega-3 supplementation on various outcomes, such as mortality. Putting all of this data together gives a good idea of what is established and what areas need more research.

Cardiovascular Health

The use of omega-3 fatty acids for heart health is no longer under question. Specifics remain to be considered. Who should be taking omega-3s, how much should they be taking, and which ones should they take? Primary prevention means trying to protect people against developing cardiovascular disease. Secondary prevention means protecting people who already have had an adverse cardiovascular event or known disease from having further damage. Prevention can be achieved by reducing risk factors.

Experts know that there is a whole host of factors that raise a person's risk for coronary heart disease, from high blood pressure to elevated cholesterol. They also know that the trigger for a heart attack may have more to do with inflammation and dysfunction in the walls of the coronary arteries than simply a plugged up pipe.[1]

From epidemiologic evidence plus clinical trials, it seems very clear that both DHA and EPA provide cardioprotective benefits by lowering triglycerides, lowering blood pressure, and decreasing inflammatory chemicals involved in heart disease. They also lower the risk of irregular heart rhythms (arrhythmias) and sudden cardiac death. Studies have been done with fish, fish oil, and specific omega-3s. Most have shown that increased fish intake and supplementation with fish oil or its components can be beneficial.

In 2004, the Agency for Healthcare Research and Quality (from the Institute of Medicine) announced to the public that fish oil can help reduce deaths from heart disease, according to all the evidence available. It detailed certain specifics of how fish oil reduces the risk of more cardiovascular problems in patients with cardiovascular disease. Fish oil lowers the risk of irregular heartbeats and sudden death. Fish oil can lower triglycerides, slightly lower blood pressure, reduce the risk of coronary arteries becoming blocked again after being surgically opened, and may increase exercise capacity.[2]

There were three reports from the AHRQ that analyzed the data in regard to fish oil and heart disease.[3,4,5] After these reports, groups like American Heart Association came out with guidelines for the use of fish oil. For example, in 2006, when treating patients with coronary or other vascular diseases, the AHA advised physicians to "encourage consumption of omega-3 fatty acids in the form of fish or in capsule form ... for risk reduction."[6] This is an example of secondary prevention.

There have been a number of large, randomized, controlled clinical trials that demonstrated the effect of omega-3s with results published since the AHRQ reports. For example, the JELIS (Japan EPA Lipid Intervention Study) study followed almost 19,000 people with elevated cholesterol over approximately five years. One group was given statin therapy (prescription medication to lower cholesterol), the other statin plus 1,800 mg of EPA a day. The EPA group had a statistically significant decrease in major coronary events, including nonfatal events.[7] A follow-up study on secondary prevention showed a significant decrease in major coronary events in patients with preexisting coronary heart disease who took 1,800 mg EPA in addition to statins.[8]

Evidence continues to be gathered about the positive effects of omega-3s on heart health. The GISSI-HF is a large, double-blind, multicenter trial in Italy, which evaluated the effect of omega n-3s on heart failure. It followed 7,000 patients for four years. A 2008 report indicated that there was a definite benefit to supplementation, with lowered risk of mortality and hospital admission. Although the benefit was small, it was statistically significant. The omega n-3 supplementation was free of serious side effects, which makes it a good addition to the treatment of patients with heart failure.[9]

Questions still remain about the best way to get the needed omega-3s, diet or supplement, which ones should be taken in the greatest amount, and what is the best amount to take for cardioprotection. There has been some evidence that DHA is more effective than EPA.[10] However, many of the studies and the large clinical trials have used fish or fish oil containing both, or used EPA.

Epidemiologic studies and clinical trials have yielded mixed results in terms of the effects of ALA, the third omega-3 fatty acid, on cardiovascular disease. At the current time, it is not recommended.[11]

Heart Rhythm Disorders

Fish oil and omega-3 fatty acids (EPA and DHA) can prevent arrhythmias. The AHRQ review collected the evidence to date that showed antiarrhythmic effects in animal studies. ALA did not confer the same protection.[5]

The AHRQ press statement also let the public know that fish oil and omega-3 fatty acids can reduce the risk of arrhythmias after a heart attack.[2] This reduces the risk of sudden cardiac death.

Cardiovascular Risk/Markers of CHD

As stated, DHA and EPA lower a number of cardiovascular risk factors. In addition to decreasing blood pressure and triglycerides, they have been shown to improve arterial and endothelial function (the workings of the artery walls and their linings) and decrease platelet clumping.

Large scale trials-have proved the usefulness of the omega-3s for both primary and secondary prevention of coronary heart disease as well as advanced heart failure. The American Heart Association recommends 1 g per day of a combination of DHA and EPA for individuals with coronary heart disease. It recommends at least 500 mg a day of the same as primary prevention, to prevent cardiovascular disease.[1,6]

Elevated triglycerides, especially after meals, are a risk factor for CHD independent of cholesterol and other factors. DHA and EPA have large effects on elevated triglycerides. This has been demonstrated in multiple clinical trials. Studies indicate that omega-3 fatty acids can help lower triglycerides by themselves, or along with commonly used statins. A lot more omega-3 needs to be taken to reduce very high triglyceride levels, some 3 to 4 g of EPA plus DHA.[1]

Asthma

As noted in "Mechanism of Action," omega-3 fatty acids, especially EPA and DHA, are metabolized into a number of chemical mediators of inflammation. Asthma is a disease of airway inflammation; substances like omega-3s involved in inflammation might help asthma. The AHRQ report reviewed a large amount of data and many studies. There was not adequate information to say that omega-3 fatty acids are of any benefit for asthma. Studies were either flawed or inconclusive. There has also been very little research done on North American populations.

It was suggested that more, well-designed, and well-controlled studies are needed. Omega-3 fatty acids do seem to be very safe when used for asthma. There was also a suggestion that a lowering of dietary omega-6 fatty acids might need to take place along with supplements of omega-3 fatty acids for benefits to occur.[12]

Central Nervous System Disorders/Neurologic Development

There have been epidemiologic studies as well as lab studies indicating that DHA may protect against Alzheimer's disease as well as ensure the proper development of the brain. For example, one population study of a group (called the Framingham group) showed that the highest levels of measurable DHA were associated with the lowest risk for developing Alzheimer's disease over the course of approximately nine years.[13]

The AHRQ report also noted that there is not enough data yet to reach definite conclusions. There is data that indicate a reduction in the risk of Alzheimer's or cognitive decline with fish or fish oil consumption, but there are not yet definitive results from clinical trials using omega-3s.

Clinical trials need to be done examining the effect of taking fish oil or omega-3 fatty acids on the risk of developing a number of neurological diseases, as well as the possibility that omega-3s may help treat these diseases.[14] There is currently a large clinical trial in progress evaluating the effect of DHA on Alzheimer's disease.[10]

It is hypothesized that adequate levels of DHA are necessary for normal neurologic development of the fetus, in infancy and childhood. Pregnant women are advised to take DHA.[15]

There have not been adequate studies to indicate a link between omega-3 fatty acids and depression, ADHD (attention-deficit hyperactivity disorder), or other neurologic or psychiatric conditions. Large well-designed studies are needed.[16,17]

Organ Transplantation

The studies reviewed by the AHRQ did not provide enough information to say whether or not omega-3 fatty acids might improve the outcome of kidney or heart transplants. Fish oil supplements do lower triglycerides in transplant patients; this might improve long-term success of kidney transplants, as well as help prevent coronary atherosclerosis from occurring after heart transplant. However, these benefits have not been found in clinical studies.[18]

Miscellaneous

DHA has anti-inflammatory properties, possibly more so than EPA, although they both are metabolized into chemicals with anti-inflammatory functions.[10] Therefore, they may be useful in treating a wide variety of diseases.

- Type II diabetes and the metabolic syndrome

  The AHRQ found no clear evidence that fish oil or omega-3 fatty acids affect diabetes. While omega-3 fatty acids clearly lower triglycerides, they do not affect other components of the metabolic syndrome. They cause no significant effect on fasting blood sugar or glycosylated hemoglobin, a way to measure sugar levels over the long term. The report also indicated that there has not been a demonstrated effect on insulin or insulin resistance.[19]

- Inflammatory bowel disease, systemic lupus erythematosus, and rheumatoid arthritis

  There is no clear evidence that omega-3 fatty acids make a difference in any of these disease states. Research continues on these and other illnesses with an inflammatory component.[19]

Cancer

The AHRQ review found that there is not enough clear evidence that fish or omega-3 fatty acids can help prevent or treat cancer. There is some evidence in animal models that omega-3s might reduce tumor growth.[20] Many of the studies to date have come to opposing conclusions. In an analysis of some 40 years of research, and many studies looking at many kinds of cancer, other reviewers agreed that there is not enough evidence to say that omega-3 fatty acids can prevent or treat cancer. This was published in the *Journal of the American Medical Association* in 2006.[21] More studies are needed.

DEFICIENCY

The only actual deficiency of polyunsaturated fatty acids occurs when there is not enough linoleic acid (LA) or alpha-linolenic acid (ALA) in the diet. These two fatty acids cannot be made by the body. LA is an omega-6 PUFA, not an omega-3.

ALA is converted to EPA and DHA. However, there may be circumstances in which there is a need for more EPA and DHA than the body can convert from ALA. In that case there would be a situational deficiency of EPA and DHA. For example, investigations have shown that 5 to 10 percent of ALA is converted to EPA, and 2 to 5 percent of ALA is converted to DHA. Some studies show even less conversion.

The International Society for the Study of Fatty Acids and Lipids (ISSFAL) has made an official statement that the conversion of ALA to DHA is 1 percent in infants and less in adults. This makes deficiency of DHA a possibility, especially for individuals who do not eat fatty fish and vegetarians who do not take supplements.[11]

EPA can also be converted via a number of steps to DHA.[10]

There is no specific deficiency disease. Rather, it is believed that enough of these fatty acids are needed for health, growth, and development.[10,16,17]

FOOD SOURCES

ALA can be found in green leafy vegetables, nuts (especially walnuts), and vegetable oils including soy, canola, and flaxseed oil. Flaxseed and flaxseed oil are the richest source of ALA. However, flaxseed oil tends to go rancid and must be kept in a cool, dark area.

EPA and DHA come from fish, especially fatty fish and their eggs, as well as oil derived from fish. Organ meats also contain EPA and DHA.[22] Some of the best fish sources are from the ocean, including salmon, herring, mackerel, halibut, and tuna. Freshwater fish with omega-3s include lake herring, lake trout, whitefish, and freshwater trout.[23]

Most fish oils contain much larger amounts of EPA than DHA; the DHA comes from algae eaten by the fish. Pure DHA comes from fermentation of microalgae. This is the only DHA allowed in infant formula in the United States.[10]

Flaxseed oil is a source of ALA for vegetarians, and it will be converted in small amounts to EPA and DHA. LA can be found in oil from algae, as well as other vegetable oils, seeds, and nuts.

The American diet contains 10 times more omega-6 fatty acids than omega-3 fatty acids. More omega-3 and less omega-6 would be beneficial. The average intake per person of DHA and EPA in North America is 0.1 to 0.2 g a day. Around 1.4 grams a day of ALA is ingested.[11]

MECHANISM OF ACTION: HOW DOES IT WORK?

Omega-3 fatty acids are absorbed in the small intestine. ALA can be converted into DHA and EPA in the body. More ALA is converted in healthy young women than men; this may be related to estrogen levels.[24] Omega-3s are used all over the body.

Omega-3 PUFAs are very important to cell membranes. They are parts of phospholipids, which help determine many properties of the cell membrane, like what the membrane will allow in, and what to keep out. More DHA is incorporated into the cell membranes in the nervous system.[24] It is the main PUFA in the brain and is believed to be critical for brain development and brain function. It may be involved with the transmission of signal from nerve cell to nerve cell. It may also be made into compounds that help reduce brain inflammation that comes from lack of blood flow.[22]

While LA is an omega-6 PUFA, it is metabolized to arachidonic acid (AA), which is metabolized like EPA into the biologically active eicosanoids. Eicosanoids are hormone-like chemicals with multiple activities, principally relating to inflammation. Eicosanoids include prostaglandins, thromboxanes, and leukotrienes. However, the specific eicosanoids differ depending on the precursor. AA-derived eicosanoids tend to be released in response to stress and increase tendencies to clot blood and constrict blood vessels. Those from EPA help decrease some of the chemicals that can actually cause injury. This gives them the ability to protect against heart attacks and inflammatory diseases, in which prostaglandins play a causative role.[22]

The more EPA in the diet, the more of its prostaglandins and other metabolites will be made. EPA metabolites can help inhibit platelet aggregation and vasoconstriction, which can reduce the damage caused in atherosclerotic vascular disease. At the same time, EPA metabolites increase vasodilation, which again helps protect against more damage.[11]

Recently, new classes of inflammatory mediators derived from ALA, EPA, and DHA have been discovered. These may be equally important to the biological activities of these PUFAs and are being studied. The names give an idea of their function, including lipoxins, resolvins, and neuroprotectins.[11]

Omega-3 fatty acids are thought lower triglycerides by reducing synthesis of triglycerides, as well as increasing clearance of triglycerides from the circulation.[23]

There are many more biologic activities of omega-3 fatty acids that are being studied. They each seem to have somewhat different mechanisms of action. At the current time, EPA and DHA are thought to be the most active in preventing cardiovascular disease as well as other conditions. Some think that DHA may be more active in the central nervous system.[10,25]

While the focus has not been on ALA, it may have beneficial activities as well. It is the main omega-3 in the North American diet, and only a small amount gets converted to DHA and EPA. It seems likely that ALA itself may have biological activity apart from DHA and EPA, but this is not well understood.[11]

PRIMARY USES

- Primary prevention of coronary heart disease and cardiovascular disease; maintaining good health.
- Secondary prevention of further cardiovascular events.
- Reduction of elevated triglycerides. This includes very high triglycerides (equal to or greater than 500 mg/dL) or high triglycerides (above 150 mg/dL).
- Supply of the essential nutrient, alpha-linolenic acid.

COMMON DOSAGES

There has only been an Adequate Intake level set for ALA by the Institute of Medicine, which is 1.1–1.6 g per day for adults, the lower dose suggested for women, the higher, for men.[26] In 2002, the IOM indicated that there were not enough data to recommend an AI for EPA and DHA.

However, in 2008 the Technical Committee on Dietary Lipids of the International Life Sciences Institute North America did come to consensus on adequate doses of EPA and DHA. Based on the evidence regarding the reduction in risk of coronary heart disease achieved by these PUFAs, it recommended a Dietary Reference Intake (DRI) of between 250 mg and 500 mg of EPA plus DHA. It further stated that since very little ALA gets converted into EPA and DHA, these requirements must be met by consuming EPA and DHA.[15]

The committee also indicated that, although evidence is being accumulated on the effect of these PUFAs and cognitive decline, there is not enough to recommend any different amount than the amount for cardiovascular protection. It also stated that there does not appear to be evidence that DHA and EPA reduce cancer. There is also no reason to suggest that the level of supplementation suggested would be dangerous.[15]

The dose recommended by the American Heart Association for primary prevention of cardiovascular disease is 500 mg a day of EPA and DHA. This can be accomplished by eating two meals a week of fatty fish, or with supplements.

For secondary prevention, the AHA recommends 1 g a day of EPA/DHA. This will probably mean taking a supplement for most people.

To reduce very high triglycerides, 3 to 4 g a day of the two omega-3 fatty acids need to be taken every day. This necessitates the consumption of a highly purified and concentrated source of fish oil. A prescription supplement can be used.[1]

There is one prescription form of omega-3 fatty acids in the United States. It is called Lovaza®, which is a 1-g capsule with 465 mg of EPA and 375 mg of DHA that have undergone a five-step purification process. The omega-3s are derived from fish and not synthesized. The usual dose for very high triglycerides is four capsules a day.[23,27]

Pregnant women are advised to take 200 mg of DHA a day. There is also DHA in infant formula, and there are suggestions the amount in infant formula should be raised.[10,15]

POTENTIAL SIDE EFFECTS

Omega-3 fatty acids are very safe. There has been no significant toxicity noted in any of the large studies. The three biggest, the JELIS, GISSI-Prevencione, and GISSI-Heart Failure, had no significant adverse events with a total of 35,000 people taking DHA and EPA.[15]

Common complaints are gastrointestinal, including dyspepsia, belching, and belching a fishy odor/flavor.

With prescription omega-3 fatty acids at the 4 g a day dose, eructation, infection, flu syndrome, and dyspepsia were observed in studies. Elevations of liver function tests have been seen.

There was a concern that omega-3s might increase bleeding in patients on anticoagulants. In fact, bleeding has been observed very rarely and has not been serious.[27]

There is also a real concern about the mercury content of some fish, for people who want to meet the omega-3 requirements without supplements. In one analysis of the risk to benefit ratio in 2008, there were a number of fish recommended for daily consumption (presuming no other contaminants). These include tilapia, pollock, flounder, shrimp, trout, herring, and salmon. Fish to be eaten twice a week include cod and canned tuna, while tuna steak should not be eaten more than once a week. Swordfish and shark should not be eaten based on mercury levels in this study.[28]

The contamination of seafood varies from place to place and should be checked before making a dietary change, if possible.

FACT VERSUS FICTION

There are lots of facts, and very little fiction, in claims made for omega-3 fatty acids in terms of cardiovascular disease. While there are differences of opinion as to dose, and DHA:EPA ratios, many regulatory agencies and health care groups around the world advocate the use of fish, fish oil, or omega-3 fatty acids to prevent cardiovascular disease. This is true for healthy people, as well as people who already have evidence of heart or vascular disease, although the dose should be higher for those who already have damage.

There may very well also be a protective effect on the central nervous system conferred by the omega-3s. Even if this is proven to be true, the recommended dose of omega-3 fatty acids will probably not change for most people.

Individuals with high triglycerides may be advised to take more EPA and DHA, even as much as 4 g a day, which can be taken in the form of a prescription capsule.

As of 2008, there were at least two dozen ongoing trials using prescription omega-3s for many different conditions listed with the National Institutes of Health. As of 2010, there were 372 trials in total investigating the use of omega-3 fatty acids on a large range of conditions, with others listed under EPA and DHA.[29]

REFERENCES

1. O'Keefe, JH, Carter, MD, Lavie, CJ. Primary and secondary prevention of cardiovascular diseases: A practical evidence-based approach. *Mayo Clin Proc.* 2009;84(8):741–757.
2. AHRQ Evidence Reports confirm that fish oil helps fight heart disease. Press release. April 24, 2004. http://www.ahrq.gov/news/press/pr2004/omega3pr.htm. Accessed April 20, 2010.
3. Institute of Medicine. Agency for Healthcare Research and Quality. Health effects of omega-3 fatty acids on cardiovascular disease. March 2004. Tufts-New England Medical Center. http://www.ahrq.gov/downloads/pub/evidence/pdf/o3cardrisk/o3cardrisk.pdf. Accessed December 29, 2010.
4. Institute of Medicine. Agency for Healthcare Research and Quality. Health effects of omega-3 fatty acids on cardiovascular risk factors and intermediate markers of cardiovascular disease. March 2004. Tufts-New England Medical Center. http://www.ahrq.gov/clinic/epcsums/o3cardrisksum.htm. Accessed December 29, 2010.
5. Institute of Medicine. Agency for Healthcare Research and Quality. Health effects of omega-3 fatty acids on arrhythmogenic mechanisms in animal and isolated organ/cell culture studies. March 2004. Tufts-New England Medical Center. http://www.ahrq.gov/clinic/epcsums/o3arrsum2.htm. Accessed December 29, 2010.
6. Smith, Jr, SC, Allen, J, Blair, SN, et al. AHA/ACC guidelines for secondary prevention for patients with coronary and other atherosclerotic vascular disease. 2006 update: Endorsed by the National Heart, Lung, and Blood Institute. *Circulation.* 2006;113:2363–2372.
7. Yokoyama, M, Origasa, H, Matsuzaki, M, et al. Effects of eicosapentaenoic acid on major coronary events in hypercholesterolaemic patients (JELIS): A randomised open-label, blinded endpoint analysis. Japan EPA Lipid Intervention Study (JELIS) Investigators. *Lancet.* 2007;369(9567):1090–1098.

8. Matsuzaki, M, Yokoyama, M, Saito, Y, et al. Incremental effects of eicosapentaenoic acid on cardiovascular events in statin-treated patients with coronary artery disease: Secondary prevention analysis from JELIS. *Circ J.* 2009;73:1283–1290.

9. GISSI-HF Investigators. The GISSI-HF Trial: A randomised, double-blind, placebo-controlled trial. *The Lancet.* 2008;372(9645):1223–1230.

10. Docosahexaenoic acid (DHA). *Altern Med Rev.* 2009;14(4):391–399.

11. Anderson, BM, Ma, DWL. Are all N-3 polyunsaturated fatty acids created equal? *Lipids in Health and Disease.* 2009;8:33:33–53.

12. Institute of Medicine. Agency for Healthcare Research and Quality. Health effects of omega-3 fatty acids on asthma. March 2004. University of Ottawa. http://www.ahrq.gov/clinic/tp/o3asthmtp.htm.

13. Schaefer, EJ, Bongard, V, Beiser, AS, et al. Plasma phosphatidylcholine docosahexaenoic acid content and risk of dementia and Alzheimer disease. *Arch Neurol.* 2006;63:1545–1550.

14. Institute of Medicine. Agency for Healthcare Research and Quality. Effects of omega-3 fatty acids on cognitive function with aging, dementia, and neurological diseases. February 2005. Southern California-Rand. http://www.ahrq.gov/clinic/epcsums/o3cognsum.htm.

15. Harris, WS, Mozaffarian, D, Lefevre, M, et al. Towards establishing dietary reference intakes for eicosapentaenoic and docosahexaenoic acids. *J Nutr.* 2009;139:804S–819S.

16. Ramakrishnan, U, Imhoff-Kunsch, B, DiGirolamo, AM. Role of docosahexaenoic acid in maternal and child mental health. *Am J Clin Nutr.* 2009; 89(Suppl):958S–962S.

17. Institute of Medicine. Agency for Healthcare Research and Quality. Effects of omega-3 fatty acids on child and maternal health. July 2005. University of Ottawa. http://www.ahrq.gov/clinic/tp/o3mchtp.htm.

18. Institute of Medicine. Agency for Healthcare Research and Quality. Effects of omega-3 fatty acids on organ transplantation. February 2005. Tufts-New England Medical Center.

19. Institute of Medicine. Agency for Healthcare Research and Quality. Health effects of omega-3 fatty acids on lipids and glycemic control in type II diabetes and the metabolic syndrome and on inflammatory bowel disease, rheumatoid arthritis, renal disease, systemic lupus erythematosus and osteoporosis. March 2004. Southern California-Rand. http://www.ahrq.gov/clinic/tp/o3lipidtp.htm.

20. Institute of Medicine. Agency for Healthcare Research and Quality. Effects of omega-3 fatty acids on cancer. February 2005, updated January 2006. Southern California-Rand. http://www.ahrq.gov/downloads/pub/evidence/pdf/o3cogn/o3cogn.pdf.

21. MacLean, CH, Newberry, SJ, Mojica, WA, et al. Effects of omega-3 fatty acids on cancer risk. A systematic review. *JAMA.* 2006;295:403–415.

22. National Institutes of Health. Office of Dietary Supplements. Omega-3 fatty acids and health. http://ods.od.nih.gov/FactSheets/Omega3FattyAcidsandHealth.asp. Accessed April 20, 2010.

23. Bays, HE, Tighe, AP, Sadovsky, R, Davidson, MH. Prescription omega-3 fatty acids and their lipid effects: Physiologic mechanisms of action and clinical implications. *Expert Rev. Cardovasc. Ther*. 2008;6(3):391–409.

24. Higdon, J. Essential fatty acids. Linus Pauling Institute. Micronutrient Research for Optimum Health. Reviewed and updated in 2009. http://lpi.oregon state.edu/infocenter/othernuts/omega3fa/. Accessed April 20, 2010.

25. Vedin, I, Cederholm, T, Levi, YF, et al. Effects of docosahexaenoic acid–rich n-3 fatty acid supplementation on cytokine release from blood mononuclear leukocytes: The OmegAD Study. *Am J Clin Nutr*. 2008;87:1616–1622.

26. Institute of Medicine. *Dietary reference intakes for energy, carbohydrate. fiber, fat, fatty acids, cholesterol, protein, and amino acids*. 2002/2005. http://www.iom.edu/Global/News%20Announcements/~/media/C5CD2D D7840544979A549EC47E56A02B.ashx. Accessed April 20, 2010.

27. Sadovsky, R, Kris-Etherton, P. Prescription omega-3-acid ethyl esters for the treatment of very high triglyerides. *Postgraduate Medicine*. 2009;121(4): 145–153.

28. Ginsberg, GL, Toal, BF. Quantitative approach for incorporating methyl-mercury risks and omega-3 fatty acid benefits in developing species-specific fish consumption advice. *Environmental Health Perspectives*. 2009;117(2): 267–275.

29. ClinicalTrials.gov. U.S. National Institutes of Health. http://clinicaltrials.gov/ct2/results?term=omega-3+fatty+acids. Accessed April 27, 2010.

27

Saccharomyces Boulardii

BRIEF OVERVIEW

Saccharomyces boulardii is a probiotic. Probiotics are live microbes that are beneficial to human health. Right now, there is a lot of advertising for probiotics on television. It seems like it must be a brand-new concept, but it is not. Scientists have known about probiotics for a long time. The first definition was written in 1989 by Robert Fuller. A probiotics is, he said, "A live microbial feed supplement which beneficially affects the host animal by improving its intestinal microbial balance."[1] According to the World Health Organization, it now includes "live microorganisms that, when administered in adequate amounts, confer a health benefit to the host."[2]

While probiotics have been in use for decades, they are now being taken by more people than ever before. Most probiotics are bacteria. These organisms can be found in yogurt and other milk products that say on the packaging that they contain probiotics. They are being sold to promote good gastrointestinal health.

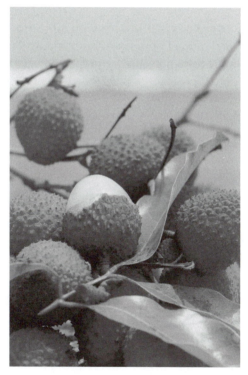

S. boulardii was originally isolated from the lychee fruit in Indonesia by Henri Boulard in the 1920s. (© Margouillat/Dreamstime.com)

S. boulardii is one of the most effective probiotics in helping prevent or treat disease. It is a yeast, not a bacteria like most of the other probiotics. There is a patented preparation of the yeast, lyophilized into powder that is placed inside a capsule. These capsules have been used for decades in Europe to treat diarrheal diseases.

THE HYPE

Saccharomyces Boulardii Can Help Treat and Prevent Most Diarrheal Illness without Any Risk

S. boulardii has been proposed as a treatment or preventative measure for almost every kind of diarrheal illness, from infectious to inflammatory. It has been used in Europe for 30 years. S. boulardii is either closely related to or a subspecies of S. cerevisiae, which is brewer's yeast and not considered dangerous.

Studies have been done and research continues to try and ascertain when treatment with S. boulardii is truly effective and also to understand what the risks might be of taking it.

Prevention of Traveler's Diarrhea

Traveler's diarrhea is usually infectious, caused by one of three known bacteria in 80 percent of cases. The remaining 20 percent are caused by viruses. S. boulardii taken in doses of 1 g per day lowered the incidence of traveler's diarrhea from 40 to 29 percent in one study of more than 1,000 travelers. Analyses of a number of separate studies came to the conclusion that S. boulardii can be successful in preventing traveler's diarrhea.[3,4]

Prevention and Treatment of Childhood Diarrhea

For children suffering from diarrhea as the result of acute gastroenteritis, adding S. boulardii to oral fluid treatment shortens the length of the diarrheal illness. Good results have been obtained treating children with acute gastroenteritis in many parts of the world.[5,6]

Most cases of gastroenteritis are from viruses or specific bacteria such as E. coli. Reports have also indicated S. boulardii can help treat diarrhea in children suffering from infection with amebiasis and giardiasis, both parasitic infections.[7]

S. boulardii can help prevent diarrhea in children at risk, in addition to treating them.[8]

Prevention of Antibiotic-Associated Diarrhea

Treatment with antibiotics frequently causes diarrhea. It has been estimated that between 5 and 30 percent of people treated with antibiotics will develop diarrhea during treatment or afterward, as many as two months after the end of treatment.[9] Children are somewhat more likely to develop diarrhea this way than adults; as many as 11 to 40 percent of children will have antibiotic-associated diarrhea.

This can happen as the result of treatment with almost any antibiotic, but certain antibiotics are more likely to cause diarrhea. These would include amoxicillin with or without clavulanate, cephalosporins, and clindamycin. The more broad spectrum the antibiotic, the more likely it is to cause diarrhea. Broad-spectrum antibiotics kill more of the good bacteria normally found in the intestinal tract. The change can cause diarrhea by allowing other bad bacteria to grow.

S. boulardii has been proven to lower the risk of antibiotic-associated diarrhea, in both adults and children. Early trials have also indicated that S. boulardii may also be effective in treating antibiotic-associated diarrhea and shortening the course of the illness.[4]

In one double-blind, randomized, placebo-controlled study, children placed on antibiotics were given either the antibiotic plus placebo, or the antibiotic plus S. boulardii. Approximately 120 children completed each part of the study. S. boulardii reduced the risk of antibiotic-associated diarrhea from 23 to 7.5 percent. This is statistically significant. The yeast also lowered the number of cases of Clostridium difficile–induced diarrhea, from 7.9 to 2.5 percent, but this was not statistically significant. The probiotic was well tolerated.[10]

Similar results have been obtained when studying adults and in other trials with children. A review of many of the studies concluded that S. boulardii is an effective way to lower the number of cases of antibiotic-associated diarrhea. It is estimated that for every 10 patients taking the two together, 1 less patient will develop diarrhea.[10]

S. boulardii also lessens the risk of diarrhea after treatment for Helicobacter pylori, the bacteria that can cause ulcers.[8]

The most severe cases of antibiotic-associated diarrhea are usually caused by the bacterium Clostridium difficile.

Prevention and/or Treatment of C. Difficile Diarrhea

The bacterium Clostridium difficile can cause diarrhea during and after antibiotic treatment. While antibiotics kill many of the bacteria that live in the intestine, C. difficile can survive, grow, and cause diarrheal disease through toxins it secretes. Some 2 percent of people carry the bacteria without symptoms, an amount that rises to 20 to 30 percent of adults who are in the hospital. Hospitalized elderly, or those in nursing homes, are more at risk for C. difficile illness.[11] The range of this disease is from a simple, diarrheal illness to something much more serious called pseudomembranous colitis, which can lead to intestinal perforation and even death. C. difficile is difficult to treat because it is resistant to many antibiotics. It is usually treated with vancomycin or metronidazole.

Some studies have shown that adding S. boulardii to treatment with antibiotics has been safe and effective therapy for treatment of recurrent cases of C. difficile.[24] In one early study, adding the yeast to antibiotic treatment of patients with recurrent C. difficile resulted in approximately twice as many treatment successes—34.6 percent recurrence with S. boulardii versus 64.7 percent without.[12] Other studies have confirmed that S. boulardii is effective in treating recurrent C. difficile, and reviews of available study data suggest that it is a reasonable choice for recurrent C. difficile infection.[3,8,11]

It has not been shown to prevent or improve treatment of an initial infection with C. difficile.[13] This is still an area of active investigation.

Prevention or Treatment of Other Adult Diarrheal Illnesses

Adults, like children, may contract infectious gastroenteritis, although it is less frequent and less severe in adults. Taking S. boulardii can lower the risk of infection, although there have not been very many studies using healthy adults.[8]

Treatment of Inflammatory Bowel Diseases

There have been small trials using S. boulardii to help treat inflammatory bowel diseases like Crohn's disease or ulcerative colitis. In one such trial, 25 patients having slight flare-ups of ulcerative colitis received S. boulardii in addition to their normal treatment; 17 patients had remission of their flare-up.[14]

In another study, 32 patients with Crohn's disease in remission were randomly assigned to take mesalamine (a standard treatment) 1 g three times a day or mesalamine two times a day plus S. boulardii. After six months, 37.5 percent of the patients taking only mesalamine had suffered relapses, as opposed to 6.25 percent of the patients who also took S. boulardii. Again, this was a very small study.[15]

Larger well-controlled trials need to be done to determine how much benefit can be gained by using S. boulardii to treat inflammatory bowel disease.

Treatment for Irritable Bowel Syndrome

There has been some success treating irritable bowel syndrome with S. boulardii, as well as other probiotics.[16] In one French controlled trial involving 34 patients with irritable bowel syndrome, treatment with S. boulardii resulted in less diarrhea but did not help other symptoms.[17]

Diarrhea in Other Situations

S. boulardii has also shown success in treating diarrhea associated with tube feedings as well as in AIDS patients.[16] However, since these patients often do not have strong immune systems, S. boulardii may not be a good choice for them (see "Potential Side Effects").

DEFICIENCY

Since S. boulardii is not an essential nutrient, there is no deficiency state. There are no symptoms specifically found in people who do not ingest S. boulardii.

FOOD SOURCES

S. boulardii was originally isolated from the lychee fruit in Indonesia by Henri Boulard in the 1920s. It is one member of the Saccharomyces species but may differ from other members of the species that are more often used in beverage fermentation, like S. cerevisiae.[16] There are investigators who believe the two are the same organism. This may be an important distinction, because many of the systemic infections caused by Saccharomyces are typed as cerevisiae, even when the yeast in use was boulardii (see "Potential Side Effects").

The yeast can be found in certain beverages and fermented foods, but not in high amounts. To be effective as a probiotic, enough yeast must be present. S. boulardii is usually taken in a capsule filled with lyophilized yeast.

MECHANISM OF ACTION: HOW DOES IT WORK?

S. boulardii works in a multitude of ways in the intestine, depending on what kind of infectious agent or inflammatory process is stimulating intestinal cells. These properties are being studied in cell cultures, in animal models, with whole yeast, and with chemicals derived from S. boulardii.

In some cases of infectious diarrhea, the yeast may simply compete with the infecting organism and win.[18] However, many of its activities are very complex.

Experimental studies have shown that S. boulardii has antimicrobial properties, as well as anti-inflammatory and antitoxic properties.[19]

S. boulardii can stimulate the immune response in the intestine.[20] It releases substances called polyamines, which may in turn stimulate enzymatic activity in the intestinal mucosa.[19]

The yeast secretes a substance that can neutralize both toxins A and B made by C. difficile, as well as digesting toxin receptors on the intestinal cells.[20] S. boulardii increases production of immunoglobulins by the intestinal cells, which help fight the infection. There are also substances made by S. boulardii that prevent the release of a whole cascade of inflammatory substances from the intestinal cells in response to C. difficile.[21]

E. coli is a common cause of infectious diarrhea around the world. S boulardii is able to prevent the release of many of the chemicals and mediators that E. coli triggers in the intestinal cells. E. coli also sticks to S. boulardii, so fewer bacteria are able to enter the intestinal cells. S. boulardii makes a substance that inactivates an inflammatory chemical released by E. coli.[21] It also reduces the ability of E. coli to cause intestinal epithelial cell apoptosis or death.[17] S. boulardii is able to inhibit protein kinases that are involved in communication between intestinal cells when they are infected.

Looking at the whole picture, investigators have surmised that the two main ways S. boulardii helps shorten disease caused by infecting organisms is by neutralizing their toxins and affecting the signaling responses between the infected cells and thereby decreasing the inflammatory response of the cells.[3]

There are similar chemical mediators involved in inflammatory bowel disease, which is why S. boulardii administration may help reduce symptoms of these diseases.[21]

PRIMARY USES

In Europe, S. boulardii has been used for decades as treatment for diarrhea. It is increasingly being accepted in the United States. Its primary uses are:

- Prevention of antibiotic-associated diarrhea.
- Prevention of recurrent C. difficile diarrhea.
- Prevention/treatment of acute diarrhea in children.
- Prevention of traveler's diarrhea.
- Prevention/treatment acute diarrhea in adults. (This use is less well accepted.)

S. boulardii may also be useful for other types of diarrhea and other intestinal ailments as indicated previously, but more research needs to be done.

COMMON DOSAGES

Doses for prevention of antibiotic-associated diarrhea are 250 to 500 mg per day.[18]

In some studies, 1 g a day has been used to prevent antibiotic-associated diarrhea.

In terms of actual numbers of live yeast, 10 to 20 billion organisms a day are usually needed to treat adults.[17] These numbers are not usually used, but rather the amount in milligrams or grams.

POTENTIAL SIDE EFFECTS

S. boulardii is very well tolerated. A few side effects have been reported, including mild abdominal discomfort or excess gas. It has not been shown to interact with prescription medications.[18]

However, in immunocompromised patients, such as people with cancer on chemotherapy or organ transplant patients, generalized infection (septicemia or fungemia) with Saccharomyces has occurred. Some of the cases have been in patients not given yeast themselves, but with central lines (direct access into the blood for medicine or nutrition) whose access lines had been contaminated by the yeast. An outbreak of this kind in 3 ICU patients was believed to have occurred secondary to contamination in the area from preparations of S. boulardii given to other patients.[22] The authors of this paper noted reports of other cases, for a total of 27 patients, 4 of whom died, probably as a result of the S. boulardii infection.

There have been a number of articles reviewing the cases of fungemia. While the amount may appear small compared to the number of patients treated, as noted, there have been deaths. In one study, 28 percent of the patients with fungemia died.[23] The serious infections have almost all occurred in patients with many other critical illnesses. Many of the infections apparently happened because of yeast contamination in the area where S. boulardii was being readied to give to other patients.[13]

Patients in intensive care units, and many others in hospital, should probably not get S. boulardii. Great care needs to be taken when preparing it for use. It should not be used in immunocompromised patients. This could include people with cancer, AIDS, and renal failure. It could also include patients with autoimmune diseases taking medicines that reduce their immune response. Fungemia has even been reported in hospitalized infants.[17] Anyone who is not sure about his or her immune system should consult a physician before taking S. boulardii.

It is still unclear if there is a subtype of the yeast that is more dangerous and pathogenic. There may be a separate fungus S. cerevisiae (brewer's yeast), or it may be a subtype of S. boulardii. There are at least two strains available in Europe, where this has been used to treat diarrhea for decades. However, many consider these to be the same yeast.[23] There is an ongoing argument of a sort over this, as new techniques are available to type yeast and new results are reported. It is probably best to view S. boulardii as a subtype of S. cerevisiae.[22]

FACT VERSUS FICTION

S. boulardii is effective in preventing and treating most antibiotic-associated diarrhea, as well as acute diarrheal illnesses in children and possibly adults. It may reduce the reoccurrence of antibiotic-associated diarrhea due to Clostridium difficile, but it has not been proven to prevent or treat initial infections. S. boulardii can prevent traveler's diarrhea. It may prove useful in treating both inflammatory bowel disease as well as irritable bowel disease, but this has not been proven.

Healthy adults and children can take S. boulardii as a preventative measure when on antibiotics or when traveling to another country. They can also take the yeast if suffering from an acute diarrheal illness. Patients with the diagnosis of irritable bowel syndrome who are otherwise healthy could consider a trial of S. boulardii to see if it lessens their symptoms. However, patients with chronic medical problems that affect the immune system should not take the probiotic unless a doctor tells them it is safe for them to do so.

It must be emphasized that not all probiotics are the same. S. boulardii has different effects than many of the bacteria used in yogurt and other milk products.

REFERENCES

1. Fuller, R. A review: Probiotics in man and animals. *Journal of Applied Bacteriology*. 1989;66:365–378.
2. Food and Agriculture Organization of the United Nations and World Health Organization. *Evaluation of health and nutritional properties of probiotics in food including powder milk with live lactic acid bacteria*. Cordoba, Argentina: FAO/WHO, 2001.
3. Czerucka, D, Piche, T, Rampal, P. Review article: Yeast as probiotics—Saccharomyces boulardii. *Aliment Pharmacol Ther.* 2007;26:767–778.
4. Marteau, PR, de Vrese, M, Cellier, CJ, Schrezenmeir, J. Protection from gastrointestinal diseases with the use of probiotics. *Am J Clin Nutr.* 2001; 73(Suppl):430S–436S.
5. Kurugol, Z, Koturoglu, G. Effects of Saccharomyces boulardii in children with acute diarrhea. *Acta Pediatr*. 2005;94:44–47.
6. Villarruel, G, Rubio, DM, Lopez, F, et al. Saccharomyces boulardii in acute childhood diarrhoea: A randomized, placebo-controlled study. *Acta Pediatr.* 2007;96:538–541.

7. Htwe, K, Yee, KS, Tin, M, Vandenplas, Y. Effect of *Saccharomyces boulardii* in the treatment of acute watery diarrhea in Myanmar children: A randomized controlled study. *Am J Trop Med Hyg.* 2008;78(2):214–216.

8. de Vrese, M, Marteau, PR. Probiotics and prebiotics: Effects on diarrhea. *J Nutr.* 2007;137:803S–811S.

9. Szajewska, H, Mrukowicz, J. Meta-analysis: Non-pathogenic yeast Saccharomyces boulardii in the prevention of antibiotic-associated diarrhea. *Aliment Pharmacol Ther.* 2005;22:365–372.

10. Kotowska, M, Albrecht, P, Szajewska, H. Saccharomyces boulardii in the prevention of antibiotic-associated diarrhoea in children: A randomized double-blind placebo-controlled trial. *Aliment Pharmacol Ther.* 2005;21:583–590.

11. Thompson, I. Clostridium difficile-associated disease: Update and focus on non-antibiotic strategies. *Age and Ageing.* 2008;37:14–18.

12. McFarland, LV, Surawicz, CM, Greenberg, RN, et al. A randomized placebo-controlled trial of Saccharomyces boulardii in combination with standard antibiotics for Clostridium difficile disease. *JAMA.* 1994;271:1913–1918.

13. Segarra-Newnham, M. Probiotics for Clostridium difficile–associated diarrhea: Focus on Lactobacillus rhamnosus GG and Saccharomyces boulardii. *The Annals of Pharmacotherapy.* 2007;41:1212–1221.

14. Guslandi, M, Giollo, P, Testoni, PA. A pilot trial of Saccharomyces boulardii in ulcerative colitis. *Eur J Gastroenterol Hepatol.* 2003;15:697–698.

15. Guslandi, M, Mezzi, G, Testoni, PA. Saccharomyces boulardii in maintenance treatment of Crohn's disease. *Dig Dis Sci.* 2000;45:1462–1464.

16. Zanello, G, Meurens, F, Berri, M, Salmon, H. Saccharomyces boulardii effects on gastrointestinal diseases. *Curr Issues Mol Biol.* 2009;11:47–58.

17. Saccharomyces boulardii. *Alternative Medicine Review Monographs.* Dover, ID: Thorne Research, 2002.

18. Kligler, B, Cohrssen, A. Probiotics. *American Family Physician.* 2008;78(9): 1073–1078.

19. Billoo, AG, Memon, MA, Khaskheli, SA, et al. Role of a probiotic (Saccharomyces boulardii) in management and prevention of diarrhea. *World J Gastroenterol.* 2006;28:4557–4560.

20. Castagliuolo, I, Riegler, MF, Valenick, L, LaMont, JT, Pothoulakis, C. Saccharomyces boulardii protease inhibits the effects of Clostridium difficile toxins A and B in human colonic mucosa. *Infect Immun.* 1999;67:302–307.

21. Pothoulakis, C. Review article: Anti-inflammatory mechanisms of action of Saccharomyces boulardii. *Aliment Pharmacol Ther.* 2009;30(8):826–833.

22. Cassone, M, Serra, P, Mondello, F, et al. Outbreak of Saccharomyces cerevisiae subtype boulardii fungemia in patients neighboring those treated with a probiotic preparation of the organism. *J Clin Microbiol.* 2003;41:5340–5343.

23. Muñoz, P, Bouza, E, Cunca-Estrella, M, et al. Saccharomyces cerevisiae fungemia: An emerging infectious disease. *Clin Infect Dis.* 2005;40:1625–1634.

24. Miller, K, Fraser, T. What is the role of probiotics in the treatment of acute Clostridium difficile-associated diarrhea? *Cleveland Clinic Journal of Medicine.* 2009;76(7):391–392.

28

S-Adenosylmethionine (SAMe)

BRIEF OVERVIEW

S-Adenosylmethionine, discovered in 1952, is an organic substance that is a key component of many biochemical reactions in humans as well as all other biological organisms. Its transferable methyl group is what makes SAMe so important. Methylation, in which a methyl group is donated to another molecule, often activates the now-methylated compound. There are more than 40 known reactions in which SAMe donates its methyl group, called transmethylation reactions. These can involve lipids, proteins, and nucleic acids, which make up DNA. The methylation of DNA is extremely important, because if it is not methylated, cells are more likely to become cancerous. DNA and also protein methylation affects inheritance of genes. A large percent of all the body's genes are methyltransferases dependent on SAMe.

S-Adenosylmethionine is formed from the amino acid methionine and ATP. Called SAM, SAMe, and AdoMet, it can also donate other components including sulfur where needed.

SAMe is distributed throughout the body. Most of its activity takes place in the liver, where 85 percent of methylation reactions occur. Therefore, much research has been devoted to understanding its actions in the liver and evaluating it as a treatment of a variety of kinds of liver damage. It is also active in the central nervous system and joints. It has been advertised as a treatment for depression, osteoarthritis, fibromyalgia, and Alzheimer's disease.

In 2002 it received a title in a journal article,[1] as follows: "S-Adenosylmethionine: A Control Switch That Regulates Liver Function." However, its importance is not confined to the liver. The many processes affected by SAMe have been called the "SAMe Empire."

THE HYPE

Osteoarthritis

In some studies, SAMe has been found to be as effective as conventional treatments for osteoarthritis, or "wear and tear" arthritis. It has been compared to placebo as well as to nonsteroidal anti-inflammatory agents (NSAIDS) and the COX-2 inhibitor celecoxib (Celebrex). Initial trials used injectable forms of SAMe because the oral form was unstable. Once a stable oral preparation was available, preliminary studies determined an effective dose to be 600 mg to 1,200 mg of SAMe. Review of early studies in the 1980s and 1990s indicated that SAMe might be useful.[2]

SAMe may be directly protecting joints, as opposed to providing a general anti-inflammatory effect. SAMe seems to cause an increase in the synthesis of a number of substances by the cells lining the joints. This would reduce damage to the cartilage lining the joints.

SAMe may also oppose the effect of tumor necrosis factor (TNF).[3] Tumor necrosis factor is a compound responsible for the symptoms of many diseases associated with inflammation. It causes the release from cells of chemicals that cause inflammation. In the case of arthritis, TNF causes the cells in the joints to release pain-causing chemicals as well as chemicals that can destroy the joints. TNF is a major cause of symptoms in rheumatoid arthritis.

A trial comparing SAMe to celecoxib over four months for osteoarthritis of the knee found SAMe to be effective, although it took longer to relieve pain.[2]

A *Cochrane Review* in 2009, in which the many studies were analyzed according to their scientific validity and findings, could not come to a definitive conclusion about the use of SAMe for osteoarthritis of the knee or hip. The studies were too small and of questionable quality. As is often the case, more high-quality research needs to be done. The authors could not recommend SAMe for osteoarthritis, also noting that there were no data on long-term side effects.[4]

The *American Family Physician* undertook a similar review and stated that although SAMe may reduce pain, its high cost and problems with the quality of the preparations must limit its use.[5]

Depression

As a methyl group donor, SAMe is involved in the synthesis of neurotransmitters, like serotonin. Neurotransmitters are chemicals in the brain that signal from one cell to another. Decreased levels of various neurotransmitters can cause many symptoms and diseases, including depression. Low SAMe could be expected to cause lower levels of some of these neurotransmitters. Lowered neurotransmitters have been found in association with lowered SAMe in the central nervous system. Logically, SAMe has been studied as a treatment for depression.[6]

There have been a number of trials using SAMe to treat depression. Many of the trials took place in the 1980s and 1990s and compared SAMe to older antidepressants. Studies of medications to treat depression, like other clinical research, need to compare the substance being studied to placebo. This is particularly important in trials of psychopharmaceutical treatments. Some studies used injectable SAMe, and they did not compare SAMe to placebo. The studies have been small, and also short term.

One of the main studies referred to when discussing SAMe and depression compared the supplement to imipramine, one of the older, so-called tricyclic antidepressants. This trial, done in 1988, compared SAMe to imipramine in 18 patients. Nine were given intravenous SAMe, and nine were given low doses of the antidepressant. The study lasted two weeks. The authors concluded that SAMe produced more improvement after one week, and that after two weeks, 66 percent of the patients treated with SAMe improved, versus 22 percent of the patients taking imipramine. They also noted fewer side effects.[7]

This is the type of study that is not a reliable predictor of actual benefit. Most antidepressants need weeks to months until their maximum benefit is achieved. SAMe intravenously may have no relationship to the oral form. It would be easy for the intravenous medication to have a placebo effect, as many people think injectable medication is "stronger." However, the fact that SAMe works more quickly than traditional antidepressants may be an advantage.[8]

SAMe has also been used to treat depressed patients with Parkinson's disease. There is less SAMe in the cerebrospinal fluid and brains of people with Parkinson's. In one small study, 13 patients with Parkinson's disease and depression who had not responded to conventional antidepressants were treated with SAMe. Ten improved and chose to continue the supplement after the trial ended. The researchers noted that the placebo effect is strong in psychiatric drug trials, and they suggested further long-term, controlled studies.[9]

In another study, 20 patients with HIV and depression were improved after eight weeks of treatment with SAMe. There was no control group, no blinding, and no long-term assessment.[10]

More research is needed, comparing SAMe to placebo, and to newer antidepressants. Long-term studies must also be done. SAMe may be of benefit for depressed adults.[11,12] However, the research does not yet exist to state that it is definitely safe and effective. There are questions about length of treatment, dosage, long-term effects, and stability of the medication, all requiring further study.[13]

Alzheimer's Disease

Research into Alzheimer's disease has uncovered a connection between SAMe and the disease. This research is in early stages. Alzheimer's disease is multifactorial, which means that many things contribute to cause it. In animals, SAMe can reverse pathology in the brain that is similar to what is seen in humans.[14]

SAMe may be able to exert a neuroprotective effect on the brain and can be given to patients with mild dementia. Recent studies have given some support to this idea, as well as using SAMe with other nutriceuticals such as PUFA, polyunsaturated fatty acids.[15]

Fibromyalgia

There is some evidence that SAMe may improve symptoms of fibromyalgia.[16] Some small trials have been done. In one, 11 of 17 patients showed improvement in depressive symptoms and also trigger-point pain after treatment with SAMe.[17]

The Liver: Alcoholic Liver Disease; Cirrhosis; Other Liver Disease; Liver Cancer

Alcohol ingestion lowers the level of SAMe in the liver via a number of pathways (see "Deficiency" below). This leaves the liver with lowered defense against damaging chemicals like free radicals. The many reactions dependent upon SAMe are down-regulated with a decrease in SAMe.[18]

In addition, many things that damage the liver inactivate the genes that code for SAMe, so there is even less SAMe available. Cirrhosis further limits the ability to make SAMe. Does that mean that SAMe might be a treatment for liver diseases? There have been studies to show benefit from SAMe in a variety of liver problems.[1]

In animals, SAMe can prevent alcohol-induced liver damage. In nonalcohol-related liver damage, animal testing has shown that SAMe can lessen liver injury and protect against cancer. There have been a number of human studies, treating both alcohol-induced liver disease as well as alcoholic cirrhosis. Some of the early animal and human studies led to predictions of SAMe as a treatment for many types of liver disease.[19]

An example of a study using SAMe to treat patients with cirrhosis was a double-blind, randomized, placebo-controlled trial following 123 patients for 24 months. SAMe was given orally. The overall mortality rate and liver transplantation rate was slightly lower in the patients taking SAMe, but it was not statistically significant. The data suggested that it was more efficacious in patients with less advanced cirrhosis. In that subgroup, there was a significantly lower mortality and transplant rate in the treated group (29% in untreated group vs. 12% in treated group). There were no adverse reactions to the supplement.[20]

There have been studies showing that supplementation either orally or intravenously with SAMe can help patients with intrahepatic cholestasis and cholestasis of pregnancy.[1] These are conditions in which the bile does not flow normally.

Although some of the initial reports of treatment benefits for patients with a variety of liver diseases are available, an overall benefit is not clear at this time.[18]

In 2006, reviewers of available research could not find definitive evidence of a benefit from treating alcoholic liver disease with SAMe; they could also find no serious risks. The reviewers agreed that more long-term, randomized, high-quality trials are needed before SAMe can be recommended outside of clinical trials.[21]

A confounding factor may be the discovery that too much SAMe can also damage the liver. Animals and humans with specific mutations in one of the methyltransferases cannot metabolize SAMe, and they can develop steatohepatitis (fatty liver), fibrosis, and liver cancer. Since too much and too little SAMe can damage the liver, more study needs to be done to try and discover how to create the right balance.[22]

It has also been suggested that SAMe might exert a chemoprotective effect and prevent hepatic cancer in patients with chronic liver disease. It seems to protect normal liver cells while stimulating apoptosis (death) of hepatic cancer cells. It is possible that these effects of SAMe are separate from its role as a methyl donor.[22,23]

DEFICIENCY

There is no specific deficiency of SAMe. The body makes all the SAMe that is needed. Deficiency of sulfur or sulfur-containing amino acids can lead to a deficiency in SAMe because it is made from methionine, a sulfur-containing amino acid. As long as a person is getting enough sulfur in the diet, SAMe will be produced and available.

Other vitamins are necessary to make and utilize SAMe, including folic acid and B12.

However, SAMe can be decreased in certain areas, like the liver or brain, with serious consequences.

Chronic alcohol exposure leads to decreased levels of SAMe in the liver in animal studies and in humans. It is unclear exactly why SAMe levels drop when the liver is exposed to alcohol. It is possible that the ethanol inactivates the enzyme needed for SAMe synthesis. Ethanol may increase SAMe usage/consumption in the liver. A third possibility is that alcohol decreases other molecules needed for SAMe synthesis.

What happens to the liver when it is deficient in SAMe?

A decrease in SAMe leads to a deficiency of glutathione in the liver. There is a two-step process by which it is synthesized, one involving SAMe. Glutathione is an antioxidant that helps protect liver cells against free radical damage. Decreased levels of SAMe can cause decreased levels of glutathione, and thereby leave the liver relatively unprotected.[18]

SAMe is the main methyl donor in all cells, required by, among other compounds, DNA, RNA, phospholipids, and proteins. It is the precursor of polyamine synthesis, necessary for cell growth and viability.

The decreases of these three—glutathione, methyl groups for donation, and precursors for polyamines—can all be part of the mechanism by which SAMe deficiency causes liver damage.

Additionally, there can be problems with the genes coding for SAMe. There are different genes in different parts of the body. There are genes associated with normal liver cells that are not active in hepatocellular carcinoma (liver cancer). In cancer, a different gene helps the cancer cells grow.[1]

SAMe regulates normal hepatocyte (liver cell) growth. SAMe deficiency can result in abnormal liver cell growth and a decreased response to growth factors that would cause normal growth. SAMe also induces apoptosis (death) of cancerous liver cells but not normal cells.[22]

FOOD SOURCES

SAMe is made in the human body from methionine and ATP. The body needs enough of the essential, sulfur-containing amino acid methionine in order to make SAMe. Enough B12 and folic acid are also needed.

SAMe is not found in any food sources in appreciable amounts.

MECHANISM OF ACTION: HOW DOES IT WORK?

SAMe anchors three metabolic pathways in humans. One, it is a source of methyl groups for many substrates. This is called transmethylation. Two, SAMe is also active in polyamine synthesis. In these cases, it donates its n-propylamine group, a process called aminopropylation. Three, the transulfuration of homocysteine makes it cysteine, which is eventually converted to glutathione. In this way, SAMe is a precursor of glutathione. Transulfuration mainly takes place in the liver.

Additionally, SAMe is needed for cell repair and growth. It donates methyl groups to nucleotides in RNA.

SAMe is necessary for the synthesis of a number of neurotransmitters and hormones, including dopamine and serotonin in the central nervous system. It donates a methyl group during the synthesis of neurotransmitters. Its effects on depression and cognition may be related to neurotransmitter synthesis. Or they may be related to SAMe's effects on cell membranes. Other effects may be secondary to SAMe's polyamine synthesis, because polyamines affect intracellular signals.[8]

Separate from its actions on the central nervous system, SAMe can be an anti-inflammatory as well as analgesic compound. Its effects on osteoarthritis may be related to its ability to stimulate proteoglycan synthesis inside the joints.[8]

In the liver SAMe is involved in growth and differentiation. The liver regulates blood methionine concentrations, to a large extent via SAMe methylation reactions. SAMe does not just donate methyl groups and regulate methionine metabolism, but also acts as a signal inside liver cells that controls their growth, differentiation, and sensitivity to injury. From other parts of the body, hormones, growth factors, and cytokines regulate the synthesis of SAMe.[1]

The mechanism by which SAMe protects the liver in animals, and possibly in humans, includes the following: SAMe causes an increase in glutathione, which protects the liver against oxidative stress. SAMe may be able to blunt the inflammatory response in the liver. It may be able to prevent normal liver cell death, while causing the death (apoptosis) of cancerous cells.[18] SAMe also regulates the growth of liver cells.[22]

PRIMARY USES

- There are people taking SAMe, and doctors recommending it, for a number of conditions. However, the effectiveness and long-term safety of SAMe has not been proven. Much of this should still be considered experimental until more data are available.

Osteoarthritis

Probably the most common use at this time is for osteoarthritis. SAMe is marketed and sold directly to people for knee and hip osteoarthritis. As noted in "The Hype," this use has not been proven completely safe and effective. It has, however, been effective in a number of clinical trials, and significant side effects have not been discovered. People who cannot take NSAIDs for their arthritis might consider SAMe for this purpose.

Liver Disease

At this time, SAMe should only be used for liver disease in clinical trials. There is too much uncertainty about it to recommend it in general.

Depression

Studies are not adequate to recommend this except as part of a clinical trial. Anyone who needs to take medication for depression should be under the care of a health practitioner. If SAMe actually does improve depression, there is the possibility for mania to be induced in people who actually have bipolar illness.[8] Long-term therapy has not been studied.

Alzheimer's Disease, Fibromyalgia

Research in both of these areas is underway, but there is not enough information to recommend its use in general clinical practice.

COMMON DOSAGES

An adequate dose to treat osteoarthritis is 400 mg three or four times a day. If it causes stomach irritation, the dose can be started lower, at 200 mg twice a day, and increased gradually. Some people start at the higher dose and find that once symptoms improve, they are able to lower the dose.

SAMe is very expensive at the recommended dose, costing more than $200 a month.[24] It also should be noted that both SAMe and its precursors can lose potency, sometimes very quickly when exposed to air at room temperature.[25] This has been noted in clinical trials and remains a concern.[8]

However, there have been some patented salts of SAMe that are said to be stable, enteric-coated SAMe-1,4-butanedisulphonate in particular.[3]

There continue to be questions about its potency and cost, as it is marketed directly to consumers.[26]

POTENTIAL SIDE EFFECTS

SAMe has very few side effects. There can be some gastrointestinal distress associated with the supplement, but there is no actual damage.

As noted above, when used for depression, SAMe has the potential for inducing mania or hypomania in people with bipolar illness.

FACT VERSUS FICTION

SAMe shows promise in treating osteoarthritis, depression, early dementia such as in Alzheimer's disease, and possibly other central nervous system disorders. It may turn out to be of great benefit for patients with certain liver diseases that have no other treatment.

At the current time, conferring with a health care practitioner before starting on a course of SAMe would be recommended, especially before taking it for depression or other problems in the nervous system, as well as before taking it for liver problems.

Taking SAMe for osteoarthritis seems to be relatively safe; people taking it can judge for themselves if it reduces their symptoms.

REFERENCES

1. Mato, JM, Corrales, FJ, Lu, SC, Avila, MA. S-Adenosylmethionine: A control switch that regulates liver function. *FASEB J.* 2002;16:15–26.
2. Najm, WI, Reinch, S, Hoehler, F, et al. S-Adenosyl methionine (SAMe) versus celecoxib for the treatment of osteoarthritis symptoms: A double-blind cross-over trial. *BMC Musculoskeletal Disorders.* 2004;5:6.
3. Bottiglieri, T. *S*-Adenosyl-L-methionine (SAMe): From the bench to the bedside—molecular basis of a pleiotrophic molecule. *Am J Clin Nutr.* 2002;76(Suppl):1151S–1157S.
4. Rutjes, AW, Nüesch, E, Reichenbach, S, Jüni, P. S-Adenosylmethionine for osteoarthritis of the knee or hip. *Cochrane Database of Systematic Reviews.* 2009;4. Art. No.: CD007321. doi: 10.1002/14651858.CD007321.pub2.
5. Gregory, PJ, Sperry, M, Wilson, AF. Dietary supplements for osteoarthritis. *Am Fam Physician.* 2008;77(2):177–184.
6. Miller, AL. The methylation, neurotransmitter, and antioxidant connections between folate and depression. *Altern Med Rev.* 2008;13:216–226.
7. Bell, KM, Plon, L, Bunney, WE, Jr, Potkin, SG. S adenosylmethionine treatment of depression: A controlled clinical trial. *Am J Psychiatry.* 1988; 145:1110–1114.
8. Crone, C, Gabriel, G, Wise, TN. Non-herbal nutritional supplements—the next wave. A comprehensive review of risks and benefits for the C-L psychiatrist. *Psychosomatics.* 2001;42:4.
9. Di Rocco, A, Rogers, J, Brown, R, Werner, P, Bottiglieri, T. S-adenosyl-methionine improves depression in patients with Parkinson's disease in an open-label clinical trial. *Movement Disorders.* 2000;15:1225–1229.
10. Shippy, RA, Mendez, D, Jones, K, et al. S-adenosylmethionine (SAM-e) for the treatment of depression in people living with HIV/AIDS. *BMC Psychiatry.* 2004;4:38. doi:10.1186/1471–244X-4–38.
11. Morgan, AJ, Jorm, AF. Self-help interventions for depressive disorders and depressive symptoms: A systematic review. *Annals of General Psychiatry.* 2008;7:13. doi:10.1186/1744–859X-7–13.
12. Williams, AL, Girard, C, Jui, D, Sabina, A, Katz, DL. S-adenosylmethionine (SAMe) as treatment for depression: A systematic review. *Clin Invest Med.* 2005;28(3):132–139.
13. Papakostas, GI. Evidence for S-adenosyl-L-methionine (SAM-e) for the treatment of major depressive disorder. *J Clin Psychiatry.* 2009;70(Suppl 5):18–22.
14. Tchantchou, F, Graves, M, Ortiz, D, Chan, A, Rogers, E, Shea, TB. S-adenosyl methionine: A connection between nutritional and genetic risk factors for neurodegeneration in Alzheimer's disease. *J Nutr Health Aging.* 2006;10(6):541–544.

15. Panza, F, Frisardi, V, Capurso, C, et al. Possible role of S-adenosylmethionine, S-adenosylhomocysteine, and polyunsaturated fatty acids in predementia syndromes and Alzheimer's disease. *J Alzheimers Dis.* 2009;16(3):467–470.

16. National Center for Complementary and Alternative Medicine. National Institutes of Health. Fibromyalgia and CAM: At a glance. Created July 2008, updated July 2009. http://nccam.nih.gov/health/pain/D413_GTF.pdf. Accessed January 20, 2010.

17. Tavoni, A, Vitali, C, Bombardieri, S, Pasero, G. Evaluation of S-adenosylmethionine in primary fibromyalgia. A double-blind crossover study. *Am J Med.* 1987;83(5A):107–110.

18. Purohit, V, Abdelmalek, MF, Barve, S, et al. Role of *S*-adenosylmethionine, folate, and betaine in the treatment of alcoholic liver disease: Summary of a symposium. *Am J Clin Nutr.* 2007;86:14–24.

19. Lieber, CS. Role of S-adenosyl-L-methionine in the treatment of liver diseases. *Journal of Hepatology.* 1999;30:1155–1159.

20. Mato, JM, Camara, J, Fernandez de Paz, J, et al. S-Adenosylmethionine in alcoholic liver cirrhosis: A randomized, placebo-controlled, double-blind, multicenter clinical trial. *Journal of Hepatology.* 1999;30(6):1081–1089.

21. Rambaldi, A, Gluud, C. S-adenosyl-L-methionine for alcoholic liver diseases. *Cochrane Database of Systematic Reviews.* 2006;2. Art. No.: CD002235. doi:10.1002/14651858.CD002235.pub2.

22. Mato, JM, Lu, SC. Role of S-adenosyl-l-methionine in liver health and injury. *Hepatology.* 2007;45:1306–1312.

23. Lu, SC, Mato, JM. *S*-Adenosylmethionine in cell growth, apoptosis and liver cancer. *J Gastroenterol Hepatol.* 2008;23(S1):S73–S77.

24. EBSCO CAM Review Board. S-Adenosylmethionine (SAMe). *Health Library: Herbs & Supplements.* Last reviewed/updated September 1, 2009. http://healthlibrary.epnet.com/GetContent.aspx?deliverycontext=&touchurl= &CallbackURL=&token=e0498803–7f62–4563–8d47–5fe33da65dd4&chun kiid=21460&docid=/tnp/pg000216#ref1. Accessed January 20, 2010.

25. Young, SN. Psychopharmacology for the clinician. *J Psychiatry Neurosci.* 2003;28(6):471.

26. Shu, L, Lee, NP. SAMe targets consumers via the Web. *West J Med.* 2000;173:229–230.

29

Selenium

Selenium is a trace mineral that is found naturally in soil. In small amounts, it is essential to good health. Ingested selenium is made by the body into selenoproteins. Between 25 and 30 selenoproteins have been identified, but not all their functions are understood. There is active research all over the world trying to define the role of selenium in health and disease.

One of the functions of selenoproteins appears to be prevention of free radical damage. When oxygen is metabolized in the body, free radicals are produced. These free radicals have been linked to cancer, heart disease, and other chronic illnesses. Antioxidants are important because they help prevent the damage that free radicals can do to cells. Some selenoproteins are antioxidant enzymes.

Selenoproteins are not just antioxidants. At least three are involved in the regulation of the thyroid gland and others help the immune system, the reproductive system, and more.[1,2,3]

The optimal amount of selenium for humans to ingest has not been conclusively determined.[1] However, in 2000, a recommended dietary allowance for the United States and Canada was set at 55 μg a day for adults.[4] Other countries have recommended different amounts.[5]

A deficiency of selenium can cause specific heart, thyroid, and immune system dysfunction. A large excess of selenium also causes symptoms. In between those two amounts is an amount that may be useful not only to prevent deficiency but also to help protect the body from free radical damage. Additionally, selenium supports immunocompetence.[5] Selenium, possibly in larger amounts, may be useful in helping to treat disease as well as prevent it.[5]

THE HYPE

Overall Use of Selenium

Generally speaking, as an antioxidant, selenium may be able to decrease the risk of cancer, cardiovascular disease, autoimmune disease, and other chronic illnesses.

Selenoproteins acting as enzymes may directly reduce the risk of cancer. For example, selenoenzymes can help remove damaged DNA.[6] In this regard, selenium is sometimes grouped and tested with other antioxidants including vitamin E, C, and others. For example, SELECT (Selenium and Vitamin E Cancer Prevention Trial) was a large trial designed to determine if selenium and/or vitamin E would reduce the risk of prostate cancer in healthy men.[7]

It is also possible that selenium can decrease the risk of chronic illness by other means than simply as an antioxidant.[8]

A lack of selenium increases the risk of cancer, and giving people adequate amounts of selenium removes that risk. Does taking more than the recommended amount of selenium increase the protective effect against cancer?[6]

Since adequate selenium provides immunocompetence, would elevated levels of selenium, "supra-nutritional" levels, increase immunocompetence further?[5] In 2002, Margaret Rayman, in an article entitled "The Argument for Increasing Selenium Intake" brought up two key points about selenium levels. One was a concern that even in Europe and the United Kingdom, there are people with low selenium intake. In fact, selenium levels are dropping.[3] The other was the idea of supra-nutritional therapy. Would higher intakes confer even more benefits? At that time, studies were being designed in an attempt to answer this second question, including SELECT, HIV and AIDS studies,[5] among others.

There are a number of basic unanswered questions that affect the interpretation of information about selenium. One is, "How should selenium levels in the body be measured?" Another is, "Is there a basic difference between giving selenium to people known to be deficient in selenium, and giving extra selenium to people thought to have a normal amount?" This is the so-called superimmunocompetence. A third is, "Do we really know how much selenium is normal and necessary for the human body?"

An equally important question to which the answer is no, is, "Do we know everything that selenoproteins do?"[9]

In 2002, Rayman believed that the correct supra-nutritional intake of selenium at 200 µg a day might optimize health, and, for example, prevent cancer.[5] Support for this theory was expected to materialize from the SELECT study, but it did not.

Researchers make certain assumptions in every study. Incorrect assumptions can lead to faulty reasoning and unclear results.

There are many ongoing studies about selenium, as there should be.

Selenium Supplementation can Decrease the Risk of Cancer

Selenium has been documented to reduce cancer rates in areas of selenium deficiency. In one study in rural China where selenium levels are low, giving people supplements with selenium, beta-carotene, and alpha tocopherol lowered gastric cancer mortality as well as all-cause mortality.[4] There is no way to know which of the supplements specifically caused the decrease.[4,10]

A trial in 1996, giving selenium to patients with treated skin cancer (not melanoma), led to an unanticipated result—a decrease in the rates of prostate, colon, and total cancers.[11,12] A third study indicated that 200 µg of selenium a day might lower the rate of prostate cancer.[13] Data from some studies have shown that the patients with the lowest selenium levels at onset benefit the most from supplementation.[5] The Nutritional Prevention of Cancer Trial (NPC) did show modest protection against some cancers, especially prostate, and also especially among people with lower selenium levels at the onset.[14]

However, other studies do not show an association between higher selenium levels and lower cancer rates. The Nurse's Health Study Cohort examined more than 120,000 women over the course of 41 months. Selenium levels, as determined from toenail clippings (which are believed to reflect selenium intake over a period of time), showed no inverse (or any other) association with the incidence of cancer.[15]

The SELECT trial was set up to answer the question in regard to selenium and/ or vitamin E. Would supplements lower the incidence of prostate cancer in healthy men? More than 35,000 men were in the study, which was stopped in 2008. After around 5.5 years, it was clear that the supplements were not decreasing the risk of prostate cancer.[16]

Further studies are being done, because this question has not been answered completely.

Increased Immunocompetence Helps Fight Viral Illnesses

Coxsackie virus has been found in patients with Keshan disease, a heart disease found in areas of China with low selenium (see "Deficiency"). This may be a cofactor that is necessary along with selenium deficiency for the development of this illness.

Selenium has been shown to inhibit HIV (human immunodeficiency virus) replication in the lab. Selenium status is a predictor of mortality as a result of HIV,[17] including that of pregnant, HIV-positive women.[18]

Some studies have shown suppression of HIV viral load in patients who are given selenium, which is inexpensive and relatively easy to do.[19]

Selenium may also help prevent the progression of disease in patients with hepatitis B and C.[5]

Some viruses, including HIV, can incorporate selenium into viral selenoproteins, which makes the selenium unavailable to help fight the infection.[5] Higher dosages may be needed in patients with severe viral infections.

Selenium Supplementation Can Help Treat Thyroid Disease

Since a number of selenoproteins are involved in iodine regulation, investigators have suggested that selenium may help treat thyroid disease. One study showed that patients with autoimmune thyroiditis given selenium supplementation made less autoantibodies and reported an improved quality of life.[20]

People with myxedematous cretinism (see "Deficiency"), whose thyroid glands do not work, can improve when given selenium along with iodine.

Selenium May Protect against Development of Type II Diabetes

Since impaired glucose metabolism is thought to be related to oxidative stress, an antioxidant such as selenium could improve glucose metabolism. However, studies have not shown this protective effect. One study provided data that suggest that selenium supplementation may increase the risk of diabetes.[21]

Selenium Supplementation can Protect against Cardiovascular Disease

Theoretically, this makes sense. It is believed that many antioxidants can lower atherosclerotic heart disease. Selenoproteins can interrupt many of the steps involved in the buildup of arterial plaque. Conversely, a deficiency of selenium can cause platelets to become stickier and blood vessels more constricted. However, studies have not shown a convincing benefit from selenium administration in terms of reducing cardiovascular events.[5]

There is a definite association between selenium deficiency and cardiomyopathy, such as in Keshan disease (see "Deficiency"). It may also play a role in a specific kind of heart problem called nonischemic dilated cardiomyopathy. This disease occurs after a viral exposure in a patient with altered immunity.[22] Low selenium levels may also be involved.

It is not yet clear what other relationships exist, if any, between selenium status and cardiovascular disease.[23]

Selenium Has Both an Antioxidant and Anti-Inflammatory Action. This Should Make Selenium Useful in Combating Any Illnesses Associated with Inflammation and/or Oxidative Stress

Illnesses of this type include rheumatoid arthritis, asthma, and pancreatitis, among others. Trials of supplementation of selenium in rheumatoid arthritis have yielded mixed results. However, a number of studies have shown benefit from giving selenium to patients with pancreatitis.[5,24] A protective benefit of selenium for patients with asthma has been found in some studies.[5] Selenium may help critically ill patients with systemic inflammatory response.[5] All of these areas continue to be studied.

Selenium Supplementation can Augment Fertility

Selenium is necessary for normal, motile spermatozoa, but too much selenium damages sperm. It seems that selenium is stored in the male reproductive system in such a way as to protect sperm from excessively high levels of selenium.[25] It also may protect against miscarriages. Studies have been inconsistent.[5]

Mood and Cognition May Be Affected by Selenium Status

Lower levels of selenium are associated with depressed mood as well as difficulties with cognition. Selenium may have an effect on neurotransmitters.[5] Studies are ongoing.

DEFICIENCY

Diseases Known to Be Associated with Deficiency

Selenium deficiency exists in some parts of the world. There are areas where there is very little selenium in the soil, including parts of China and Russia, as well as New Zealand[1] and parts of Africa.[26] People living in areas where selenium is low seem to be more susceptible to certain illnesses. Selenium deficient individuals are more likely to develop certain types of heart disease, osteoarthritis, hypothyroidism (low thyroid), and weakness in their immune system.

One illness associated with severe selenium deficiency is called Keshan disease. This is a cardiomyopathy that is endemic in China, where selenium soil levels are very low. However, this disease may only occur when children who are deficient in selenium are exposed to a second stress, which might be a viral illness or a toxin.[1,4] WHO has suggested that the amount of selenium necessary to prevent Keshan disease as the basal requirement for selenium (the amount needed to prevent deficiency). That is 21 µg per day for men and 16 µg a day for women.[1] Administering selenium to people in the affected area has markedly reduced the number of new cases of Keshan disease.[5]

A second endemic deficiency disease in China, Tibet, and Siberia is called Kashin-Beck disease, which is a type of cartilage damage that leads to osteoarthritis.[1] It occurs in the same age group as Keshan disease[1,4] and may also require a second trigger. In this case, the trigger may be iodine deficiency, toxins from fungus, or fulvic acid.[4,26] In China, supplementation of salt with selenium has decreased the incidence of this disease in the endemic areas.

In areas such as parts of Africa where selenium intake is low along with low iodine intake, pregnant women given iodine but not supplemental selenium give birth to babies with "myxedematous cretinism." These children have small, damaged thyroids,[20] as well as abnormal skeletal and neurological development.[26] Treatment of this condition can only be accomplished by giving both iodine and selenium.

How to Diagnose Deficiency Outside of Geographic Areas with Low Selenium

There are many questions about the best way to measure selenium in humans, in order to detect deficiency. It can be found in blood, nails, and hair. A blood level may reflect the amount of selenium currently available while the amount in red cells or nails may reflect stores of selenium.[1] Most of the research has measured blood levels of selenium.

There are five selenoproteins that are glutathione peroxidases (GPx), including cellular GPx (GPx1). The United States and Canada use the level of selenium in the blood that maximizes the functioning of GPx as the best estimate of daily requirements.[1,4] They have set the rate at 55 μg a day.

The World Health Organization set the requirements at 30 μg a day for women and 40 for men. Australia set its RDI at 85 μg per day for men and 70 for women. Different countries in Europe recommend different amounts of selenium.[1]

Selenium deficiency occurs when none is ingested, such as when a patient is getting all of his or her diet through hyperalimentation, either by feeding tube or intravenously. When this was first done, for patients who could not take in food normally, selenium was not recognized as essential. These patients developed muscle weakness and tenderness, cardiomyopathy, and nail bed abnormalities. These problems were largely reversible with selenium administration.[26] Similar problems can occur in patients whose gastrointestinal tract is so damaged that selenium cannot be absorbed.

It has also been suggested that critically ill, hospitalized patients may be relatively low in selenium and need supplementation way above the 50 μg suggested for healthy people, to the 400 μg suggested as an upper level, and even beyond.[27]

Selenium deficiency in patients with celiac disease, who cannot absorb enough, may be responsible for the development of autoimmune thyroid disease in these patients.[28]

FOOD SOURCES

Selenium occurs naturally in the soil. The amount in soil varies from almost nothing in some areas of China, Russia, and New Zealand, among other places, to areas of very high concentration, such as the high plains of northern Nebraska and the Dakotas in the United States. Plants growing in selenium-rich soil can be a good source of selenium in the diet.

Animals, like people, need selenium. Now that the importance of selenium is understood, many governments have tried to make sure that there is enough in the foot chain. In New Zealand, for example, chicken feed has added selenium as do the foods given to other animals. New Zealand also imports a lot of wheat from Australia, which has selenium-rich soil.[29]

In the United States there are areas of high and low selenium. Action has been taken to prevent selenium deficiency or toxicity. In the United States, animals are not raised for meat in the high plains areas of the Dakotas where there is too much selenium in the soil.[4]

Because so much food is transported around the world, most people in many countries get enough selenium in their diet to prevent obvious deficiency disease.

However, people who live in low selenium areas like parts of China, and who do not have enough money to buy anything but local, plant-derived food, can and do become selenium deficient.

The only selenium-fortified food of any kind in the United States is baby formula. Selenium is included in many kinds of multivitamins. It has been estimated by many groups that Americans have enough selenium in their diet already.[4]

Ingested selenium is well absorbed. Excess selenium is stored in some of the selenoproteins used in enzymatic reactions.

Because selenium is a trace element and is also used in manufacturing as a semiconductor, because so many humans are deficient, and there is a finite amount of selenium in the world, there may actually one day be worldwide selenium deficiency.[30]

MECHANISM OF ACTION: HOW DOES IT WORK?

The mechanism of action of selenium in the body is being studied, and new properties are discovered frequently. One very interesting fact is that selenium is the only trace element that is specified in the genetic code, as selonocysteine, which is like the amino acid cysteine but with the selenium attached. In certain kinds of protein synthesis, human genes specify the incorporation of selenocysteine into protein to make a selenoprotein. Selenocysteine is the 21st amino acid. Selenocysteine has different chemical properties than cysteine, which allow selenoproteins to act as enzymes.[5]

Indeed, much of the action of selenium occurs via selenoproteins that act as enzymes. These are still being identified and characterized. There are five glutathione peroxidases dependent on selenoproteins. These peroxidases are defenses against oxidative stress. Other selenoproteins also defend against oxidative stress[4] via other pathways. There are three known selenoproteins that help regulate thyroid metabolism. There is selenoprotein necessary to synthesize selenophosphate, which is the precursor of selenocysteine. In this way, selenium is necessary to use selenium. Multiple selenoproteins are associated with spermatozoa.[5] Selenoprotein P is an antioxidant that may protect endothelial cells.

Other selenoproteins may operate outside the enzymatic processes. It is thought that some of the protective effects against cancer and chronic disease may come from selenium-containing molecules that are not enzymes. Selenoprotein W seems to be involved in the metabolism of both skeletal and cardiac muscle.[5] There is a selenoprotein called 18kDa, found in the kidneys and many other places, which is preserved even in selenium deficiency, so it is presumably a very important protein.

Selenium deficient animals as well as humans seem to be susceptible to certain viruses and other vitamin deficiencies that they could otherwise tolerate.[4] How this happens is still not clear.

Current evidence suggests that a plasma level of around 120 µg per liter may be optimal for cancer protection, at least against some cancers,[31] as well as beneficial in terms of immunocompetence.[5] People may have to take as much as 400 µg daily to reach this level.

PRIMARY USES

- Selenium is used to treat deficiency diseases, including Keshan disease, Kashin-Beck disease, and myxedematous cretinism.

- It is used to prevent deficiency in patients who receive all of their nutrition intravenously. This is called total parenteral hyperalimentation (TPR), and at one time patients on TPR became selenium deficient because the need for selenium was not known. It is now added to TPR solutions. It is added to liquid nutrition given by tube into the intestinal tract.

- Selenium is also given to people whose gastrointestinal tract cannot absorb enough nutrients because of extensive disease. It can be given intravenously.

- Selenium is being given to boost immunity in patients sick with viral illness, and sometimes other illnesses.[5,31]

- Because of the inconsistency of dietary selenium, and the limitations in the process of trying to establish the best amounts of selenium for good health, many multivitamins contain selenium.

COMMON DOSAGES

The RDA for selenium in the United States is 55 µg a day. That is the recommended dietary allowance for adults. The definition of RDA is "The RDA recommends the average daily dietary intake level that is sufficient to meet the nutrient requirements of nearly all (97–98%) healthy individuals in each age and gender group."[2]

The FDA, on the other hand, quotes a Daily Value for selenium of 70 µg a day.

The DRIs (Dietary Reference Intakes) refer to the following values, when quoted by the National Academy of Sciences in the United States: the Recommended Dietary Allowance (RDA), the Adequate Intake (AI), the Tolerable Upper Intake Level (UL), and the Estimated Average Requirement (EAR). These numbers are not always easy to determine. Other countries use different terminology and methods. They are also different for different ages, as well as sometimes being different by sex.

The RDA for selenium was calculated by measuring the amount necessary to maximize synthesis of the selenoprotein glutathione peroxidase, using the plateau in activity of the enzyme. Other countries have used other methods for determining adequate intake.[4]

There are researchers and clinicians using higher doses to boost immunity.[5,31] This is especially true for critically ill, hospitalized patients. There are no clear studies of how much selenium these patients need.[32]

POTENTIAL SIDE EFFECTS

In the normal range, selenium is very well tolerated.

There is a known state of chronic excess selenium in the body, called selenosis. It happens rarely to people living in areas with high levels of selenium. There have also been reports of an area in China with selenosis. The affected individuals were consuming 3,200–6,690 µg of selenium a day.[31] It has also happened accidentally because of supplements containing too much selenium. The symptoms of chronic selenosis include garlic breath odor, gastrointestinal complaints, white, blotchy nails and lined nails, brittleness and loss of hair, irritability, fatigue, skin rash, and mild nerve damage. The symptoms usually go away when selenium levels become normal.[2,4,29] There is no treatment or way to remove selenium.

Acute poisoning is very rare. There have been documented cases of accidental or suicidal ingestion of large amounts of selenium, which would have to be grams. There have also been murder attempts using selenium. Gun blue, a lubricant, contains large amounts of selenium and has been used. Symptoms include severe gastrointestinal and neurological disturbance, acute respiratory and renal failure, and heart attack.[33] If the person does not survive, autopsy shows necrosis of kidney and intestines, a damaged heart, and fluid in the lungs.

Chronic selenosis is rare in the United States. It has happened with industrial accidents and manufacturing errors. The tolerable upper level of ingestion for adults is considered to be 400 μg per day. That means there is a wide range between what is suggested daily and what is considered excessive.

FACT VERSUS FICTION

The fact is that there is still a lot unknown about selenium.

It should definitely be given to people with known deficiency diseases such as Keshan disease.

It should definitely be added to solutions of total parenteral nutrition, or any similar diet.

More should be given to people with diseased gastrointestinal tracts who may have trouble absorbing it.

It is reasonable to give supplements to people sick with viral or other diseases, which may use up the selenium they already have. This would include patients with HIV, hepatitis B, hepatitis C, and probably tuberculosis.

There are no reasons not to try a supplement in the 200-μg range to see if it will boost immunity, on a person-by-person basis. Even higher ranges are probably safe.

However, since it is not clear that selenium protects against cancer or cardiovascular disease, and may cause more diabetes, it seems premature to recommend its use to people in general for those reasons.

REFERENCES

1. Thompson, CD. Assessment of requirements for selenium and adequacy of selenium status: A review. *European Journal of Clinical Nutrition.* 2004; 58:391–402.
2. Office of Dietary Supplements. *Dietary Supplement Fact Sheet: Selenium.* NIH Clinical Center, National Institutes of Health. http://ods.od.nih.gov/fact sheets/selenium.asp#en16. Accessed October 15, 2009.
3. Brown, KM, Arthur, JR. Selenium, selenoproteins and human health: A review. *Public Health Nutr.* 2001;4:593–599.

4. Institute of Medicine. Food and Nutrition Board. *Dietary reference intakes for vitamin C, vitamin E, selenium, and carotenoids*. Washington, DC: National Academies Press, 2000.

5. Rayman, MP. The argument for increasing selenium intake. *Proceedings of the Nutrition Society*. 2002;61:203–215.

6. Combs, GF, Lu, J. Selenium as a cancer preventative agent. Chapter 17 in: Hatfield, DL. (Ed). *Selenium: Its molecular biology and role in human health*. Boston: Kluwer Academic Publishers, 2001, 205–219.

7. Lippman, SM, Goodman, PJ, Klein, EA, et al. Designing the Selenium and Vitamin E Cancer Prevention Trial (SELECT). *Journal of the National Cancer Institute*. 2005;97(2):94–102.

8. Papp, LV, Lu, J, Holmgren, A, et al. *Antioxidants & Redox Signaling*. 2007;9(7):775–806.

9. Arthur, JR, McKenzie, RC, Beckett, GJ. Selenium in the immune system. *Journal of Nutrition*. 2003;133:1457S–1459S.

10. Blot, WJ, Li, JY, Taylor, PR, et al. Nutrition intervention trials in Linxian, China: Supplementation with specific vitamin/mineral combinations, cancer incidence, and disease-specific mortality in the general population. *J Natl Cancer Inst*. 1993;85:1483–1492.

11. Combs, GF, Clark, LC, Turnbull, BW. Reduction of cancer risk with an oral supplement of selenium. *Biomed Environ Sci*. 1997;10(2–3):227–234.

12. Clark, LC, Combs, Jr, GF, Turnbull, BW, et al. Effects of selenium supplementation for cancer prevention in patients with carcinoma of the skin. A randomized controlled trial. *J Am Med Assoc*. 1996;276:1957–1963.

13. Yoshizawa, K, Willett, WC, Morris, SJ, et al. Study of prediagnostic selenium level in toenails and the risk of advanced prostate cancer. *J Natl Cancer Inst*. 1998;90:1219–1224.

14. Duffield-Lillico, AJ, Reid, ME, Turnbull, BW, et al. Baseline characteristics and the effect of selenium supplementation on cancer incidence in a randomized clinical trial: A Summary Report of the Nutritional Prevention of Cancer Trial. *Cancer Epidemiology, Biomarkers & Prevention*. 2002;11:630–639.

15. Garland, M, Morris, JS, Stampfer, MJ, Colditz, GA, Spate, VL, et al. Prospective study of toenail selenium levels and cancer among women. *J Natl Cancer Inst*. 1995;87:497–505.

16. Lippman, SM, Klein, EA, Goodman, PJ, Lucia, MS, Thompson, IM, Ford, LG, et al. The effect of selenium and vitamin E on risk of prostate cancer and other cancers: The Selenium and Vitamin E Cancer Prevention Trial (SELECT). *JAMA*. 2009;301:39–51.

17. Baum, MK, and Shor-Posner, G. Micronutrient status in relationship to mortality in HIV-1 disease. *Nutr Rev*. 1998;56:S135–S139.

18. Kupka, R, Msamanga, GI, Spiegelman, D, et al. Selenium status is associated with accelerated HIV disease progression among HIV-1–infected pregnant women in Tanzania. *J Nutr*. 2004;134:2556–2560.

19. Hurwitz, BE, Klaus, JR, Llabre, MM, et al. Suppression of human immunodeficiency virus type 1 viral load with selenium supplementation: A randomized controlled trial. *Arch Intern Med.* 2007;167(2):148–154.

20. Gartner, R, Gasnier, BC, Dietrich, JW. Selenium supplementation in patients with autoimmune thyroiditis decreases thyroid peroxidase antibodies concentrations. *J Clin Endocrinol Metab.* 2002;87(4):1687–1691.

21. Stranges, S, Marshall, JR, Natarajan, R, et al. Effects of long-term selenium supplementation on the incidence of type 2 diabetes. *Ann Intern Med.* 2007;147:217–223.

22. Cooper, LT, Rader, V, Ralston, NVC. The roles of selenium and mercury in the pathogenesis of viral cardiomyopathy. *Congestive Heart Failure.* 2007;13(4):193–199.

23. Neve, J. Selenium as a risk factor for cardiovascular diseases. *J Cardiovasc Risk.* 1996;3:42–47.

24. McCloy, R. Chronic pancreatitis at Manchester, UK. Focus on antioxidant therapy. *Digestion.* 1998;59:36–48.

25. Hawkes, WC, Alkan, Z, Wong, K. Selenium supplementation does not affect testicular selenium status or semen quality in North American men. *J Androl.* 2009;30(5):525–533.

26. Coppinger, RJ, Diamond, AM. Selenium deficiency and human disease. Chapter 18 in: Hatfield, DL. (Ed). *Selenium: Its molecular biology and role in human health.* Boston: Kluwer Academic Publishers, 2001, 219–233.

27. Vincent, JL, Forceville, X. Critically elucidating the role of selenium. *Current Opinion in Anesthesiology.* 2008;21(2):148–154.

28. Stazi, AV, Trinti, B. Selenium deficiency in celiac disease: Risk of autoimmune thyroid diseases. *Minerva Med.* 2008;99(6):643–653.

29. New Zealand Medicines and Medical Devices Safety Authority. Selenium. July 2000. http://www.medsafe.govt.nz/Profs/PUarticles/Sel.htm. Accessed October 15, 2009.

30. Haug, A, Graham, RD, Christophersen, OA, Lyons, GH. How to use the world's scarce selenium resources efficiently to increase the selenium concentration in food. *Microb Ecol Health Dis.* 2007;19(4):209–228.

31. Combs, GF. Selenium in global food systems. *British Journal of Nutrition.* 2001;85:517–547.

32. Angstwurm, MW, Gaertner, R. Practicalities of selenium supplementation in critically ill patients. *Curr Opin Clin Nutr Metab Care.* 2006;9(3):233–238.

33. Ruta, DA, Haider, S. Attempted murder by selenium poisoning. *BMJ.* 1989; 299:31.

30

Vitamin A

BRIEF OVERVIEW

In the early 1900s, researchers began to discover that animals needed substances other than proteins, carbohydrates, and fats to live. Vitamin A, first called "fat-soluble factor A," was the second recognized vitamin. Vitamin A is necessary for many normal functions, including reproduction, growth and development, immunologic competence, and vision, among others.

Vitamin A deficiency can be deadly. While most people in Western countries get enough vitamin A, in poor countries, millions of children, perhaps as many as 10 million, are deficient in the vitamin enough to cause xeropthalmia, an eye condition that can lead to blindness. Vitamin A deficiency makes children more susceptible to infectious illnesses and can lead to death at a young age.

Too much vitamin A can also prove deadly. An early description of hypervitaminosis A was penned by an explorer named Gerrit de Veer, who was attempting to find the Northern Passage to Indonesia in 1597. During the winter in Nova Zembla, he and his men were forced to eat polar bear for food, and all the men almost died after eating polar bear liver. They survived, and he very accurately described their symptoms of vitamin A toxicity.[1]

Liver has an extremely high concentration of vitamin A. It can be fatal if eaten in large amounts. In addition to an acute toxic reaction, there is also an illness caused by taking in too much vitamin A over long periods of time.

Vitamin A, also called retinol, is part of a group of compounds called retinoids. In addition to vitamin A, there is beta-carotene, a pro-vitamin that the body can convert into retinol, giving it vitamin A activity. The amount of beta-carotene that is actually converted into vitamin A is dependent on how much retinol is already in the body, among other factors. It appears that people cannot get vitamin A toxicity from too much beta-carotene, because the body stops converting it when there is enough retinol. There are other carotenoids, some of which have vitamin A activity, others that do not. The information herein pertains to beta-carotene and vitamin A only.

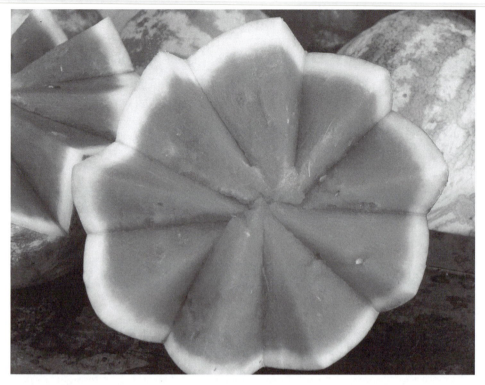

This vibrant red watermelon, shown at a makeshift fruit stand near Los Fresnos, Texas, is the leading source of lycopene, an antioxidant believed to have cancer prevention benefits. Watermelons are also are high in vitamins C and A. The fruit can be a tasty base for salsas, jams, and chutneys. (AP Photo/Joe Hermosa)

Vitamin A has been known in one form or another for centuries. Long before they knew its name, people recognized that there was something of nutritional value in liver. They also connected carrots (and therefore beta-carotene) with good eyesight.

THE HYPE

Supplementation with Vitamin A or Beta-Carotene Will Lead to an Overall Decrease in Chronic Diseases and Mortality

Both vitamin A and beta-carotene are antioxidants, like vitamin E and selenium. Since antioxidants can counteract free radicals in the body, it is thought they might prevent damage to DNA and blood vessels. If this is true, then supplementation should help prevent cancer and cardiovascular disease as well as other diseases in which oxidation plays a role. Much of the research about vitamin A has been done with beta-carotene, because high doses of vitamin A can cause toxicity. Some investigations have used both.

Many observational studies show an inverse relationship between various diseases and beta-carotene levels. With an inverse relationship, the higher the beta-carotene levels, the lower the incidence of certain diseases. Studies also show an inverse relationship between mortality and beta-carotene level. For example, in one study, blood samples were drawn from a group of men and women, and they were followed for approximately eight years. There was an inverse relationship between beta-carotene and cardiovascular and cancer mortality, as well as all-cause mortality.[2]

However, prospective studies do not seem to confirm these results. A well-designed, double-blind, placebo-controlled primary prevention trial called the Beta-Carotene and Retinol Efficacy Trial, or the CARET trial, studied 18,314 smokers, former smokers, and people exposed to asbestos (also a cancer risk). The treated group got vitamin A and beta-carotene. After four years, no benefit was seen from the supplements, and there were adverse effects, with an increased risk of lung cancer, death from lung cancer, cardiovascular disease, and death from all causes. This trial was discontinued early.[3]

Supplementation can Protect against Cardiovascular Disease

There have been observational studies showing a higher risk of cardiovascular disease in patients with low carotenoids and/or vitamin A.[4]

However, many trials using a variety of antioxidant vitamins as supplements have shown no benefit from most. The Women's Antioxidant Cardiovascular Study, the results of which were published in 2007, tested a number of antioxidants to see if they would provide cardiovascular protection over approximately 10 years. There was no effect of beta-carotene on any cardiovascular disease or cause of death.[5]

One review of all the available research trials concluded that vitamin A and beta-carotene may increase mortality and do not decrease the risk of cardiovascular disease or cancer.[6]

The American Heart Association's position on beta-carotene and other antioxidants was stated in an article in *Circulation* in 2004, and it remains the same in 2009. The association does not advise giving high doses of any antioxidants, including beta-carotene and vitamin A, as supplements to reduce cardiovascular disease risk.[7]

Vitamin A (or Beta-Carotene) Will Decrease the Risk of Certain Cancers

In one study in rural China where selenium levels are low, giving people supplements with selenium, beta-carotene, and alpha tocopherol lowered gastric cancer mortality as well as all-cause mortality. There is no way to know which of the supplements specifically caused the decrease.[8,9]

There are hundreds of observational studies looking at the relationship between beta-carotene and cancer. Many show an inverse relationship between beta-carotene levels and/or consumption and development of cancer.[9,10]

The ATBC study of Finnish smokers found the opposite from what was expected based on the observational studies. Supplementation with beta-carotene increased the number of new lung cancers in this group and had no effect on numbers of other cancers. The beta-carotene part of the study was stopped because of the increased cancer risk.[11]

Similar results were found in the CARET study as noted above. In the CARET study, participants were given both beta-carotene and vitamin A daily, compared with a group given placebo. This study showed no benefit from the vitamins, but there were excess lung cancer cases and mortality, so that the study was stopped early.[12,13]

In 2003, the U.S. Preventive Services Task Force recommended against routine supplementation with vitamin A and beta-carotene, based on all the available evidence.[14]

DEFICIENCY

Vitamin A deficiency is uncommon in the United States. It can happen to people who are chronically ill and malnourished, especially the elderly in the United States and children in other parts of the world. Vitamin A deficiency can occur as a result of inadequate intake of vitamin A and beta-carotene, impaired absorption in the gastrointestinal tract, or altered metabolism of the vitamin. It can also occur if there is an increased need for the vitamin because of illness.[15] Causes of secondary vitamin A deficiency include any intestinal diseases that cause chronic diarrhea including celiac sprue and cystic fibrosis, among others. Cirrhosis of the liver, surgical bypass of the small intestine, and pancreatic insufficiency can all reduce the absorption of vitamin A.

There is no beta-carotene deficiency state. The only time a person needs a certain level of beta-carotene is if he or she is vitamin A deficient. Enough beta-carotene can be converted into vitamin A and prevent deficiency disease.[4]

The metabolism of vitamin A and beta-carotene is very complex. Both are absorbed as are other fats into the intestinal cells. Some beta-carotene is transformed into retinol in the cells of the intestinal lining. The retinol and carotene are released into the lymphatic system and eventually delivered to the liver in chylomicrons remnants. Retinol is bound to cellular retinol-binding protein (RBP) in the liver. It is released into the circulation as necessary, in combination with RBP. In addition to the liver, where 80 to 90 percent of the vitamin is stored, excess retinol and beta-carotene may also be stored in kidney, lung, and fat. It is believed beta-carotene can be converted into retinol in multiple places in the body.[4,15,16,17,18]

Anything that interrupts the absorption of vitamin A and beta-carotene, or prevents the conversion to retinol, or inhibits the delivery of the vitamin to tissues can cause deficiency.

Adults can store about a year's worth of vitamin A if they have been taking in enough. Children can usually only maintain storage of enough vitamin A to last a couple of weeks. If the diet is low in vitamin A and beta-carotene, retinol will be released from the liver, and beta-carotene will be converted to retinol. Since vitamin A needs retinol-binding protein (RBP) to travel, problems with RBP can affect vitamin A status. Zinc deficiency is thought to lower vitamin A by interfering with RBP synthesis. Lowered iron stores also can contribute to vitamin A deficiency.[15,19,20]

The first symptom of vitamin A deficiency is a loss of night vision. If the deficiency is not corrected, the eyes become more damaged. Xeropthalmia occurs as a result of lack of vitamin A. The front parts of the eye including the covering layers, called the conjunctiva, and the clear part of the center of the eye, called the cornea, become dry and thickened. There may be spots on the eye. The cornea can develop ulcers and holes. Eventually, this may lead to blindness.

Children who are vitamin A deficient as well as severely calorie deficient and protein deficient are the most at risk for xeropthalmia and blindness. This is a significant problem in parts of the world where children and others do not get enough to eat.

The lining of multiple systems in the body can weaken without enough vitamin A. The hair becomes dry, as does the skin. The skin will also be scaly. Linings of the urinary tract, intestinal tract, and lungs get stiff and lose proper function. Blood cells may not be made normally. A weakened immune system secondary to vitamin A deficiency makes infectious diseases a serious problem for people with vitamin A deficiency, especially children. They may die from measles, gastrointestinal viruses, HIV/AIDs, or other infections. Children may not grow and develop normally.[15,18,19,20] The mortality rate of severe vitamin A deficiency may be as high as 50 percent in children.

Vitamin A deficiency can be diagnosed in patients with night blindness and xeropthalmia. There are specific vision tests to ascertain if vitamin A deficiency is present. Plasma retinol level can be measured, but this does not always reflect the amount of vitamin A in the body. Sometimes, giving vitamin A and seeing improvement can make sure that it is the right diagnosis.

The dosages of vitamin A needed to treat deficiency are high; such amounts can cause toxicity in a patient with adequate stores of vitamin A.[18,20]

FOOD SOURCES

Retinol is found in foods derived from animals, including meat, eggs, and milk and fish. There are very large amounts of vitamin A in liver. Three ounces of cooked beef liver contains 245 percent of the daily value for vitamin A, which is 5,000 IU. The vitamin A naturally found in milk is removed when fat is removed. Milk is then fortified with vitamin A, so that a cup of skim milk has about 10 percent of the daily value. Vitamin A is readily absorbed and used. People who eat meat and animal products usually do not need any more vitamin A.[20] Too much vitamin A can cause disease.

Beta-carotene is found in plant-derived foods, especially certain darkly colored vegetables and fruit. One raw carrot contains about 175 percent of the daily value for vitamin A. Spinach, cantaloupe, papaya, and apricots all contain significant amounts, as do other fruits and vegetables. Beta-carotene is not well absorbed and has to be converted in the body to retinol. For vegetarians, that means a significant amount of beta-carotene foods must be eaten, or supplements must be taken.[20]

MECHANISM OF ACTION: HOW DOES IT WORK?

Vitamin A is essential for many normal functions in humans. It is especially important to maintaining vision. It is also essential for reproduction and immune function.[19] It has effects on bone growth and helps maintain the linings of the intestinal tract, as well as the urinary tract and respiratory tract. During fetal development, vitamin A is necessary, and it has a regulatory effect on some genes.[15,19]

Vitamin A is needed to make rhodopsin, a pigment in the retina that is a photoreceptor. As levels of vitamin A fall, the retina suffers. Vitamin A is necessary for the health of the eyes' conjunctival cells, as well as protective goblet cells that secrete mucin.

Vitamin A also helps keep epithelial cells intact, so that there are skin abnormalities with vitamin A deficiency. Lowered numbers of white blood cells have been associated with vitamin A deficiency, including cells necessary to mount an immune response to illness and tumors. Vitamin A has a complex effect on multiple components of the immune system, so that deficiency leads to increased rates of severe illness and death from measles, diarrheal disease, and other infections.[19,21]

Both vitamin A and beta-carotene do act as antioxidants in the body and help prevent damage to cells and DNA.[17]

Beta-carotene may increase cell-to-cell communication, improve immunity, lower the risk of certain cancers, and lower mortality rates.[4] It is difficult to separate actions of beta-carotene from actions of retinol, because ingested beta-carotene is converted to retinol at variable rates.

All of the functions of vitamin A and beta-carotene are not completely understood. There are complex interactions and reactions in the body involving these vitamins and many pathways in many systems.

PRIMARY USES

- Vitamin A is used to treat clinically obvious deficiency of vitamin A, meaning people with symptoms due to lack of the vitamin.

- It is also used as a dietary supplement for people who may not get enough from their diet. Beta-carotene can be used for the same purpose.

- Large doses of beta-carotene are used to treat a condition called erythropoietic protoporphyria, a disease in which people develop reactions to sunlight.[4]

- In terms of supplementation, vitamin A can cause toxicity and is not considered a safe supplement in high doses. High doses of beta-carotene are better tolerated. Most of the testing to see if the antioxidant properties of these compounds could help prevent chronic disease has been done with beta-carotene. As previously indicated, there has not yet been clear evidence that supplementation prevents disease. To the contrary, there is evidence that beta-carotene can cause excess mortality in certain groups of people, for example, cigarette smokers.

COMMON DOSAGES

Despite continued attempts to standardize measurements for vitamin A, the amounts needed by the body are still confusing. Vitamin A and beta-carotene are not equivalent. Furthermore, there is different absorption of natural versus synthetic versions of these compounds, as well as different absorption depending on the way the vitamin is delivered.

Vitamin A

The Food and Nutrition Board (FNB) at the Institute of Medicine (IOM) of the National Academies sets the recommendations, such as the Recommended Dietary Allowances (RDAs) and Tolerable Upper Intake Levels (ULs).[19,20] The levels for vitamin A are expressed as Retinol Activity Equivalents (RAEs) because vitamin A and beta-carotene are not equivalent microgram for microgram. The following table lists the RDAs in microgram REAs, and also International Units. 1 RAE equals 3.3 IUs. The IUs are listed on food labels.

Vitamin A

Age (years)	Children	Males	Females	Pregnancy	Lactation
1–3	300 µg (1,000 IU)				
4–8	400 µg (1,320 IU)				
9–13	600 µg (2,000IU)				
14–18		900 µg (3,000 IU)	700 µg (2,310 IU)	750 µg (2,500 IU)	1,200 µg (4,000 IU)
19+		900 µg (3,000 IU)	700 µg (2,310 IU)	770 µg (2,565 IU)	1,300 µg (4,300 IU)

The Food and Drug Administration also sets a target for vitamins, called the Daily Value (DV). For vitamin A, that level is 5,000. When a container of food says on the label 20% DV for vitamin A, it has 1,000 IU of the vitamin. Most foods, however, do not have labels including vitamin A.

These are the amounts of vitamin A considered to be best to keep healthy people healthy. These amounts do not apply to treating patients who are deficient in vitamin A. Both too much and too little vitamin A are dangerous. For healthy individuals, the Tolerable Upper Intake Levels are approximately three times the RDA for vitamin A (see "Potential Side Effects").

Beta-Carotene

There is no RDA for beta-carotene or other carotenes. Beta-carotenes and some but not all other carotenes are converted to retinol in the body. The IOM has stated that 3 to 6 mg of beta-carotene a day may be reasonable because that amount of intake leads to levels in the blood that are associated with lower risks of chronic disease.[9] There is no deficiency disease from low beta-carotene in people getting enough vitamin A. There is also no toxic amount of beta-carotene. People who eat large amounts of beta-carotene may have yellow skin, called carotenemia, but it is not dangerous.[9] If this happens, the person just needs to eat fewer vegetables if concerned about the color.[16]

People treated for erythropoietic protoporphyria at doses of approximately 180 mg a day of beta-carotene have shown no evidence of toxicity.[9]

In terms of beta-carotene, the Dietary Reference Intakes (DRI) is recommending at least five servings of fruit and vegetables a day for good health, but not suggesting supplementation.

There is also the risk to smokers demonstrated in the ATBC trial.

There are questions about supplemental beta-carotene in certain circumstances, as discussed in "The Hype" section.

For Vitamin A Deficiency

For treatment of vitamin A deficiency, large doses must be given. Usually vitamin A in oil is used, because the oil increases absorption of the vitamin.[15,18] A sample regimen would be 60,000 IU for two days, then 4,500 IU daily. If the person is vomiting or has intestinal problems that decrease absorption, or if xerophthalmia is present, as much as 200,000 IU may be given to adults, for two days, and then a third dose two weeks later. Infants and children born to HIV-positive mothers and children with measles need large amounts of vitamin A.

In countries where many people are malnourished, large doses of vitamin A are often given to a mother after she gives birth, and again a number of months later. This is to improve the health of the mother, as well as get vitamin A to breast-fed babies.

Care must be taken as deficiency is corrected not to give excessive vitamin A.[18]

POTENTIAL SIDE EFFECTS

The body cannot eliminate excess vitamin A. Too much can cause toxicity, immediately in large doses, and also over a long period of time. Vitamin A is thought to be teratogenic, meaning it can cause birth defects. Since most people in the United States get enough vitamin A in the diet, supplementation with excessive amounts of vitamin A (not beta-carotene) can cause toxicity. The exact amount of vitamin A that causes acute and chronic toxicity is not absolute. It may depend on the source of the vitamin, what else was ingested at the same time, and many other factors. Alcohol use may potentiate the damage of vitamin A.[22]

Someone taking about 25,000 IU vitamin A per kilogram of body weight all at one time, usually by accident, can suffer acute vitamin A toxicity.[16,18] If this happens, the person may have many symptoms, including loss of appetite, nausea, vomiting, and abdominal pain. Someone with vitamin A toxicity may be sleepy, irritable, or demonstrate what is called altered mental status, which can appear as confusion and forgetfulness. Other symptoms include headache, muscle pain and weakness, and blurred vision. If a doctor examines a patient in this condition, he or she may find tenderness over long bones, as well as an abnormal neurologic exam. This type of acute toxicity usually occurs with accidental ingestion of vitamin A by children, or in adults exploring the Arctic who eat either polar bear or seal liver, which does actually still happen.[18]

Some of the same symptoms can be seen in someone who is taking 25,000 to 100,000 IU a day of vitamin A over a long period. Toxicity has been reported with lower doses over a longer period of time. This can occur in individuals taking excessive amounts of supplemental A. Large doses are occasionally prescribed for acne or other skin problems.[18]

There are additional problems with chronic toxicity. There may be dry mucus membranes in the mouth and cracks in the lips. The person may lose hair and may lose weight. There may be itching and fever and difficulty sleeping. Chronic overdoses of vitamin A can cause fractures of bone, low blood count (anemia), pain in the bone and joints, nosebleeds, diarrhea, and abnormal menstruation. Some of these things will be apparent to an examining doctor. The doctor might also find that the skin is red and peeling. There may be inflammation of the outer eye coverings (conjunctivitis) and tiny pinpoints of bleeding under the skin. The liver and spleen may be large; later the liver may be scarred and small (cirrhotic). Many abnormalities of the nervous system will be visible, from obvious serious eye problems, to difficulty walking and trouble controlling the limbs. These are just some of the things a person might experience and a doctor might see.

There are a number of blood tests, x-rays, and scans that can confirm that someone has vitamin A toxicity. The main treatment is supportive, in addition to stopping the ingestion of vitamin A. If a person is very sick, he or she would be admitted to the hospital for monitoring and to administer a number of medications that can help. People with vitamin A toxicity usually recover.[16,18] However, since vitamin A is teratogenic, infants can be born with a birth defect as the result of excess vitamin A in the mother's system.

It is important to note that too much vitamin A can cause bone fractures. There is a possibility that excess vitamin A can contribute to osteoporosis. There have been many studies showing that people who have high levels of retinol also have a higher incidence of osteoporosis and fractures.[1,16,22,23]

Beta-carotene is very well tolerated and not converted enough to vitamin A to cause toxic reactions. Side effects, not proven but associated with beta-carotene intake, include allergic reactions, possible increase in prostate cancer, retinopathy, low white blood cells, and trouble with reproduction.[9]

As stated previously, beta-carotene supplementation may be associated with increased mortality and increased cancer in certain groups. Other analyses have shown that treatment with a number of antioxidants, including vitamins E and A as well as beta-carotene, may increase mortality.[24]

FACT VERSUS FICTION

At the current time, supplementation with large doses of either vitamin A or beta-carotene does not seem wise. With vitamin A, there is a risk of toxicity as well as the possible negative effects on cardiovascular disease, cancer, and mortality. While beta-carotene does not cause toxicity, it is associated with the other negative outcomes.

The doses in commonly used multivitamins may even be too high. Anyone who feels he or she does not get enough retinol in the diet should pick a vitamin supplement that includes a dose of vitamin A close to the RDA or DV. While supplements are not recommended for beta-carotene, beta-carotene supplements may be a safer way to get vitamin A. The best choice is to eat a well-balanced diet and get these nutrients from food sources.

REFERENCES

1. Lips, P. Hypervitaminosis A and fractures. *New England Journal of Medicine.* 2003;348(4):347–349.
2. Greenberg, ER, Baron, JA, Karagas, MR, et al. Mortality associated with low plasma concentration of beta carotene and the effect of oral supplementation. *JAMA.* 1996;275(9):699–703.
3. Omenn, GS, Goodman, GE, Thornquist, MD, et al. Effects of a combination of beta carotene and vitamin A on lung cancer and cardiovascular disease. *New England Journal of Medicine.* 1996;334:1150–1155.
4. Office of Dietary Supplements. *Dietary Supplement Fact Sheet: Selenium.* NIH Clinical Center, National Institutes of Health. http://ods.od.nih.gov/fact sheets/selenium.asp#en16. Accessed November 6, 2009.
5. Cook, NR, Albert, CA, Gaziano, JM, et al. A randomized factorial trial of vitamins C and E and beta carotene in the secondary prevention of cardiovascular events in women. *Arch Intern Med.* 2007;167(15):1610–1618.
6. Bjelakovic, G, Nikolova, D, Gluud, LL, Simonetti, RG, Gluud, C. Antioxidant supplements for prevention of mortality in healthy participants and patients with various diseases. *Cochrane Database of Systematic Reviews.* 2008;2. Art. No.: CD007176. doi:10.1002/14651858.
7. Kris-Etherton, PM, Lichtenstein, AH, Howard, BV, et al. Antioxidant vitamin supplements and cardiovascular disease. *Circulation.* 2004;110:637–641.
8. Blot, WJ, Li, J-Y, Taylor, PR, et al. Nutrition intervention trials in Linxian, China: Supplementation with specific vitamin/mineral combinations, cancer incidence, and disease-specific mortality in the general population. *J Natl Cancer Inst.* 1993;85:1483–1492.
9. Institute of Medicine. Food and Nutrition Board. *Dietary reference intakes for vitamin C, vitamin E, selenium, and carotenoids.* Washington, DC: National Academies Press, 2000.
10. Micozzi, MS, Beecher, GR, Taylor, PR, Khachik, F. Carotenoid analyses of selected raw and cooked foods associated with a lower risk for cancers. *J Natl Cancer Inst.* 1990;82:282–285.
11. The Alpha-Tocopherol, Beta Carotene Cancer Prevention Study Group. The effect of vitamin E and beta carotene on the incidence of lung cancer and other cancers in male smokers. *N Engl J Med.* 1994;330:1029–1035.

12. Omenn, GS, Goodman, GE, Thornquist, MD, et al. Risk factors for lung cancer and for intervention effects in CARET, the Beta-Carotene and Retinol Efficacy Trial. *J Natl Cancer Inst.* 1996;88(21):1550–1559.

13. Albanes, D, Heinonen, OP, Taylor, PR, et al. Alpha-tocopherol and beta-carotene supplements and lung cancer incidence in the Alpha-Tocopherol, Beta-Carotene Cancer Prevention Study: Effects of base-line characteristics and study compliance. *J Natl Cancer Inst.* 1996;88(21):1560–1570.

14. U.S. Preventive Services Task Force. Routine vitamin supplementation to prevent cancer and cardiovascular disease: Recommendations and rationale. *Ann Intern Med.* 2003;139:51–55.

15. Ansstas, G, Thakore, J, Gopalswamy, N. Vitamin A deficiency. *eMedicine.* http://emedicine.medscape.com/article/126004-overview. Accessed November 9, 2009.

16. Eledrisi, MS, McKinney, K, Shanti, MS. Vitamin A toxicity. *eMedicine.* http://emedicine.medscape.com/article/126104-overview. Accessed November 9, 2009.

17. Boileau, TW, Moore, AC, Erdman, JW. Carotenoids and vitamin A. Chapter 8 in: Papas, AM. (Ed). *Antioxidant status, diet, nutrition, and health.* Boca Raton, FL: CRC Press, 1999, 133–158.

18. The Merck Manuals Online Medical Library. Vitamin A. For healthcare professionals. Last full review/revision April 2007 by Larry E. Johnson, MD, PhD. http://www.merck.com/mmpe/sec01/ch004/ch004g.html. Accessed November 10, 2009.

19. Institute of Medicine. Food and Nutrition Board. *Dietary reference intakes for vitamin A, vitamin K, arsenic, boron, chromium, copper, iodine, iron, manganese, molybdenum, nickel, silicon, vanadium, and zinc.* Washington, DC: National Academies Press, 2001.

20. Office of Dietary Supplements. *Dietary Supplement Fact Sheet: Vitamin A and carotenoids.* NIH Clinical Center, National Institutes of Health. http://dietary-supplements.info.nih.gov/factsheets/vitamina.asp#en1. Accessed November 9, 2009.

21. Villamor, E, Fawzi, WW. Effects of vitamin A supplementation on immune responses and correlation with clinical outcomes. *Clinical Microbiology Reviews.* 2005;18(3):446–464.

22. Penniston, KL, Tanumihardjo, S. The acute and chronic toxic effects of vitamin A. *Am J Clin Nutr.* 2006;83:191–201.

23. Michaelsson, K, Lithell, H, Vessby, B, et al. Serum retinol levels and the risk of fracture. *New England Journal of Medicine.* 2003;348:4:347–349.

24. Bjelakovic, G, Nikolova, D, Gluud, LL, Simonetti, RG, Gluud, C. Mortality in randomized trials of antioxidant supplements for primary and secondary prevention: Systematic review and meta-analysis. *JAMA.* 2007;297:842–857.

31

Vitamin B12

BRIEF OVERVIEW

Vitamin B12, also called cobalamin, is an essential factor in the production of red blood cells. People who do not have enough B12 in their systems suffer from anemia. B12 is also necessary for the production of other blood cells, as well as normal neurologic function. Someone with severe B12 deficiency may have anemia as well as a variety of neurologic and psychiatric problems. These symptoms can be as mild as irritability, a slight memory loss, and the sensation of pins and needles in the extremities. They can be severe, including, among other things, shaky, unsteady gait, weakness, incontinence, peripheral neuropathy, dementia, and psychosis.

One disease associated with low levels of B12 was known even before the specific vitamin was discovered. It was called pernicious anemia. Doctors knew that something collected in animal livers cured the disease, so people with pernicious anemia were effectively treated with large amounts of liver. Eventually the vitamin was isolated and its chemical composition understood.

Research has led to much greater knowledge of B12 and its role in health as well as disease.

Vitamin D is necessary for normal DNA synthesis. It works along with folic acid in a wide variety of ways. Normal amounts of both B12 and folic acid are necessary to prevent a substance called homocysteine from accumulating in the body. Elevated homocysteine levels are implicated in many common medical problems, including cardiovascular disease, neurologic disorders, and cancer.[1,2]

It is somewhat difficult to look at Vitamin B12 in isolation from folic acid.

THE HYPE

The Pick-Me-Up Injection

B12 became known as a pick-me-up for a whole generation of people. People with pernicious anemia given B12 injections started making more red blood cells,

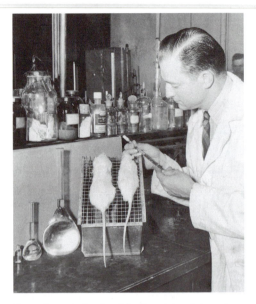

Experiments in the biochemistry laboratory at the University of Wisconsin established that one gram—about two thousandths of a pound—of the new vitamin would supply the daily requirements of 20 million rats. A millionth of a gram daily is used to tread pernicious anemia in humans. The rat at right, whose diet lacked B12, besides being smaller is also more nervous than his "brother." U. D. Register, graduate student in biochemistry at the university, is drawing a quantity of the vitamin from a tiny vial, August 10, 1949. (AP Photo)

and as their anemia went away, they got back their normal energy. What worked for one person feeling tired seemed like it might work for other people that were tired. Patients would go to the doctor and ask for their monthly B12 shot. Most doctors do not give B12 injections for this reason anymore, but it was not that long ago when they did.

B12 and Homocysteine

Elevated homocysteine levels have been found in a wide range of common and less common medical problems. B12, with or without folic acid, can lower levels of homocysteine. There is a lot about this that is not well understood yet. Are elevated homocysteine levels the cause of these diseases or just a marker for some other problem? Will giving B12 to people with elevated homocysteine levels actually lower the risk or even help cure some of these diseases? Is this hype, or are there actually studies to answer these questions? Here are some of the problems associated with both low B12 and high homocysteine.

Alzheimer's Disease, Depression, and Other Psychiatric and Neurologic Problems

Since a lack of B12 is known to cause dementia, depression, and other neurologic and psychiatric disorders, researchers have considered the possibility that low B12 levels might be found in patients with these conditions. Researchers have found low levels of B12 in elderly patients with depression,[3,4] patients with Alzheimer's disease and other cognitive disorders,[5,6] and even psychosis.[7,8]

In many studies, such as the Rotterdam study published in 2002,[4] participants were found to have elevated homocysteine levels along with lowered levels of B12. There is a Homocysteine Hypothesis of Depression, which postulates that elevated homocysteine levels may cause depression.[9,10] Anything decreasing homocysteine might help patients with depression, including supplements of B12 (and folic acid).

A similar mechanism involving elevated homocysteine may contribute to symptoms of Alzheimer's disease and dementia.[2,5] However, some studies have found lower B12 levels, but not elevated homocysteine levels, associated with declining cognitive function.[11]

Even if patients with low B12 levels and/or high homocysteine levels are more likely to be depressed or have difficulty with cognition, such as what is found in Alzheimer's disease, does that mean that supplements will improve their symptoms? This is the question that has to be answered in relationship to B12 and many neurologic and psychiatric conditions.

Cardiovascular Disease and Stroke

Since the level of B12 affects the level of homocysteine, and high homocysteine levels are associated with higher risk of cardiovascular disease, including coronary heart disease and stroke, it has been suggested that B12 supplementation might lower the risk of these conditions, in patients with elevated homocysteine.[1,12]

Cancer

Since B12 is necessary for DNA synthesis, low levels of the vitamin might hinder cell repair and lead to higher incidence of cancer. Perhaps supplemental B12 can reduce the risk of cancer. Lower rates of colon cancer and cervical cancer may be related to higher B12 levels.[12]

Other Possibilities

There are a number of other conditions that may be related to low B12 levels. They are also often associated with low folic acid levels and elevated homocysteine levels.

Folic acid is known to be necessary to prevent defects in the neural tube of the developing embryo. In some people, vitamin B12 may also be necessary.[12]

High levels of homocysteine may be related to early pregnancy loss and preeclampsia. This may be secondary to insufficient B12.[1]

Macular degeneration, a deterioration of the retina that can lead to blindness, is associated with high levels of homocysteine. It is possible that B12 might help treat this condition.[13]

There are many other conditions that may be related to elevated homocysteine levels and/or low B12 levels.

MECHANISM OF ACTION: HOW DOES IT WORK?

There are two specific enzymatic reactions in the body that are dependent on B12. The one that has received the most attention is the conversion of homocysteine to methionine. When there is a lack of B12, homocysteine levels rise. Elevated homocysteine levels are being discovered in a wide variety of diseases, as noted elsewhere in this chapter. The other reaction involves the conversion of methylmalonic acid to succinyl-CoA.[14,2]

B12 is needed for normal DNA synthesis. It is needed to make blood cells. When there is not enough B12, not enough red blood cells are made. Eventually, with severe deficiency, other blood cells will also decrease. The nervous system needs B12 and will show the effects of deficiency.

Vitamin B12 and folic acid work together in the body. In many cases it is difficult to separate their effects.

PRIMARY USES

B12 Deficiency (of All Types)

It is clear that vitamin B12 is necessary to all people for good health. It is indicated as a supplement for anyone who is deficient in B12.

Who develops a B12 deficiency? B12 exists in nutrients that come from animal tissues. Normally, B12 in food must be separated from the food in the stomach. It is there that intrinsic factor, made by parietal stomach cells, attaches to B12. The combination B12-intrinsic factor continues down the intestinal tract to the end of the small intestine called the terminal ileum. It is absorbed through the lining of the ileum, and from there, into the bloodstream. It binds to transcobolamin II and can then travel to the rest of the body.

The original understanding of B12 came from the study of people with pernicious anemia. Pernicious anemia is an autoimmune disorder, a disease in which the body mistakenly attacks itself. In this case, the body makes antibodies against the cells in the stomach that make intrinsic factor. People without intrinsic factor have trouble absorbing food-bound B12. They develop pernicious anemia.

Other Causes of B12 Deficiency

Most people get enough B12 in their diet, and in fact, have enough stored in their body that it takes years to develop a deficiency. Strict vegans can become low on B12 if they never eat anything from an animal source, as can the elderly and alcoholics, who may not be ingesting enough B12. More commonly, people who do not have enough hydrochloric acid in their stomachs develop B12 deficiency. The acid is needed to dissolve the B12 from its food source. Elderly people can become B12 deficient because they develop atrophic gastritis, and the stomach does not make enough acid. People of all ages take histamine blockers and proton-pump inhibitors to stop heartburn. These medicines are available over the counter, in generic and brand forms, from Zantac to Prilosec. With acid suppressed over a long period of time, people can develop a deficiency of B12 because it does not get separated from food.

Other less common causes include other causes of malabsorption in general, such as inflammation in the intestine from Crohn's disease, tapeworm, and bacterial overgrowth. Surgery involving removal of parts of the stomach or small bowel can also contribute to B12 deficiency.

It is possible for vitamin B12 deficiency to occur without anemia, and even with apparently normal blood levels of B12.[14] It may be necessary for other blood tests to be done in order to diagnose B12 deficiency, including checking homocysteine and methylmalonic acid levels. It is also possible for psychiatric and neurologic disease to be present without anemia. Anyone who might be at risk for B12 deficiency needs to keep this in mind.

Elderly Patients at Risk for Dementia and Vitamin B Deficiency

In one study, 20 percent of elderly patients had undiagnosed vitamin B12 deficiency.[6] Some doctors give B12 and folic acid to elderly patients for this reason.

Depression

There is evidence that people with higher levels of B12 improve faster when treated for depression.[15] Some psychiatrists are giving B12 to patients treated for depression.[16]

Macular Degeneration

One study showed that giving women at risk for cardiovascular disease supplements of B vitamins, including B12, lowered the risk of macular degeneration.[13]

COMMON DOSAGES

For Deficiency

Injections are not necessary for B12 deficiency or pernicious anemia. Large doses by mouth work just as well.[17,14] There are apparently other pathways by which B12 is absorbed in small amounts. If enough is take in, enough will be absorbed.

Oral doses of 1,000 to 2,000 µg per day are enough to correct deficiency but have to be taken for life if the cause is pernicious anemia or something else that cannot be corrected. Alternatively, B12 can be given by injection into muscle; 100 to 1,000 µg must be given every day or every other day for one to two weeks, followed by shots of 100 to 1,000 µg every one to three months for life.[14]

The Recommended Dietary Allowance (RDA) for B12 is 2.4 µg per day for healthy adult males and females. This goes up to 2.6 µg a day for pregnant and breast-feeding women. Most people consume much more than this in their diet. If, however, they are not absorbing B12 as explained above, they need to take a supplement containing large amounts of B12.

POTENTIAL SIDE EFFECTS

B12 is very safe to use and well tolerated by most people.

There are no established adverse effects from taking too much B12.

There have been reports of itching and rash following ingestion of B12, and also reports of diarrhea. B12 and pyridoxine together have been associated with rosacea fulminans, which may need to be treated with steroids. Vascular thrombosis has been reported. B12 replacement can make other hidden illnesses apparent, including polycythemia vera. B12 should not be taken by patients who are going to have coronary artery stents placed or who have Leber's disease—hereditary optic nerve atrophy.[23]

FACT VERSUS FICTION

There is proof that people with cardiovascular diseases, heart attacks, and strokes have elevated homocysteine levels. Vitamin B12 deficiency can cause elevated homocysteine levels. However, there is no proof at the current time that using B12 to lower homocysteine levels will actually lead to less cardiovascular disease, strokes, heart attacks, or death from cardiovascular causes.[18,19,20] It may be that further studies with larger groups of people over longer periods of time will show that B12 supplements do improve cardiovascular health. Or it may be that homocysteine is a marker for something else that is actually causing the damage, and that something else may need to be addressed.

There are conflicting studies about B12 supplements for neurologic or psychiatric problems.[21] Some have shown benefit to giving patients with Alzheimer's disease B12, with or without folic acid. Some have not.[18] There is evidence that many elderly patients are deficient in B12 without being anemic and go undiagnosed. So it may be that B12 supplements are really helping patients whose memory problems and other difficulties are actually caused by vitamin B12 deficiency.

Adding B12 has been shown in some studies to help people recover more quickly from depression.

Considering the fact that B12 is very safe to use and inexpensive, it seems reasonable to try supplements for people with depression or Alzheimer's disease and other similar conditions.[16] It also is important to make sure that vitamin B12 deficiency is not overlooked, especially in the elderly.[2]

The data in regard to neural tube defects are conflicting, and it is difficult to separate folic acid, B12 deficiency, and elevated homocysteine levels.[22,1] This is also true for a lot of the studies looking at cancer and B12 levels. There is a possibility that genetics may determine whether or not a B12 deficiency poses greater risks for certain people than others.[12]

It may be some time before there is more certainty regarding the use of supplementary B12 for a variety of conditions.

REFERENCES

1. Selhub, J. Public health significance of elevated homocysteine. *Food Nutr Bull*. 2008 Jun;29(2 Suppl):S116–S125.
2. Miller, AL. The methionine-homocysteine cycle and its effects on cognitive diseases. *Altern Med Rev*. 2003 Feb;8(1):7–19.
3. Penninx, Brenda WJH, Guralnik, JM, Ferrucci, L, Fried, LP, Allen, RH, and Stabler, SP. Vitamin B12 deficiency and depression in physically disabled older women: Epidemiologic evidence from the Women's Health and Aging Study. *Am J Psychiatry*. 2000;157:715–721.

4. Tiemeier, H, Ruud van Tuijl, H, Hofman, A, Meijer, J, Kiliaan, AJ, Breteler, MMB. Vitamin B12, folate, and homocysteine in depression: The Rotterdam Study. *Am J Psychiatry*. 2002;159:2099–2101.

5. Clarke, R, Smith, AD, Jobst, KA, Refsum, H, Sutton, L, Ueland, PM. Folate, vitamin B12, and serum total homocysteine levels in confirmed Alzheimer disease. *Arch Neurol*. 1998;55(11):1449–1455.

6. Hin, H, Clarke, R, Sherliker, P, Atoyebi, W, Emmens, K, Birks, J, Schneede, J, Ueland, PM, Nexo, E, Scott, J, Molloy, A, Donaghy, M, Frost, C, Evans, JG. Clinical relevance of low serum vitamin B12 concentrations in older people: The Banbury B12 Study. *Age & Ageing*. 2006 Jul;35(4):416–422.

7. Chronic psychosis associated with vitamin B12 deficiency. *J Assoc Physicians India*. 2008 Feb;56:115–116.

8. Durand, C, Mary, S, Brazo, P, Dollfus, S. Psychiatric manifestations of vitamin B12 deficiency: A case report. *Encephale*. 2003 Nov–Dec;29(6):560–565.

9. Folstein, M, Liu, T, Peter, I, Buel, J, Arsenault, L, Scott, T, Qiu, WW. The homocysteine hypothesis of depression. *Am J Psychiatry*. 2007;164:861–867.

10. Bjelland, I, Tell, GS, Vollset, SE, Refsum, H, Ueland, PM. Folate, vitamin B12, homocysteine, and the MTHFR 677C->T polymorphism in anxiety and depression: The Hordaland Homocysteine Study. *Arch Gen Psychiatry*. 2003;60(6):618–626.

11. Clarke, R, Birks, J, Nexo, E, Ueland, PM, Schneede, J, Scott, J, Molloy, A, Evans, JG. Low vitamin B-12 status and risk of cognitive decline in older adults. *Am J Clin Nutr*. 2007;86:1384–1391.

12. Ryan-Harshman, M, Aldoori, W. Vitamin B12 and health. *Can Fam Physician*. 2008;54:536–541.

13. Christen, WG, Glynn, RJ, Chew, EY, Albert, CM, Manson, JE. Folic acid, pyridoxine, and cyanocobalamin combination treatment and age-related macular degeneration in women: The Women's Antioxidant and Folic Acid Cardiovascular Study. *Arch Intern Med*. 2009;169(4):335–341.

14. Oh, RC, Brown, DL. Vitamin B12. *Am Fam Physician*. 2003 Mar 1; 67(5):993–994.

15. Hintikka, J, Tolmunen, T, Tanskanen, A, Viinamäki, H. High vitamin B12 level and good treatment outcome may be associated in major depressive disorder. *BMC Psychiatry*. 2003;3:17.

16. Coppen, A, Bolander-Gouaille, C. Treatment of depression: Time to consider folic acid and vitamin B12. *J Psychopharmacol*. 2005 Jan;19:59–65.

17. Kuzminski, AM, Del Giacco, EJ, Allen, RH, Stabler, SP, Lindenbaum, J. Effective treatment of cobalamin deficiency with oral cobalamin. *Blood*. 1998;92:1191–1198.

18. Lonn, E, Yusuf, S, Arnold, MJ, et al. Homocysteine lowering with folic acid and B vitamins in vascular disease. *N Engl J Med*. 2006;354(15):1567–1577.

19. Albert, CM, Cook, NR, Gaziano, JM, Zaharris, E, MacFadyen, J, Danielson, E, Buring, JE, Manson, JE. Effect of folic acid and B vitamins on risk of cardiovascular events and total mortality among women at high risk for cardiovascular disease: A randomized trial. *JAMA*. 2008;299(17):2027–2036.

20. Ebbing, M, Bleie, O, Ueland, PM, Nordrehaug, JE, Nilsen, DW, Vollset, SE, Refsum, H, Pedersen, EKR, Nygard, O. Mortality and cardiovascular events in patients treated with homocysteine-lowering B vitamins after coronary angiography: A randomized controlled trial. *JAMA*. 2008;300(7):795–804.

21. Malouf, R, Evans, JG. Folic acid with or without vitamin B12 for the prevention and treatment of healthy elderly and demented people. *Cochrane Database of Systematic Reviews*. 2008 Oct 8;4. Art. No.: CD004514. doi:10.1002/14651858.

22. Ray, JG, Blom, HJ. Vitamin B12 insufficiency and the risk of fetal neural tube defects. *QJM*. 2003;96(4):289–295.

23. Medline Plus review. Vitamin B12. http://www.nlm.nih.gov/medlineplus/druginfo/natural/patient-vitaminb12.html. Accessed December 30, 2010.

32

Vitamin D

BRIEF OVERVIEW

Vitamin D is a fat-soluble vitamin that is made in human skin when it is exposed to ultraviolet light. It can also be found naturally in a few foods and added as a supplement to other foods. Vitamin D is not active until it has been metabolized in the body. It must undergo two processes called hydroxylation, one in the liver and one in the kidney. The active form of vitamin D is 1,25-dihydroxyvitamin D [1,25(OH)$_2$D], also called calcitriol.

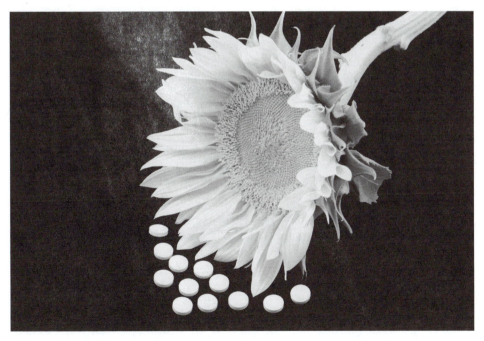

Very few foods have significant amounts of vitamin D; the best source is exposure to sunlight. (© Boomfeed/Dreamstime.com)

Vitamin D is absolutely essential for bone health. The most obvious conditions related to serious deficiency of vitamin D involve bone—the bony deformities of childhood rickets, the painful soft bones of adult osteomalacia, or the thin, easy-to-fracture bones of older adults with osteoporosis. However, vitamin D does much more in the body than was initially thought, and new actions of the vitamin are being discovered and described by current researchers. At the same time, it is becoming clear that many people have less-than-optimal levels of the vitamin, which in addition to damaging bones, makes them susceptible to a large range of other health problems. Many experts consider vitamin D insufficiency a worldwide epidemic.[1]

Vitamin D made in the human body is D_3, also called cholecalciferol. This is also the form of vitamin D found in animal-derived food. There is another form, called D_2, or ergocalciferol, made from yeast. While supplements used to contain either form, it is now known that D_3 is many times more potent than D_2.[2] Most supplements now contain D_3. It is important to try and see which form of the vitamin is in any supplement.[3] In this chapter, vitamin D will mean D_3 unless otherwise noted.

THE HYPE

The first question is—who should take vitamin D? The answer might turn out to be just about everyone. The next question is—how much should they take?

Many people know that they need vitamin D in addition to calcium for good bone health. However, there is a lot more to vitamin D than that. For example, there is "the vitamin D hypothesis." It has been observed that the occurrence and mortality rates of many diseases increase the farther away from the equator the population is. In North America, there is increased mortality from cancer, cardiovascular disease, and diabetes traveling north. Additionally, patients survive longer if they are diagnosed with cardiovascular disease and certain cancers during the summer as opposed to the winter.

The vitamin D hypothesis is that decreased skin synthesis of vitamin D at higher latitudes causes the increased incidence of these diseases and the increased mortality. This hypothesis has received support from the discovery of vitamin D receptors in cells all over the body; these receptors have many important functions (see "Mechanism of Action" below). It follows that people with higher levels of vitamin D should have lower mortality rates. At least one review of multiple studies that included mortality data showed a decreased risk of overall mortality with vitamin D supplementation, 400 to 830 IU of vitamin D per day.[4]

The following information about vitamin D's possible connection to a wide variety of diseases is not exhaustive. There are investigators looking at other possibilities, including but not limited to, depression, Alzheimer's disease, specific kinds of cancer, heart failure, autism, chronic pain, and longevity.

Osteoporosis

When doctors started treating osteoporosis, the first thing given was calcium. Even though the function of vitamin D was known, since it is made in human skin, it did not seem necessary. However, it has become clear that many people are vitamin D deficient. They need supplementary vitamin D along with calcium to build bones, to prevent osteoporosis in the first place, and to treat it if it occurs.

Studies of supplementation have been done to verify that osteoporosis is being prevented or improved by treatment. Scans of bone density can tell if supplements appear to be working. However, since the reason to treat osteoporosis is to prevent fractures, that is the endpoint that trials need to evaluate.

Some trials of calcium with lower doses of vitamin D do not show evidence of fracture prevention, whereas with higher doses of vitamin D, fracture risk is usually decreased. And 400 IU of vitamin D may not be enough; at least 1,000 to even 5,000 IU's may be needed, depending on what one's vitamin D level is.

In one trial done in the United Kingdom, vitamin D alone was used. The dose was 100,000 IU, once every four months, given to half the study participants at random. This trial lasted five years. The 100,000 IU given every four months is about 833 IU a day; vitamin D is retained in the body. The group given vitamin D had a 33 percent lower rate of fractures of the hip, wrist, forearm, or vertebra. The investigators checked vitamin D levels for a portion of each of the two groups, placebo and treated. It was 74.3 nmol/L (nanomoles per liter) in those given vitamin D, and 53.4 in the group given placebo.[5] While these numbers may not seem worth remembering, the amount of vitamin D measured in the blood is at the center of the debate about how much vitamin D to take. In this case, according to many experts, the 74.3 nmol/L would be in the range necessary to prevent fractures.

An analysis of vitamin D dose and fracture prevention, reviewing many available trials, published in 2005 clearly showed that 400 IU was an inadequate amount of vitamin D for this purpose. It was found that 700 to 800 IU vitamin D was associated with a 26 percent reduction of hip fracture risk and a 23 percent lower risk of any nonvertebral fracture (any fracture except the backbone). The authors noted that in addition to strengthening bone, vitamin D has also been shown to prevent falls, which may contribute to the decrease in fractures.[6] Most, but not all, other reviewers have come to similar conclusions.

Despite the evidence that 400 IU of vitamin D are probably not sufficient to prevent fractures, studies already in progress were using this dose. For example, in a placebo-controlled, randomized trial reported in the *New England Journal of Medicine* in 2006, more than 36,282 women were studied over approximately seven years. Half received placebo; the other half were given 1,000 mg calcium carbonate and 400 IU vitamin D. This did slightly reduce the incidence of fractures, but it was not statistically significant. The authors of this study noted that more vitamin D was probably needed.[7]

This was part of the U.S. Women's Health Initiative Study designed approximately 20 years earlier, at which time 400 IU of vitamin D seemed enough. Despite this information, there were still news reports that vitamin D and calcium did not reduce fractures in people with osteoporosis; this kind of information most likely had an effect on both doctors' and patients' decisions about vitamin D.[8]

While fracture risk has not been lowered with 400 IU vitamin D, there is fairly wide consensus that 700 IU to 800 IU of vitamin D, along with calcium, can be an effective way to prevent and treat osteoporosis. A number of studies have shown increases of bone density and decreases in fractures. Studies that have shown little benefit tend to be community-based and with a demonstrated compliance problem. Studies of institutionalized patients who definitely took the supplements have more consistently shown benefits.[6,9,10]

Some advocate supplementing all people at risk for osteoporosis or with measured, low vitamin D levels.[9]

Unanswered questions revolve around exact vitamin D doses and who should take supplements.

Falls

There are multiple studies demonstrating that vitamin D by itself lowers the risk of falls. The most common cause of injury leading to death in the elderly is a fall. Falls lead to fractures and functional decline in the elderly. Falls lead to 40 percent of admissions to nursing homes.[11]

An analysis done in 2004 indicated that vitamin D may reduce the risk of falls in elderly patients both in institutions and at home by more than 20 percent. The authors of this review suggested the need for more study, especially in regard to vitamin D dose and calcium supplementation. There is also a need for more study involving men.[11]

Some of the clinical trials evaluating vitamin D (with or without calcium) for osteoporosis found a significant decrease in falls even if not fractures. There tend to be more falls and more fractures when vitamin D levels are below 25–30 nmol/L.[9]

Considering the high cost of falls, in terms of the health, longevity, and quality of life of the elderly, vitamin D should be considered for all older people for this reason alone. The dose suggested in this study was 800 IU.[11]

Muscle Strength

It is believed that the effect of vitamin D on falls has at least in part to do with improving muscle strength. Active vitamin D binds to receptors in muscles. This leads to improved function and reduced falls. Muscular weakness tends to occur at levels of 25(OH)D less than 50 nmol/L.[9]

Hypertension

Studies have shown an association between higher levels of vitamin D and lower levels of systolic blood pressure. The association of hypertension with vitamin D status is very strong.[2] One study reported the association in white persons without hypertension, another in non-Hispanic white as well as black persons. This deserves further investigation.[12]

Diabetes

Children treated with vitamin D have a lower incidence of type 1 diabetes. Conversely, vitamin D deficient children have an increased risk of developing type 1 diabetes.[13]

Vitamin D may also help prevent type 2 diabetes. Multiple studies have shown an inverse relationship between vitamin D levels and incidence of type 2 diabetes.[14] This may be due to a direct effect of vitamin D on insulin action, or it may be due to its effects on inflammation.

Cardiovascular Disease

There also appears to be an increased risk of cardiovascular disease in patients with low vitamin D levels. For example, a study of a group of 1,739 individuals in 2008 found an association between low vitamin D levels and cardiovascular disease.[15]

Increased vitamin D blood levels have been shown to decrease the risk of cardiovascular disease. In one study of 9,400 patients, most female, the participants whose vitamin D levels rose above 43 ng/mL over the course of a year had 47 percent less risk of cardiovascular disease than those whose vitamin D levels did not get that high.

The same group of investigators evaluated 31,000 people, who they placed into three groups depending on their vitamin D levels. Participants in each group who raised their levels above 43 ng/mL had lower rates of cardiovascular disease, as well as high blood pressure, kidney failure, heart attack, heart failure, diabetes, depression, and death. The researchers suggested that 1,000 to 5,000 IU of vitamin D might be the right amount of vitamin D to take, for people with low levels.[16]

Cancer

Multiple epidemiologic studies have shown a higher rate of colon and breast cancer at higher latitudes, where vitamin D levels are lower. There may be a two-fold increased risk of colon cancer when levels are less than 50 nm/L. Similar observations have been made about prostate cancer and cancer in general in northern Europe.[13]

In a double-blind, placebo-controlled trial of calcium (1,400–1,500 mg) and vitamin D (1,100 IU) designed to look at fracture rates, cancer incidence was also noted. There were approximately 1,800 postmenopausal women in the study, which ran for four years. Vitamin D status was also checked at the beginning and after a year, which showed a significant rise in the women taking vitamin D. There was a statistically significant reduction (60%–75%) in all cancer rates in the groups of patients taking D alone, or vitamin D and calcium, as opposed to the placebo group. The researchers also found that baseline and treatment-induced vitamin D levels were good indicators of cancer risk.[17]

Infection

At least one group of investigators has suggested that the reason for the increase in influenza (flu) during the winter is vitamin D deficiency from decreased sun exposure.[18] Low vitamin D levels may contribute to reduced resistance to many types of infection, including tuberculosis.

Multiple Sclerosis

The association between high latitudes with less sun exposure and multiple sclerosis is well known.[13]

Wheezing

There is an association between lower maternal intake of vitamin D during pregnancy and wheezing of children at ages 3 and 5. This may result in more children with asthma.[19,20]

DEFICIENCY

There is a spectrum of vitamin D deficiency, from childhood rickets, to adult osteomalacia, to adult osteoporosis, as well as increased risk of many diseases and problems throughout life.

Severe deficiency of vitamin D in children causes rickets. Rickets was first described as a disease in the middle of the 17th century in England. The main defect in rickets is soft bones. This leads to characteristic deformities of the skeleton. It took centuries before the cause of rickets was ascertained. Cod liver oil was noted to reverse rickets. About 100 years ago, vitamin D, a fat-soluble vitamin in cod liver oil, was identified.

Milk has been fortified with vitamin D for many years. However, there are still cases of rickets in the United States, as well as the United Kingdom and other European countries. It is most commonly seen in breast-fed infants who are not getting supplements and whose mothers are not getting supplements. This is especially true of dark-skinned infants and mothers, as well as those with less sun exposure.[3]

In adults, lack of vitamin D also causes softened bones, a condition called osteomalacia. Weak muscles often go along with the weak bones. Adults often have bone pain.[3]

Insufficiency

Inadequate levels of vitamin D, as opposed to little-or-no vitamin D (insufficiency as opposed to deficiency), increase the risk of a wide range of problems in adults, from osteoporosis to many of the other problems described in this chapter.

Many groups of people are at risk for vitamin D insufficiency.[1,3]
These include:

- Older adults, 50 years of age and up. About 40 to 100 percent of the elderly in the United States and Europe who live at home, in some surveys, are vitamin D deficient. The skin is less able to make vitamin D and the kidneys are less able to activate it.
- Pregnant and breast-feeding women in most areas of the world, as well as breast-fed infants. There is not enough vitamin D in breast milk (see "Common Dosages" below).

- Children and young adults. Estimates place anywhere from 40 to 50 percent or so of young adults and children as vitamin D deficient, regardless of race or ethnicity. In one study, 32 percent of healthy students and physicians at a Boston hospital were vitamin D deficient even when drinking a glass of milk a day, taking a multivitamin, and eating salmon once a week.[30]

- People with trouble absorbing fat, since vitamin D is a fat-soluble vitamin. This could include people with cystic fibrosis as well as Crohn's disease. After gastric bypass surgery, vitamin D absorption is reduced.

- Obesity. Vitamin D is stored in fat, and with large amounts of fat, large amounts of the vitamin can be in the fat and not available to the body for use.

- People with dark skin. Groups with darker skin because of increased pigmentation make less vitamin D in the skin. Vitamin D deficiency is seen more frequently in ethnic groups with darker skin.

- Residents at higher latitudes, where there may not be enough sun exposure during part of the year to make vitamin D.

- People who avoid the sun.[21] The amount of sunlight necessary varies depending on location. It has been estimated that it takes 5 to 30 minutes of sun exposure between 10 A.M. and 3 P.M., leaving uncovered the face, arms, legs or back, without sunscreen, at least twice a week to meet the necessary requirements for vitamin D. Many people do not do this. In countries where they are shielded from the sun due to cultural practices, for example, Saudi Arabia and India, 30 to 50 percent of children and adults are deficient.[3]

There have been articles like one from the American Society for Nutrition in which it was argued that vitamin D deficiency is a widespread nutritional disorder and that the old recommended amounts of vitamin D supplements are not correcting the problem.[22] This article included a plea for action on the part of health care providers.

How Do You Determine Vitamin D Status?

People need to take enough vitamin D to avoid insufficiency symptoms, but some of these are not obvious. Researchers are trying to calibrate blood tests to be very consistent and correct in detecting low, normal, and high, potentially toxic levels of vitamin D.

The best blood test at the current time to assess vitamin D status is the serum concentration of 25(OH)D, or hydroxyvitamin D. This gives an indication of D status as it is produced in the skin or taken in with food or supplements. There is ongoing research to determine if the cut-off levels in use currently are actually best. This test was designated as the best indicator of vitamin D status by the National Institutes of Health in 1997, making further work easier.[23]

There was also a great amount of variation between different laboratories performing the same test. As of 2009, there is a reference sample of vitamin D that labs can use to validate the accuracy of their testing, provided by the National Institute of Standards and Technology.[24]

Hydroxyvitamin D concentrations of less than 37.5 nmol/L (nanomoles per liter) are too low. Concentrations equal to or greater than 37.5 nmol/L have been considered adequate in the past, and they are currently "officially" considered normal.[23]

Levels in that range may not be high enough to maintain bone health as well as other D-dependent functions. Levels greater than75 nmol/L have been suggested as best. The Food and Nutrition Board indicated in 2006 that it might be recommending something in the range of this level in its next official publication.[25]

In 2007, an article in the *New England Journal of Medicine* suggested that 52 to 72 nmol/L (or 21 to 29 ng/mL) might be adequate.[1] Using this or similar cut-offs, there may be as many as 1 billion people who are at least partially deficient in vitamin D.

Others have suggested levels equal to or greater than 75 nmol/L,[22] or approximately 78 nmol/L. At this level, vitamin D causes the maximum efficiency of calcium transport in the intestine.[13]

Yet other experts suggest a cut-off at 80 nmol/L. That would mean an even higher dietary intake.[2]

FOOD SOURCES

Very few foods have significant amounts of vitamin D.[13] Fish liver oils contain a lot of vitamin D, including cod liver oil, which was first used to cure rickets. Cod liver oil has 1,360 IU of vitamin D per tablespoon. The flesh of fatty fish such as salmon has vitamin D, as do the liver and fat from mammals living in and around cold water, including seals and polar bears. Hens that are fed vitamin D will produce eggs with vitamin D, but the amount is variable. The vitamin is in the yolk.

Most fish can contain 200 to 600 IU vitamin D per 100 grams. Atlanta herring have even more. Other fish are also good sources of vitamin D, including salmon, mackerel, and tuna.

Most vitamin D–fortified foods are breakfast cereals and milk products as well as orange juice. Reading labels can give an idea of what is supposed to be in the product.[3]

While milk is supposed to contain 400 IU a quart in the United States, sampling has shown that not all milk contains near that amount.[25]

A list of foods with vitamin D content can be found on the USDA Web site,[26] at http://www.ars.usda.gov/SP2UserFiles/Place/12354500/Data/SR22/nutrlist/sr22a324.pdf.

MECHANISM OF ACTION: HOW DOES IT WORK?

Vitamin D is absolutely necessary for bone health. Deficiency causes rickets in children and osteomalacia in adults, both conditions with very weak bones.

Vitamin D facilitates calcium absorption in the small intestine. Calcium and phosphate levels in the blood need to be in the right range for bones to be normal and to prevent symptoms of low calcium. This is vitamin D's well-known endocrine function.

Human bone is constantly being remodeled. That means that some bone is being absorbed, and some is being formed, so that old bone is replaced by new bone. Vitamin D is necessary for these processes to proceed normally. While vitamin D deficiency causes rickets in children and osteomalacia in adults, in older adults, both D and calcium are needed to prevent osteoporosis.

When calcium in the diet is low, vitamin D activates osteoclasts so that calcium comes out of the bone to maintain blood levels of calcium. If vitamin D is also low, as calcium levels lower, parathyroid hormone (PTH) is stimulated, which causes a number of processes to try and elevate calcium levels, including activating more osteoclasts to get calcium out of bone.[3]

After being consumed, vitamin D reaches the liver where it is hydroxylated; 25(OH)D then enters the bloodstream. That is when it can be measured. It is hydroxylated again in the kidney, becoming the active form of vitamin D. In the kidneys, this step is regulated by parathyroid hormone.

The second hydroxylation can also take place in certain cells, such as activated macrophages, some cancerous lymphoma cells, cultured skin, and bone cells.[23] Other cells that can accomplish the second hydroxylation include cells in the placenta, colon, brain, and prostate, and cells in the parathyroid glands. The other sites besides the kidney may play an important role in vitamin D's action outside of bone; the conversion outside of the kidney is not regulated by PTH or related to calcium concentrations.

Many cells have a vitamin D receptor (VDR) for activated vitamin D, including much of the intestine, activated T and B lymphocytes (parts of the immune system), pancreatic islet cells (which make insulin), and most organs, including breast, prostate, gonads, skin, brain, heart, and mononuclear cells. Because of the VDR in skin cells, topical vitamin D is an effective treatment for psoriasis.[13]

In addition to vitamin D's endocrine function, working as a hormone to regulate calcium metabolism, it also has an autocrine function, through which it facilitates gene expression in many cells.[2] The expression of genes can cause cell proliferation, differentiation, and even apoptosis (planned death). It is by the autocrine pathway, attached to VDRs in cells, that vitamin D causes many effects, including modulation of immune function and neuromuscular function and reduction of inflammation.

It is believed that the VDR activity may be the key to why vitamin D deficiency is associated with so many diseases. Activated vitamin D is one of the strongest regulators of the growth of both normal and cancerous cells. It is possible that the local production of activated vitamin D may prevent cells from becoming cancerous. Vitamin D may also work via activated T and B lymphocytes, which are very important in the immune system.[13]

When activated, VDR can cause cell differentiation while decreasing metastatic potential, cell growth, invasiveness, and blood vessel growth. This combination of effects may be involved in the beginnings of cancers and in cardiovascular disease. Activated vitamin D is known to affect the transport of bile acids, rennin production (which affects blood pressure), the lining and walls of blood vessels, and the endocrine system.[4]

PRIMARY USES

- To prevent rickets: In 2008, the American Academy of Pediatrics (APA) changed its guidelines, based on the understanding of the prevalence of vitamin D deficiency in infants, children, and adolescents. This is due to limited dietary sources of vitamin D, children getting less sun exposure, and the knowledge that previous guidelines were too low. The APA still recommends that children should minimize direct sunlight exposure to prevent skin cancer, even though this means children must take vitamin D supplements.[27] The APA recommends giving all infants, children, and most adolescents vitamin D supplements (see "Common Dosages").

- For generally good health in children: The American Academy of Pediatrics recommends supplemental vitamin D for all children. While this will prevent rickets, the APA also believes it may help maintain good health. The APA recommends that adolescents who don't drink enough milk with vitamin D should have their status assessed, and D given if needed.

- Treatment of osteoporosis: Vitamin D along with calcium is needed to treat osteoporosis. The dose of vitamin D is still being investigated. Any individual at risk of osteoporosis should be taking vitamin D and calcium. Blood levels of vitamin D can be used to check adequacy of vitamin D supplementation.

- To prevent osteoporosis: Vitamin D and calcium should also be taken to prevent osteoporosis in patients at risk. The amount of vitamin D can be assessed by using blood levels.

- For elderly patients: to treat or prevent osteoporosis and to limit falls.

- For general good health: While no adult organization similar to the APA for children has endorsed supplemental vitamin D for everyone, there are many groups and experts that think that more than half of many populations are D deficient. Many doctors will recommend supplements for people at risk (see above), or order vitamin D levels to get an idea of what is needed. There is a need to educate both health care professionals and the general public. Many people are not getting needed vitamin D.

- It used to be assumed that people got their vitamin D from the sun, so supplements were not needed. At this time, even at the old guidelines (see below), most people are not getting enough D without supplements.

COMMON DOSAGES

It may seem simple, but in order to know how much vitamin D people should take, it has to be determined how much they need. At the current time, these recommendations are in flux as new data and information become available.

As stated previously, when noted here, vitamin D means D_3. And 40 IU of vitamin D is equal to 1 μg.[3]

The last official set of guidelines from the Food and Nutrition Board at the Institute of Medicine in 1997 suggests dosages of vitamin D that most experts consider too low. It is expected that it will revise the values in 2010 or 2011. The AIs (Adequate Intakes) set in 1997 for Vitamin D were:

- 200 IU from birth to 50 years of age
- 400 IU from age 51 to 70 years of age
- 600 IU for those over 71 years of age

In an update from a workshop published in 2006, the FNB indicated that the level of 25(OH)D likely to prevent fractures should be set at around 75 nmol/L. This would probably mean doses of 800–2,000 IU should be taken. It was also noted that daily doses of as much as 1,000 to 4,000 IU a day had been taken for five months with no toxicity.[25]

Supplementation may be more important during the winter months in some areas.[21]

The American Pediatric Association recommends that pregnant women take enough vitamin D to achieve blood levels of greater than 80 nmol/L. This would be more than the amount (400 IU) in standard prenatal vitamins. For breast-feeding women, very large amounts of vitamin D must be taken to increase the amount of the vitamin taken in by the baby in a significant way. The APA supports giving supplements to breast-fed infants, 400 IU of vitamin D soon after birth and through childhood. Many infant preparations contain 400 IU in a drop. All infant formulas sold in the United States have enough vitamin D to deliver about 400 IU a day to infants.[27]

Once a baby is weaned from formula, supplemental D must be given. Adolescents who do not eat/drink enough vitamin D–enriched milk and food should also take 400 IU vitamin D. Some children and teenagers need more than this; their vitamin D levels should be checked.[27]

With a dose of 400 IU suggested for infants, it seems very likely that the recommended dose for adults will be raised to the 800 IU area.

It is estimated that for each additional 100 IU a day ingested, the vitamin D level will go up approximately 2.5 nmol/L.[2] This information can be used to guide supplementation when the D level is known.

POTENTIAL SIDE EFFECTS

Since vitamin D is fat soluble, too much vitamin D can accumulate in the body and cause toxicity. Serum concentrations of hydroxyvitamin D that stay above 500 nmol/L can be toxic.[3]

Some experts say levels greater than 374 nmol/L can be toxic.[1]

Most often, the level of vitamin D that causes an increase in serum calcium is considered too high. The serum level of 25(OH)D needed to cause hypercalcemia is greater than 600 nmol/L.[28]

In 2007, a review suggested using 220 nmol/L as the Upper Level (UL) where there is No Observed Adverse Effect (NOAEL). This corresponds to a dose of

10,000 IU of vitamin D_3.[28] Others have agreed that a safe upper limit of 10,000 IU is appropriate.[2]

In 2008, different reviewers suggested 250 nmol/L as the upper limit. However, they also noted that evidence does suggest that levels up to 750 nmol/L may in fact be safe.[29]

Most reports of actual toxicity involve accidental ingestions of large quantities of vitamin D. Symptoms can include high serum calcium, hypertension, pain, conjunctivitis, thirst, nausea, vomiting, weight loss, anorexia, fever, chills, excess urination, and difficulty concentrating. The serum 25(OH)D levels in these cases range from 700 to greater than 1,600 nmol/L. A review of multiple studies found that there is not an increased risk of kidney stones with vitamin D and calcium, even at the higher levels of D along with calcium.[28]

If the Upper Limit (UL) of supplement intake is 10,000, even considering the small amounts of vitamin D in the diet and some D that might be in a multivitamin, 800 IU more would result in a serum level much less than the amount that causes hypercalcemia.[28]

FACT VERSUS FICTION

Vitamin D should be taken by pregnant women, and all breast-fed babies. Formula-fed babies need vitamin D once weaned off formula. From that point on, all children of all ages through adolescence should be taking 400 IU vitamin D.[27]

The dose in adults recommended by the IOM is 400 IU for adults and 600 IU for the elderly. This is almost certainly too low, and new recommendations are expected; 800 IU is probably the best dose for most adults and older people.

For those at risk of vitamin D deficiency, which is essentially all elderly people, measuring vitamin D levels may be needed to establish that the D intake is sufficient. This is important to prevent or treat osteoporosis in the elderly as well as help prevent falls.

If you are at risk of osteoporosis, or have osteoporosis, you should be taking at least 800 IU of vitamin D, plus appropriate levels of calcium. If you are not sure what you should be taking, it is best to have your serum 25(OH)D level checked.

Elderly patients should be taking vitamin D to prevent falls.

Having your vitamin D level checked, and taking enough of the vitamin to get the blood level into the desired range, is always a reasonable idea, especially if you are at risk for vitamin D insufficiency. The correct range is still under investigation. It should almost certainly be above 50 nmol/L and probably above 75 nmol/L, but below 220 nmol/L. You can discuss this with your health care provider, and watch for announcements about new recommendations.

There is a lot of evidence that sufficiency of vitamin D may reduce the risk of many common diseases, from cardiovascular disease to cancer. Many studies have shown an association with low levels of vitamin D and higher risk of disease, and also the opposite, high levels of vitamin D and lower risk of disease. These studies do not prove cause and effect.

Large controlled trials using vitamin D still need to be done to see if raising vitamin D levels does in fact lower the risk of any of the diseases under question.

With osteoporosis and falls, most, but not all, trials have shown a decreased risk if enough vitamin D is ingested. There is enough information for most doctors to conclude that supplements will work to treat osteoporosis and lower the risk of falls in the elderly.

However, for most of the other diseases, the studies have not been done, or there are conflicting results. Some experts worry that giving everyone large doses of vitamin D might turn out to cause other problems. They are thinking of other vitamins, like vitamin E, that were associated with lower disease risk in observational studies but were found not as helpful in clinical trials. In fact, supplemental vitamin E seems to increase the risk of some of the diseases researchers were trying to treat. Experts point to this example as a reason to be cautious.

But there are two key differences. One, vitamin D is known to be necessary for health; absolute deficiency or very low levels cause significant disease, rickets in children. Second, enough work has been done to establish guidelines about vitamin D levels in blood serum. If there is a question about insufficiency versus sufficiency, or unsafe high levels, a blood test can answer the question. Not everyone can or will get this test. But on an individual basis, you can talk to your doctor about this test if you are not sure what to do.

Research will provide better guidelines in the future.

REFERENCES

1. Holick, MF. Vitamin D deficiency. *New Engl J Med* 357(3):266–281 (2007).

2. Heaney, RP. Vitamin D in health and disease. *Clan J Am Soc Nephrology.* 2008;3:1535–1541.

3. National Institutes of Health. Office of Dietary Supplements. *Dietary Supplement Fact Sheet: Vitamin D. Health Professional Fact Sheet.* Last updated November 13, 2009. http://dietary-supplements.info.nih.gov/factsheets/vitamind.asp#en4. Accessed April 5, 2010.

4. Augier, P, Gemini, S. Vitamin D supplementation and total mortality. *Arch Intern Med.* 2007;167(16):1730–1737.

5. Thrived, DP, Doll, R, Chaw, KT. Effect of four monthly oral vitamin D3 (cholecalciferol) supplementation on fractures and mortality in men and women living in the community: Randomized double blind controlled trial. *BMJ.* 2003;326:469–475.

6. Bischoff-Ferrari, HA, Willett, WC, Wong, JB, et al. Fracture prevention with vitamin D supplementation: A meta-analysis of randomized controlled trials. *JAMA.* 2005;293:2257–2264.

7. Jackson, RD, Labroid, AZ, Gas, M, et al. Calcium plus vitamin D supplementation and the risk of fractures. *N Engl J Med.* 2006;354:669–683.

8. Brown, SE. Vitamin D and fracture reduction: An evaluation of the existing research. *Altern Med Rev.* 2008;13(1):21–33.

9. Lips, P, Bouillon, R, van School, NM, et al. Reducing fracture risk with calcium and vitamin D. *Clinical Endocrinology.* Accepted article. July 20, 2009. doi:10.1111/j.13652265.2009.03701.x.

10. Cranny, A, Horsley, T, O'Donnell, S, et al. Effectiveness and safety of vitamin D in relation to bone health. *Avid Rep Techno Assess (Full Rep).* 2007; 158:1–235.

11. Bischoff-Ferrari, HA, Dawson-Hughes, B, Willett, WC, et al. Effect of vitamin D on falls: A meta-analysis. *JAMA.* 2004;291:1999–2006.

12. Judd, SE, Names, MS, Ziegler, TR, et al. Optimal vitamin D status attenuates the age-associated increase in systolic blood pressure in white Americans: Results from the third National Health and Nutrition Examination Survey. *Am J Clin Nutr.* 2008;87:136–141.

13. Hoosick, MF. Sunlight and vitamin D for bone health and prevention of autoimmune diseases, cancers, and cardiovascular disease. *Am J Clin Nutr.* 2004;80(Suppl):1678S–1688S.

14. Kylie, T, Groff, A, Remer, J, et al. Vitamin D: An evidence-based review. *J Am Board Fam Med.* 2009;22:698–706.

15. Wang, TJ, Pembina, MJ, Booth, SL, et al. Vitamin D deficiency and risk of cardiovascular disease. *Circulation.* 2008;117:503–511.

16. Intermountain Healthcare. Press release, March 17, 2010. Presented at the American College of Cardiology 59th Annual Scientific Session on March 15, 2010, Atlanta, GA.

17. Lapped, JM, Travers-Gustafson, D, Davies, KM, et al. Vitamin D and calcium supplementation reduces cancer risk: Results of a randomized trial. *Am J Clin Nutr.* 2007;85:1586–1591.

18. Cannel, JJ, Castoff, M, Garland, CF, et al. On the epidemiology of influenza. *Virology Journal.* 2008;5:29. doi:10.1186/1743–422X-5–29.

19. Devereuz, G, Litonjua, AA, Turner, SW, et al. Maternal vitamin D intake during pregnancy and early childhood wheezing. *Am J Clin Nutr.* 2007;85:853–859.

20. Camargo, CA, Rifas-Shiman, SL, Litonjua, AA, et al. Maternal intake of vitamin D during pregnancy and risk of recurrent wheeze in children at 3 y of age. *Am J Clin Nutr.* 2007;85:788–795.

21. Vitamin D. *Altern Med Rev.* 2008;13(2):153–164.

22. Vieth, R, Bischoff-Ferrari, H, Boucher, BJ, et al. The urgent need to recommend an intake of vitamin D that is effective. *Am J Clin Nutr.* 2007;85:649–650.

23. Institute of Medicine. *Dietary reference intakes for calcium, phosphorus, magnesium, vitamin D, and fluoride.* Washington, DC: National Academies Press, 1997. http://books.nap.edu/openbook.php?record_id=5776&page=250. Accessed April 5, 2010.

24. National Institute of Standards and Technology. NIST releases vitamin D standard reference material. *NIST Tech Beat.* July 14, 2009. http://www.nist.gov/public_affairs/techbeat/tb2009_0714.htm. Accessed April 5, 2010.

25. Institute of Medicine. Food and Nutrition Board. *Dietary reference intakes research synthesis: Workshop summary.* Washington, DC: National Academies Press, 2006. http://books.nap.edu/openbook.php?record_id=11767&page=R1. Accessed April 5, 2009.

26. U.S. Department of Agriculture. USDA National Nutrient Database for Standard Reference, Release 22. http://www.ars.usda.gov/SP2UserFiles/Place/12354500/Data/SR22/nutrlist/sr22a324.pdf. Accessed April 6, 2010.

27. Wagner, CL, Greer, FR. Prevention of rickets and vitamin D deficiency in infants, children, and adolescents. *Pediatrics.* 2008;122:1142–1152.

28. Hathcock, JN, Shao, A, Vieth, R, Heaney, R. Risk assessment for vitamin D. *Am J Clin Nutr.* 2007;85:6–18.

29. Jones, G. Pharmokinetics of vitamin D toxicity. *Am J Clin Nutr.* 2008;88 (Suppl):582S–586S.

30. Tangpricha, V, Pearce, EN, Chen, TC, Holick, MF. Vitamin D insufficiency among free-living healthy young adults. *Am J Med.* 2002;112:659–662.

33

Vitamin E

BRIEF OVERVIEW

Vitamin E was discovered over 80 years ago as a substance necessary for female rats to reproduce. Many years of research have answered some questions about this fat soluble vitamin and its actions in humans. Its antioxidant properties have been studied and analyzed, leading to the use of the vitamin to prevent a number of diseases.[1]

With vitamin E, however, there is still much to learn. It was assumed that its antioxidant properties were its most important activities in the human body. Consequently, it could be expected to protect against the kind of oxidative damage that can cause cancer and cardiovascular disease. A number of observational studies seemed to suggest that large doses of vitamin E did indeed help prevent cancer and cardiovascular disease. However, once controlled studies were undertaken, the results did not always confirm these benefits of vitamin E. In some cases, vitamin E seemed to have caused harm.[1,2,3]

It is very likely that vitamin E in its various forms does more than just prevent oxidative damage. Other roles may be equally important and may vary from person to person based on his or her own genetics and how much vitamin E he or she takes. There may be differences between individuals resulting in differential absorption and use of the vitamin.[3]

Additionally, while most of vitamin E's activity has been attributed to one of its eight natural forms, α-tocopherol, the other forms may also have functions in the body.

There is evidence accumulating for another possibility. As the data are reanalyzed, studies have been done looking at the blood levels of vitamin E in relationship to various diseases. It seems that people with low vitamin E levels may be at greater risk for cardiovascular disease and cancer than people with higher levels. The amount of vitamin E needed for this kind of protection may be relatively small. Most people in the United States do not consume enough vitamin E to get

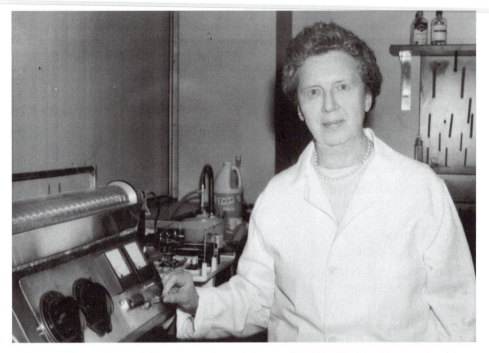

Gladys Emerson in the labs at the UCLA School of Public Health. She conducted research leading to the isolation and discovery of the nutritional value of vitamin E. (National Library of Medicine)

this benefit.[4] Consequently, it is certainly reasonable to take a supplement that has the recommended daily dose of vitamin E.

Nevertheless, many people take much larger doses of vitamin E for general health, to prevent cancer and cardiovascular disease, and to promote eye health and prevent what is called macular degeneration. However, individuals should discuss high-dose vitamin E supplementation with their doctors, to determine if it is more likely to be beneficial or harmful in each case.[1,2]

Studies continue to try and define all of the vitamin's reactivity and functions.

THE HYPE

Vitamin E is an antioxidant. It scavenges free radicals in the body and prevents DNA damage and blood vessel damage. Supplementation with large doses of vitamin E should help prevent cancer and atherosclerotic cardiovascular disease as well as other diseases in which oxidation plays a role.[1,2] Since the body is subjected to so much stress, high doses of supplements should work best.

Supplementation can Protect against Cardiovascular Disease

This theory found support in many studies during the 1990s. For example, as part of the Iowa Women's Health Study, postmenopausal women were followed and their intake of vitamin E was assessed by questionnaire. This observational study showed that the risk of cardiovascular disease decreased with higher vitamin E intake.[5]

Similar results had been found with male health professionals ages 40 to 75; those who reported higher vitamin E intake had less coronary disease risk.[6]

But further study did not support these conclusions. Researchers began to question the observational studies and also suggest that there may be other reasons for the results, stating that there was no evidence of a clinically significant effect.[7] Perhaps healthier people were taking vitamin supplements.

The Physician's Health Study II, a randomized trial giving men aged 50 and over 400 IU of vitamin E daily, for 10 years, found no benefit from the vitamin. There was no reduction of significant cardiovascular events in the group given vitamin E.[8]

The American Heart Association's position on vitamin E and other antioxidants was stated in an article in *Circulation* in 2004, and it remains the same in 2009. The association does not advise giving high-dose vitamin E supplements to reduce cardiovascular disease risk.[9]

Vitamin E Will Decrease the Risk of Certain Cancers

There have been studies associating vitamin E supplementation with lowered incidence of prostate and other cancer. Some of these studies were observational in nature—they looked at patients with cancer and then assessed their vitamin status.

Others were controlled trials assessing results after supplementation. In the ATBC Study (Alpha-Tocopherol, Beta-Carotene Cancer Prevention Study), male smokers in Finland were given daily supplements of vitamin E 50 mg and beta-carotene 20 mg. They were followed for five to eight years. Both the number of cases of prostate cancer and the number of deaths were significantly lower in the vitamin E group.[10]

One prospective study followed men for eight years, looking at the incidence of prostate cancer. Vitamin E from dietary sources as well as supplements was recorded, as was beta-carotene ingestion, and many other variables. The only correlation about vitamin E that emerged was that recent or current smokers taking vitamin E supplements may have developed less highly aggressive prostate cancer and more nonadvanced prostate cancer.[11]

The SELECT Trial (The Selenium and Vitamin E Cancer Prevention Trial) was a well-designed and much-anticipated study, hoping to finally answer the questions about the two supplements and cancer. SELECT found no evidence that vitamin E supplements lower the occurrence of prostate cancer.[12]

Some studies looked at both cancer and cardiovascular mortality. For example, the Women's Health Study, conducted between 1992 and 2004, was a randomized trial giving some women 600 IU vitamin E every other day. The data from this study revealed no overall health benefit for vitamin E. There was no effect on overall major cardiovascular events or cancer or on total mortality.[13]

The HOPE Trial selected people at least 55 years of age with either diabetes or vascular disease, supplemented them with 400 IU vitamin E daily and followed them for about seven years. They found no decreased risk of cancer or major cardiovascular events, but a possibility of increased risk of heart failure.[14]

Mortality

It was believed that vitamin E would lower mortality because of its effect on cardiovascular disease and cancer. However, some studies found the opposite to be true. One review in 2005 found increased mortality among people taking high-dose (400 IU) supplements.[15]

Other studies have come to similar conclusions. (See "Possible Side Effects" below for more information.)

Vitamin E May Protect the Retina of the Eye against Macular Degeneration

Macular degeneration is an age-related deterioration of the retina, at the back of the eye, that causes loss of vision. There have been studies showing that antioxidants might help prevent this, including vitamin E. For example, high-dose vitamin E (400 IU) along with various other antioxidants and zinc were compared with placebo to see how patients who already had macular degeneration would do over time. After six years, the antioxidants plus zinc slowed the development of degeneration in people who already had significant abnormalities. This benefit did not extend to people at low risk for advanced macular degeneration. The researchers suggested that people over the age of 55 who have their eyes examined by an eye doctor and who have certain abnormalities might benefit from the antioxidant combination.[16]

However, a review of all the research to date, conducted in 2008, revealed no benefit for consuming any of the high-dose antioxidant supplements, including vitamin E.[17] There are trials ongoing to look for more evidence of its effect on macular degeneration.

Alzheimer's Disease

Many researchers have looked at vitamin E to see if it could help slow the decline in cognitive function seen with Alzheimer's disease and similar conditions. There has been no proof that vitamin E helps the symptoms of Alzheimer's disease or improves cognitive function.[18,19]

DEFICIENCY

Actual vitamin E deficiency is very rare.[1,2] It is not manifested in otherwise healthy people, even those apparently not consuming enough E.

Vitamin E is absorbed in the intestine. Anything that decreases the body's ability to absorb fats affects vitamin E absorption. Vitamin E leaves the intestinal cells as chylomicrons, remnants of which reach the liver, which is the location of the rate-limiting step in vitamin E absorption and distribution. In the liver, α-TTP (hepatic α-tocopherol transfer protein) transfers α-tocopherol to VLDL (very low density lipoproteins). The liver breaks down and eliminates the other tocopherols, while returning α-tocopherol into the blood in VLDL. The most important part of this is that the liver controls the amount of vitamin E, via the transport protein.

Deficiency of vitamin E is seen in people with abnormalities of the transport protein, α-TTP,[2] and possibly other genetic diseases. It can also be seen in people who have serious intestinal disorders and cannot absorb fats or fat-soluble vitamins. In these cases, the affected individuals do not have a simple vitamin E deficiency.

Clusters of the α-TTP deficient patients have been found and analyzed in a number of countries. When vitamin E levels are measured, they are low. Many of the individuals have skeletal abnormalities, as well as multiple abnormalities of the nervous system that progress over time. The sensory nerves are affected, and individuals have peripheral neuropathy (problems with the nerves in the arms and legs), ataxia (difficulty with balance and walking), and if there is no way to get them vitamin E, they die of the deficiency.[4] One of the most described disorders is called AVED (ataxia and vitamin e deficiency).

If people with some of these problems get sufficient vitamin E early in life, such as by treating intestinal malabsorption syndromes, a lot of the neurologic damage can be prevented.

Diseases Known to Be Associated with Deficiency

Very small, premature babies may be deficient in vitamin E and need supplementation.[1]

As noted, abnormalities of α-TTP cause vitamin E deficiency, such as AVED. AVED can be treated with large doses of vitamin E.

Other diseases of fat absorption include Crohn's disease, cystic fibrosis, chronic cholestatic and hepatobiliary disease (liver and gall bladder problems in which fats are not absorbed). There are water-soluble types of vitamin E that can be given to patients with these disorders.[1]

Patients with abetalipoproteinemia can be given extremely large doses of vitamin E to prevent deficiency.[1]

FOOD SOURCES

Natural vitamin E comes from plants. It can be found in seeds, nuts, and many vegetable oils, including canola, corn, and soybean. There is also vitamin E in leafy green vegetables and fruits. Many people get most of their dietary vitamin E from vegetable oils used in cooking. Plant-derived vegetable oils have vitamin E, but this is rarely seen on the labels.

The Daily Value, or DV, which is supposed to guide consumers, is 30 IUs a day. The only foods required to list their vitamin E content are those that are supplemented with extra vitamins, such as cereals.

Most people in the United States get their vitamin E from oils and other food products. A tablespoonful of wheat germ oil has 100 percent of the DV for vitamin E; 2 tablespoonfuls of peanut butter have 15 percent.

MECHANISM OF ACTION: ANTIOXIDANT VERSUS OTHER MECHANISM

Vitamin E is the name of a group of naturally occurring, related, fat-soluble compounds with similar properties. There are eight known naturally occurring forms of vitamin E, including α-tocopherol, β-tocopherol, γ-tocopherol, δ-tocopherol, and four corresponding tocotrienols, which have slightly different chemical structures. Only α-tocopherol is maintained in human plasma (blood) and believed to be the most biologically active.

Synthetic vitamin E is composed of α-tocopherols, some of which are other "stereoisomers" of the vitamin, half of which are biologically active. Vitamin E sold as a supplement usually has a chemical group attached to keep the oil from going bad. In the human body, the extra group is removed.

It was not always clear that α-tocopherol was the biologically active vitamin E. There have also been different ways of naming and labeling, as well as measuring the tocopherols. It has now been standardized so that vitamin E means α-tocopherol.

Vitamin E is an antioxidant. It is this property that made vitamin E extremely interesting as a nutrient and as a supplement. Any substance that acts as an antioxidant and may be able to protect the body from free radicals may be extremely important in disease prevention.

It also acts in other ways that are being investigated. It is possible that other actions of the vitamin are actually more important than its role as an antioxidant. Vitamin E boosts an enzyme in a reaction that ultimately increases the amount of a chemical called prostacyclin in the lining of blood vessels. This inhibits the clumping of platelets and also dilates blood vessels.[1] This particular action may explain the increased incidence of hemorrhagic stroke and other bleeding found in people taking high doses of vitamin E.

Vitamin E inhibits protein kinase C, which has many functions in the body.[1] This may be how the vitamin inhibits increases in smooth muscle cells. It also has an effect on some gene regulation.[20] It is involved in many other reactions in the body that are being studied.

PRIMARY USES

- As noted, vitamin E can be used to treat any of the genetic disorders that prevent absorption in adequate amounts. Large doses may be needed, for example, 5 to 10 g a day for people with abetalipoproteinemia.[1]
- Excluding the rare genetic and intestinal problems that cause difficulty in vitamin E absorption and usage in the body, vitamin E is prescribed not as a treatment or replacement, but based on its presumed ability to prevent disease. These uses are experimental. The correct amounts have not been determined. In some cases, the use of vitamin E may actually make conditions worse.

- Nevertheless, some 11 percent of Americans choose to take vitamin E supplements in the range of 400 IU daily.[21] This is as the result of the publicity surrounding early reports about vitamin E's antioxidant capabilities. It was marketed in multivitamins specifically targeted at patients with eye problems, as well as the general public.

COMMON DOSAGES

Since there is no known deficiency state, it is hard to estimate the requirements of vitamin E for normal people. The Food and Nutrition Board (FNB) at the Institute of Medicine of the National Academies sets the recommendations. For vitamin E, it used an amount of the vitamin needed to prevent damage to red blood cells exposed to free radicals.[2] There may be a better way found in the future to set these values.

The FNB set the RDA (Recommended Dietary Allowance) for vitamin E or α-tocopherol at 15 mg a day for everyone ages 14 years and up. Breast-feeding mothers need 19 mg. Babies and children need less, from 4 mg the first six months of life, gradually up to the 15 mg at 14.

Vitamin E is often listed as international units (IUs). These represent biological activity instead of weight, so 1 mg of natural α-tocopherol is equal to 1.49 International Units (IU) of natural vitamin E, or 2.22 International Units of the synthetic α-tocopherol.[1]

After converting, the RDA for adult is 22.4 IUs of α-tocopherol a day.

The Food and Drug Administration also sets a target for vitamins, called the Daily Value (DV). The DV of vitamin E is 30 IU. If a labeled package says it contains 20 percent of the DV, it has 6 IU of vitamin E.

It has been estimated that most people in the United States do not ingest sufficient vitamin E to meet the RDA. However, it is also clear that there are enough sources for people to get enough in their diet. As explained, they may in fact be getting it from oil used in cooking, which may contain vitamin E but is not labeled as such.[22]

As noted previously, many people are also taking supplements. Supplements contain significantly more, usually as α-tocopherol, although there are products available with other tocopherols. Supplements of vitamin E usually contain at least 100 IUs of vitamin E, and often more, at least 400 IUs. The amount of vitamin E in general multivitamins, however, is usually closer to the RDA.

POTENTIAL SIDE EFFECTS

There is a tolerable upper limit set by the FNB for vitamin E at 1,000 mg or 1,500 IU. This is based on the side effect of hemorrhage.

Vitamin E interacts with a lot of medications in a variety of ways. The risk of bleeding increases if vitamin E is taken with warfarin or other anticoagulants (blood thinners). When E and other antioxidants are taken with the combination of simvastatin and niacin (to improve cholesterol values), they may not cause as great a rise in HDL (good cholesterol) as without the antioxidants.[1]

Vitamin E is usually not recommended during chemotherapy.[1]

Excess Mortality

The risk of excess mortality from taking high doses of vitamin E has been determined in a number of studies. An analysis of data from 19 trials using vitamin E to prevent various conditions (primarily cardiovascular disease and cancer) showed that all-cause mortality rose when doses of vitamin E equal to or greater than 400 IU were taken for at least a year.[15]

Another analysis came to the conclusion that treatment with a number of antioxidants, including vitamins E and A as well as beta-carotene, may increase mortality.[23]

A review of 67 trials that included young healthy people as well as older, chronically ill people came to the conclusion that vitamin E was not beneficial in terms of decreasing mortality.[24]

Since there is no definite benefit to the use of high doses, and there is possible risk, people should consider all of this when deciding how much vitamin E to take.

FACT VERSUS FICTION

At this point in time, it does not appear that large doses of vitamin E are protective against cancer, cardiovascular disease, or all causes of death taken together. It is even possible that taking large doses of vitamin E can increase mortality.

However, there is evidence that people with low intake of vitamin E and low levels in their body may benefit from taking a smaller amount of E, something like the RDA of 15 mg. Studies have shown that smokers whose blood levels of α-tocopherol are in the high normal range have lower rates of mortality than smokers with lower levels of α-tocopherol.[25] Men with higher vitamin E levels develop less prostate cancer.[26]

Until there is more information, it seems reasonable to take vitamin E to supplement what is missing from the diet, but not at anywhere near the 400 IU levels used in many studies.

REFERENCES

1. Office of Dietary Supplements. NIH Clinical Center, National Institutes of Health. *Dietary Supplement Fact Sheet: Vitamin E.* http://dietarysupplements. info.nih.gov/factsheets/vitamine.asp#en41. Accessed October 28, 2009.
2. Institute of Medicine. Food and Nutrition Board. *Dietary reference intakes for vitamin C, vitamin E, selenium, and carotenoids.* Washington, DC: National Academies Press, 2000.
3. Brigelius-Flohé, R, Kelly, FJ, Salonen, JT, et al. The European perspective on vitamin E: Current knowledge and future research. *Am J Clin Nutr.* 2002;76:703–716.
4. Traber, MG. How much vitamin E? ... Just enough! *Am J Clin Nutr.* 2006; 84:959–960.
5. Kushi, LH, Folsom, AR, Prineas, RJ, et al. Dietary antioxidant vitamins and death from coronary heart disease in postmenopausal women. *N Engl J Med.* 1996;334(18):1156–1162.

6. Rimm, EB, Stampfer, MJ, Ascherio, A, et al. Vitamin E consumption and the risk of coronary heart disease in men. *N Engl J Med.* 1993;328(20):1450–1456.

7. Eidelman, RS, Hollar, D, Hebert, PR, et al. Randomized trials of vitamin E in the treatment and prevention of cardiovascular disease. *Arch Intern Med.* 2004;164:1552–1556.

8. Sesso, HD, Buring, JE, Christen, WG, et al. Vitamins E and C in the prevention of cardiovascular disease in men. *JAMA.* 2008;300(18):2123–2133.

9. Kris-Etherton, PM, Lichtenstein, AH, Howard, BV, et al. Antioxidant vitamin supplements and cardiovascular disease. *Circulation.* 2004;110:637–641.

10. Heinonen, OP, Albanes, D, Virtamo, J, et al. Prostate cancer and supplementation with a-tocopherol and beta-carotene: Incidence and mortality in a controlled trial. *Journal of the National Cancer Institute.* 1998;90(6):440–446.

11. Kirsh, VA, Hayes, RB, Mayne, GL, et al. Supplemental and dietary vitamin E, β-carotene, and vitamin C intakes and prostate cancer risk. *Journal of the National Cancer Institute.* 2006;98(4):245–254.

12. Lippman, SM, Klein, EA, Goodman, PJ, Lucia, MS, Thompson, IM, Ford, LG, et al. The effect of selenium and vitamin E on risk of prostate cancer and other cancers: The Selenium and Vitamin E Cancer Prevention Trial (SELECT). *JAMA.* 2009;301:39–51.

13. Lee, IM, Cook, NR, Gaziano, JM, et al. Vitamin E in the primary prevention of cardiovascular disease and cancer. *JAMA.* 2005;294(1):56–65.

14. The HOPE and HOPE-TOO Trial Investigators. Effects of long-term vitamin E supplementation on cardiovascular events. *JAMA.* 2005;293(11):1338–1347.

15. Miller, ER, Pastor-Barriuso, R, Dalal, D, et al. Meta-analysis: High-dosage vitamin E supplementation may increase all-cause mortality. *Ann Intern Med.* 2005;142(1):37–46.

16. Age-Related Eye Disease Study Research Group. A randomized, placebo-controlled, clinical trial of high-dose supplementation with vitamins C and E, beta carotene, and zinc for age-related macular degeneration and vision loss: AREDS Report No. 8. *Arch Ophthalmol.* 2001;119(10):1417–1436.

17. Evans, JR, Henshaw, KS. Antioxidant vitamin and mineral supplements for preventing age-related macular degeneration. *Cochrane Database of Systematic Reviews.* 2008;1. Art. No.: CD000253. doi:10.1002/14651858.CD000253.pub2.

18. Isaac, MG, Quinn, R, Tabet, N. Vitamin E for Alzheimer's disease and mild cognitive impairment. *Cochrane Database of Systematic Reviews.* 2008 Jul 16;3. Art. No.: CD002854. doi:10.1002/14651858.

19. Kang, JH, Cook, N, Manson, J, et al. A randomized trial of vitamin E supplementation and cognitive function in women. *Arch Intern Med.* 2006;166(22):2462–2468.

20. Azzi, A, Breyer, I, Feher, M, et al. Cellular responses to α-tocopherol. *J Nutr.* 2000;130:1649–1652.

21. Ford, ES, Ajani, UA, Mokdad, AH. Brief communication: The prevalence of high intake of vitamin E from the use of supplements among U.S. adults. *Ann Intern Med.* 2005;143:116–120.

22. Gao, X, Wilde, PE, Lichtenstein, AH, et al. The maximal amount of dietary á-tocopherol intake in U.S. adults (NHANES 2001–2002). *J Nutr.* 2006;136:1021–1026.

23. Bjelakovic, G, Nikolova, D, Gluud, LL, Simonetti, RG, Gluud, C. Mortality in randomized trials of antioxidant supplements for primary and secondary prevention: Systematic review and meta-analysis. *JAMA.* 2007;297:842–857.

24. Bjelakovic, G, Nikolova, D, Gluud, LL, Simonetti, RG, Gluud, C. Antioxidant supplements for prevention of mortality in healthy participants and patients with various diseases. *Cochrane Database of Systematic Reviews.* 2008 Apr 16;2. Art. No.: CD007176. doi:10.1002/14651858.

25. Wright, ME, Lawson, KA, Weinstein, SJ, et al. Higher baseline serum concentrations of vitamin E are associated with lower total and cause-specific mortality in the Alpha-Tocopherol, Beta-Carotene Cancer Prevention Study. *Am J Clin Nutr.* 2006;84:1200–1207.

26. Weinstein, SJ, Wright, ME, Lawson, KA, et al. Serum and dietary vitamin E in relation to prostate cancer risk. *Cancer Epidemiol Biomarkers Prev.* 2007;16(6):1253–1259.

34

Vitamin K

BRIEF OVERVIEW

Vitamin K is a fat-soluble vitamin discovered in 1929. It was found to be necessary for the function of several proteins causing blood clotting, and was named K for the German term, *Koagulationsvitamin*.

More has been learned about the exact role of vitamin K in the clotting process. It is also now known to be a cofactor in bone metabolism and a candidate for the treatment of osteoporosis. It may also be important in the prevention and treatment of other diseases, including cancer and cardiovascular disease.

There is actually not one vitamin K, but rather a group of related chemicals (see "Mechanism of Action"). They may not all be identical in function. In the United States and Europe, vitamin K1 has been most studied and used as a supplement. In Japan, vitamin K2 is part of the normal diet as well as the focus of investigation.

THE HYPE

Vitamin K can Prevent and/or Treat Osteoporosis

Vitamin K is definitely needed for the activation of a number of proteins necessary for good bone health (see "Mechanism of Action"). Studies have shown a benefit to vitamin K, at higher doses than needed for clotting. It may help keep bones strong more effectively when used along with vitamin D.[1]

Researchers in Japan have studied vitamin K2 extensively, one particular form also called menatetrenone (MK-4). It is used to treat osteoporosis in Japan, with or without other substances including vitamin D and calcium. The most-studied substance in bone that vitamin K activates is called osteocalcin. Vitamin K helps carboxylate osteocalcin (see "Mechanism of Action"); carboxylated osteocalcin is a measure of adequate vitamin K intake.

There have been studies showing an association between the risk of hip fracture and vitamin K intake, many in Japan, and some in other countries. There have been

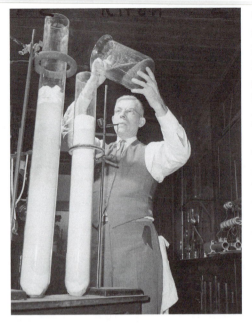

Dr. Edward A. Doisy, professor of biochemistry at St. Louis University School of Medicine, demonstrates his work in his laboratory in St. Louis, Missouri, on November 30, 1944. Dr. Doisy won the 1943 Nobel Prize in Medicine for his work on discovering the chemical properties of vitamin K. Vitamin K is vital for blood coagulation in the body. (AP Photo)

studies indicating that oral vitamin K can increase bone density. In one trial, for example, vitamin K1 at doses of 200 μg a day increased the bone mineral density (BMD) of the distal wrist bone in Scottish women 60 or more years of age.[2]

There have also been studies demonstrating what vitamin K can do in a laboratory setting. There have been tests done on samples of bone and on tissue cultures, as well as trials using animals. Vitamin K can prevent bone loss in animals.

It has also been established that taking oral vitamin K can increase the levels of the vitamin as well as the levels of carboxylated osteocalcin in normal people. For example, one group of investigators in Japan gave vitamin K2 in the form of supplemented, fermented soybean (called *natto*) to a group of healthy individuals and demonstrated an increase in the amount of the vitamin and carboxylated osteocalcin in the serum over a two-week period.[3] In another study, oral doses of only 1.5 mg a day caused measurable increases in vitamin K levels as well as the amount of carboxylated osteocalcin in postmenopausal Japanese women.[4]

Results of randomized, placebo-controlled, double-blind studies using vitamin K to prevent bone loss or fracture have yielded mixed results. The ECKO study (Evaluation of the Clinical Use of Vitamin K Supplementation), done in Canada, followed 440 postmenopausal women who had osteopenia (bone loss but not osteoporosis) on bone density scan for two to four years. They were randomly assigned to get 5 mg of vitamin K1 or placebo. They were evaluated at two years and four years. The investigators were looking primarily at the BMD of the lumbar spine and hip. They were looking secondarily at BMD at other sites, fractures, other adverse events, and quality of life. All of the women had adequate levels of vitamin D.

There were no significant differences in BMD at any site between the two groups at two and four years, despite elevated vitamin K levels and decreased markers of bone turnover in the blood. In the vitamin K group, women had fewer fractures (9 versus 20) and fewer cancers (3 versus 12). These numbers were low; the study was not set up to evaluate the statistical significance of small differences. There were no adverse events or differences in quality of life.

The ECKO study suggests more studies need to be done to examine these specific outcomes, cancer, and fracture.[5]

A comprehensive review of all the available studies using vitamin K to treat osteoporosis, done in the United Kingdom, included the ECKO trial, as well Japanese studies of high quality. A number of trials have been done in Japan using menatetrenone, compared with placebo, calcium, and/or prescription medication in postmenopausal women. Using standard eligibility criteria to select trials for analysis, such as having a control group, allowed only four Japanese trials to be included in the analysis. Three relatively recent trials showed a decrease in vertebral fracture with 45 mg of menatetrenone a day. Pooling the data from the menatetrenone studies showed no reduction in the general risk of vertebral fracture using menatetrenone.[6] There was, however, a decreased risk of a subsequent vertebral (backbone) fracture in women who had already suffered five or more fractures.[6,7]

The numbers of other fractures (nonvertebral) were either not reported or the numbers were so small that they are not statistically significant. The authors of this review could not draw any other conclusions.[6]

A previous review looked at many of the same studies and concluded that there was a decreased risk of hip fracture, all found in Japanese trials using menatetrenone. This review also noted that studies using both vitamin K1 and menatetrenone have showed reduced bone loss. While they included studies excluded by the other reviewers, they also commented that the quality of the trials was "not high" and recommended large, randomized, controlled trials on other populations.[8]

It should be noted most (if not all) of the above studies were done on postmenopausal women with osteopenia or osteoporosis. Only the ECKO trial was done outside of Japan.

One trial looking at the effects of vitamin K on BMD in older men and women ages 60 to 80 found no effect. This was a three-year, double-blind, controlled trial with 452 people in the United States. They received 600 mg elemental calcium plus 400 IU vitamin D, as well as either placebo or 500 μg of phylloquinone.[9]

An analysis in the *Alternative Medicine Review* looked at all the menatetrenone data in a more positive light, including small studies that show it may prevent or slow bone loss as the result of Parkinson's disease, steroid use, biliary cirrhosis, and stroke. The researchers also noted that vitamin K's effect on bone may be even more pronounced if it is given with adequate calcium and vitamin D.[1]

However, an article in *Nutrition Review* in 2008 concluded, "However, there are emerging data that suggest the efficacy of vitamin K supplementation on bone loss is inconclusive."[10]

Vitamin K and Cancer

The ECKO study above, which was designed to look at bone density, found a decrease in cancer: 3 in the group treated with 5 mg of K1 versus 12 in the group not treated. These numbers are too small for statistical analysis, but they do indicate the need to further evaluate the possible role of vitamin D in cancer prevention.[5]

There have been large-scale studies showing that a decreased risk of all cancer is associated with increased intake of vitamin K. The EPIC-Heidelberg study (European Prospective Investigation into Cancer and Nutrition) found that the risk of cancer decreases with increased intake of menaquinones (K2). This was especially pronounced in men and related to their incidence of prostate and lung cancer. There was no association between cancer and K1 intake.[11]

Multiple in vitro studies have shown anticancer effects of K1 and K2 on a variety of cancer cell lines.[1]

There have been Phase I and II clinical trials in humans using K1 to treat hepatocellular carcinoma with some success. It has shown no obvious toxicity.[12]

There are also case studies of successful cancer therapy with vitamin K2, mainly in patients with leukemia and other cancers derived from blood cells or abnormal bone marrow. Remission was induced with vitamin K in a number of separate individuals.[1]

Subsequently, there have been a number of controlled trials in Japan using K2 (menatetrenone) to treat cancer. One multicenter pilot study looked the vitamin's effect on myelodysplastic syndrome (MDS) and post-MDS leukemia. There was some improvement in patients taking just vitamin K2, as well as when using the vitamin with other chemotherapy. Another Japanese trial involved 121 patients with liver cancer, all getting conventional therapy. Adding 45 mg a day of menatetrenone increased survival and decreased specific complications of this cancer.[1,12]

In the United States and Europe, vitamin K3 has been studied more extensively as an anticancer agent. Studies on cell cultures and using lab animals show antitumor activity. In vitro, the effects of vitamin K3 are synergistic with traditional chemotherapy agents. Vitamin C also seems to enhance the antitumor effect of K3.

While all forms of vitamin K have been extensively tested in cell cultures and lab animals with success, to date, there have only been very limited human trials. There seems to be some success in treating liver cancer and blood cancers, but this has only been done on small numbers of people.[12] The exact mechanism by which vitamin K causes the death of cancer cells is not clear.

Vitamin K and Cardiovascular Disease

K2 inhibits calcification of arterial plaque (fatty accumulations on artery walls) in animals. At least one study has shown an association between higher K2 intake and lower coronary artery calcification.[1]

Vitamin K does not just activate proteins in the clotting cascade. As stated, it carboxylates and activates proteins in bone. It also activates proteins involved in arterial calcifications. One of these is called Matrix Gla-protein (MGP), which is found in atherosclerotic plaque. It is believed that activation of this protein prevents calcium precipitation in plaque.[13] This may lead to less cardiovascular disease.

In one study in Rotterdam, higher menaquinone intake was associated with lower risk of death from coronary heart disease, lower risk of death from all causes, and fewer severe aortic calcifications. Menaquinones are found in cheese and other dairy products, meat, eggs, and fish in the Dutch diet. Phylloquinones showed no relationship to any risk factors.[14]

Phylloquinone intake is considered to be indicator of a healthy diet and lifestyle, but not necessarily an active agent in lowering risk.[15] If vitamin K1 intake reflects a healthier lifestyle, some of its "effects" may actually be due to other components of that lifestyle.

DEFICIENCY

Vitamin K deficiency is not common except in newborn infants. Vitamin K is not transported across the placenta. Therefore, at birth, babies are deficient in vitamin D and must be given supplementation. This will prevent vitamin K-deficiency bleeding both soon after birth and in the subsequent weeks, because there is also not enough K in breast milk.[16]

There was a concern in the past that intramuscular injections of vitamin K were associated with cancer; this has been proven untrue. The later bleeding disease in newborns can be prevented only with the injection and not oral vitamin D. The American Academy of Pediatrics recommends injections of vitamin K at birth, as well as informing parents of the risk of vitamin K deficiency in newborns. Its 2003 statement has been reaffirmed in 2009.[17]

Vitamin K deficiency was originally defined as vitamin K-dependent hypoprothrombinemia, which means a low prothrombin as a result of vitamin K deficiency. Defined in this way, vitamin K deficiency is very uncommon, as well as very serious. It can result in severe bleeding.

The level of prothrombin can be measured by the INR (International Normalized Ratio for Prothrombin Activity). This is a way of assessing adequacy of vitamin K in its classical role as part of blood clotting.

Since it has become apparent that vitamin K is involved with calcium deposition in bone, deficiency of vitamin K may be a cause of osteoporosis. Levels of the vitamin may be high enough for normal clotting, but not high enough for bone health. This has not been universally accepted as a deficiency syndrome or disease. Although low intake of vitamin K has been associated with hip fractures in epidemiologic studies, this may be an indicator that the observed populations have poor overall nutrition.[6]

The activity of vitamin K as it concerns bone health can be assessed by measuring either the amount of carboxylated osteocalcin in blood or the amount of uncarboxylated osteocalcin (see "Mechanism of Action"). However, these tests are not in clinical use but are used in research settings.[18,19]

Very little vitamin K is stored in the body. Deficiency can occur as a result of decreased intake, as well as when the bacteria in the intestine that make vitamin K are reduced, for example, after long treatment with antibiotics taken by mouth. People with malabsorption of fat due to intestinal illnesses can develop vitamin K deficiency.[6]

Estrogen levels may affect vitamin K levels.[6]

FOOD SOURCES

Vitamin K1 is found in green, leafy vegetables. There is a lot of available vitamin K even after cooking many of these, such as kale, collard greens, and spinach. For example, there are 514 µg in a serving of cooked spinach.

K2 actually comprises a group of menaquinones. Currently there are seven known menaquinones. While they may be derived from bacteria, they are also found in animal protein, including meat, liver, and fermented foods, especially cheese in many countries. A food called *natto*, made from fermented soybeans, is the food richest in menaquinone, in this case, menaquinone-7 (MK-7). *Natto* is consumed in eastern Japan, where it is a traditional food.[6]

MECHANISM OF ACTION: HOW DOES IT WORK?

Vitamin K is part of a family of chemicals, all fat-soluble napthoquinones. They include phylloquinone (K1), menaquinones (K2), and menadione (synthetic, K3). The skeletons of these molecules are the same, but the side chains are different. Phylloquinone, found in algae and higher plants, was named because of its relationship to photosynthesis. Menaquinones are made by many types of bacteria. They are probably made by animals including humans and are found in foods of animal origin as well certain fermented foods (see "Food Sources"). The designation for menaquinone is MK-n, where *n* means the number of specific side chains.

K1 from plant sources is absorbed and metabolized to menaquinones, principally MK-4. The pathway for this conversion is not yet known. Menaquinones (or K2) have higher potency and more gamma carboxylation activity than K1.[1] K3 can also be converted to MK-4 in the body.[6]

Menaquinone-4 (MK-4) is also called menatetrenone. It is unclear how much MK-4 from intestinal bacteria gets into the body; it is also unclear how it is made from K1 or other forms of vitamin K in humans.

The best-known function of vitamin K is its role in vitamin K-dependent carboxylation reactions. Vitamin K helps carboxylate glutamic acid–containing proteins, which are part of the blood clotting cascade. It is a cofactor for the enzyme, gamma-glutamyl carboxylase. Since it can go through an oxidation-reduction cycle of its own, vitamin K can be reused.[16] Warfarin (an anticoagulant) inhibits one of the enzymes that recycles vitamin K; there is then not enough to carboxylate certain blood clotting factors.[12]

Vitamin K also is important to maintain bone health. It helps gamma-carboxylate osteocalcin, a protein necessary for calcium uptake and bone mineralization. Other proteins in the bone are dependent on vitamin K to be carboxylated and thus activated. They are called Matrix Gla-protein and anticoagulant protein S.[1]

PRIMARY USES

- Vitamin K is used to treat deficiency of prothrombin (hypoprothombinemia), one of the proteins involved in the blood clotting sequence.
- Patients with clotting problems who are treated with the blood thinner warfarin can get too much warfarin (Coumadin®). This leads to the risk of abnormal bleeding. Vitamin K can reverse the anticoagulant effect of warfarin more

quickly than just withholding warfarin. Studies have shown there are less bleeding complications if vitamin K is given to people with too much warfarin. The level of prothrombin is measured by the INR (International Normalized Ratio for Prothrombin Activity). Levels can be normalized by oral vitamin K more quickly than by injected vitamin K.[16]

- Supplemental vitamin K must be taken in deficiency states. There is a water-soluble K called menadiol sodium phosphate that can be taken by people who have trouble absorbing fats.

- An injectable form is used to prevent hemorrhagic disease of the newborn, which is caused by vitamin K deficiency.[6,17]

- Vitamin K can be used to increase bone density and prevent fractures; it helps treat osteoporo from many different causes. Osteocalcin is dependent on vitamin K.[1,16]

COMMON DOSAGES

The Adequate Intake (AI) for vitamin K1 is 90 µg a day for women (including pregnant and lactating) and 120 µg for men. Adolescents need 75 µg.[1,16]

In the United Kingdom, 1 µg per kilogram of body weight is the suggested daily requirement, which would be 64 µg for an average-weight woman. Vitamin supplements in the United Kingdom usually contain 45 µg.[6]

In Japan, 45 mg of menatetrenone a day in divided doses is the usual amount used to treat osteoporosis.[6] In the United States, no official recommendations have been made about K2 doses.

People who are not absorbing fat need about 10 mg a day of menadiol sodium phosphate.

Full-term newborn infants need a 1-mg injection. Premature infants need 0.5 mg; infants weighing less than 2 pounds should get 0.3 mg/kg of body weight.[16]

K1 is available in a topical, oral, and injectable form. K2 is available as a capsule.

POTENTIAL SIDE EFFECTS

No Tolerable Upper Intake Level (UL) has been set for vitamin K. Some experts put the highest safe amount at 32.5 mg per day of K1; others suggest 1 mg per day of K1.[6]

Very few side effects of vitamin K1 have been reported. One review noted an association between high dose vitamin K (higher than 1 mg a day) and periodontal disease.[6] There have been no bleeding or clotting problems reported.[1]

One company, Esai Co., makes menatetrenone in Japan. The preparation is called Glakay, and all the information about side effects of K2 come from a pamphlet that comes with the capsules. These types of package inserts are required to contain all reported side effects, but they do not necessarily prove cause and effect. In total, 81 of 1,885 patients reported side effects to the manufacturer. About 0.1 to 5 percent of patients taking menatetrenone reported headache, rash, itching and skin redness, stomach pain or discomfort, dyspepsia, nausea, diarrhea, elevation of liver enzymes, elevation of BUN (a laboratory value related to kidney function or state of hydration), edema, or eye abnormalities. Less than 0.1 percent of those taking this preparation complained of thirst, lack of appetite, glossitis (tongue inflammation), constipation, lightheadedness, and increase in blood pressure. Vomiting, dizziness, palpitations, urinary frequency, joint pains, and malaise bothered an unspecified number of people.[6] Despite this information, menatetrenone is considered to be nontoxic and has been used throughout Japan. It is approved there as a treatment for osteoporosis.

Vitamin K interacts with a large number of medications. In some cases the other medicines interfere with vitamin K; in other cases vitamin K interferes with the other medicines. These include aspirin, antibiotics, anticoagulant/antiplatelet medications, doxyrubicin, laxatives, weight-loss medications, antiseizure medicines, fat-binding medicines, and warfarin. Anyone taking these medications or with significant medical problems should discuss taking vitamin K with a health care provider.[16]

Vitamin K should not be taken by people who are on anticoagulants as treatment. The babies born to women on warfarin, anticonvulsants, rifampin, or isoniazid are at higher risk for vitamin K deficiency at birth.[1]

FACT VERSUS FICTION

It seems certain that one or another form of vitamin K is necessary for normal bone health. In at least some populations, using vitamin K seems to prevent bone loss and probably prevent fractures. The majority of studies relating to vitamin K and bone have been done in Japan, and the human trials have been done there on postmenopausal women. Vitamin K2, specifically menatetrenone, has been approved there for the treatment of osteoporosis.

It is not clear if vitamin K1 can help as much with bone health as K2. It is also not clear if the effects are the same in all populations.

Women at risk for osteoporosis without serious medical problems can certainly try vitamin K. It will probably be some time before there are enough data to be sure it will work. It should not be used instead of medication or other vitamins recommended by a personal physician.

People with trouble absorbing fat may become deficient in vitamin K and will need to take it. Newborn babies are deficient and need vitamin K injections.

Anyone who is being anticoagulated with warfarin and is taking too much should take vitamin K along with temporarily stopping the warfarin. This reduces the risk of bleeding.

The role of vitamin K in reducing cancer risk or cardiovascular risk is very far from certain. Patients with liver cancer or cancer in the blood might consider participating in clinical trials if available. Anyone with medical problems who decides to take in larger doses than the AI should probably discuss it with a health care provider.

Large-scale clinical trials will help define the role of vitamin K further.

REFERENCES

1. Vitamin K2. *Altern Med Rev.* 2009;14(3):284–293.

2. Bolton-Smith, C, McMurdo, ME, Paterson, CR, Mole, PA, Harvey, JM, Fenton, ST, Prynne, CJ, Mishra, GD, Shearer, MJ. Two-year randomized controlled trial of vitamin K1 (phylloquinone) and vitamin D3 plus calcium on the bone health of older women. *J Bone Miner Res.* 2007;22(4):509–519.

3. Yamaguchi, M. Regulatory mechanism of food factors in bone metabolism and prevention of osteoporosis. *Yakugaku Zasshi.* 2006;126(11):1117–1137.

4. Koitaya, N, Ezaki, J, Nishimuta, M, et al. Effect of low dose vitamin K2 (MK-4) supplementation on bio-indices in postmenopausal Japanese women. *J Nutr Sci Vitaminol.* 2009;55:15–21.

5. Cheung, AM, Tile, L, Lee, Y, Tomlinson, G, Hawker, G, Scher, J, et al. Vitamin K supplementation in postmenopausal women with osteopenia (ECKO Trial): A randomized controlled trial. *PLoS Med.* 2008;5:e196.

6. Stevenson, M, Lloyd-Jones, M, Papaioannou, D. Vitamin K to prevent fractures in older women: Systematic review and economic evaluation. *Health Technology Assessment.* 2009;13(45):1–174.

7. Esai Company News Release. Eisai announces the intermediate analysis of anti-osteoporosis treatment post-marketing research to investigate the benefits of menatetrenone as part of the Ministry of Health, Labour and Welfare's Pharmacoepidemiological Drug Review program. February 25, 2005. http://www.eisai.co.jp/enews/enews200506.html. Accessed April 16, 2010.

8. Cockayne, S, Adamson, J, Lanham-New, S, Shearer, MJ, Gilbody, S, Torgerson, DJ. Vitamin K and the prevention of fractures: Systematic review and meta-analysis of randomized controlled trials. *Arch Intern Med.* 2006;166(12): 1256–1261.

9. Booth, SL, Dallal, GG, Shea, MK, et al. Effect of vitamin K supplementation on bone loss in elderly men and women. *J Clin Endocrinol Metab.* 2008;93(4):1217–1223.

10. Shea, MK, Booth, SL. Update on the role of vitamin K in skeletal health. *Nutr Rev.* 2008;66(10):549–557.

11. Nimptsch, K, Rohrmann, S, Kaaks, R, Linseisen, J. Dietary vitamin K intake in relation to cancer incidence and mortality: Results from the Heidelberg cohort of the European Prospective Investigation into Cancer and Nutrition (EPIC-Heidelberg). *Am J Clin Nutr.* 2010 Mar 24. http://www.ajcn.org/content/early/2010/09/29/ajcn.110.002345.citation. Accessed December 30, 2010.

12. Lamson, DW, Plaza, SM. The anticancer effects of vitamin K. *Altern Med Rev.* 2003;8(3):303–318.

13. Berkner, KL, Runge, KW. The physiology of vitamin K nutriture and vitamin K-dependent protein function in atherosclerosis. *Journal of Thrombosis and Haemostasis.* 2004;2:2118–2132.

14. Geleijnse, JM, Vermeer, C, Grobbee, DE, et al. Dietary intake of menaquinone is associated with a reduced risk of coronary heart disease: The Rotterdam Study. *J Nutr.* 2004;134:3100–3105.

15. Braam, L, McKeown, N, Jacques, P, Lichtenstein, A, Vermeer, C, Wilson, P, Booth, S. Dietary phylloquinone intake as a potential marker for a heart-healthy dietary pattern in the Framingham Offspring cohort. *J Am Diet Assoc.* 2004;104(9):1410–1414.

16. Sarubin-Fragakis, A, Thomson, C. *The health professional's guide to popular dietary supplements.* 3rd edition. Chicago: American Dietetic Association, 2007.

17. American Academy of Pediatrics. Policy Statement. Controversies concerning vitamin K and the newborn. *Pediatrics.* 2003;112(1):191–192. Reaffirmed and updated August 1, 2009.

18. McCormick, RK. Osteoporosis: Integrating biomarkers and other diagnostic correlates into the management of bone fragility. *Altern Med Rev.* 2007; 12(2):113–145.

19. Leaf, AA. Vitamins for babies and young children. *Arch Dis Child.* 2007;92: 160–164.

35

Zinc

BRIEF OVERVIEW

The mineral zinc is the 10th most common element in the body and helps with the functioning of more than 300 hormones and enzymes, one of which is copper/zinc superoxide dismutase (Cu/Zn SOD)—an antioxidant and detoxifier. It is also essential for proper growth and development as well as the regulation of genetic activity and DNA synthesis. The human body needs a daily dose of zinc to maintain a steady state, as the body has no specialized zinc storage system. Zinc is found naturally in many food sources, but animal foods are the richest sources of zinc. Zinc is a common additive to many nutritional supplements but often appears as a stand-alone supplemental mineral.

THE HYPE

Zinc is probably best known for its role in fighting flu symptoms and is a common addition to immune-boosting formulations. Zinc supplements are used in many antiaging and antioxidant supplement formulations. Zinc also helps with proper hormone production and zinc supplements are often used as fertility boosters.

Zinc is toxic at high doses, so supplementation needs to be targeted to avoid toxic doses. Zinc is also present in many different supplements, so people taking multiple supplements, along with extra zinc or an immune-boosting concoction containing zinc, may end up with toxicity issues if used continuously.

DEFICIENCY

Zinc deficiency is common in developing countries, but severe zinc deficiency is rare in the United States.[1] Mild zinc deficiency, however, has been reported as common in the United States, according to data from the Third National Health and Nutrition Examination Survey (NHANES III).[2] Zinc deficiency is characterized by growth retardation, loss of appetite, and impaired immune function. In more severe cases, zinc deficiency causes hair loss, diarrhea, delayed sexual maturation, impotence, and hypogonadism in males.[3,4] Delayed healing of wounds, skin abnormalities, and taste abnormalities are also typical of zinc deficiency.[3,5,6,7]

The bioavailability of zinc from vegetarian diets is lower than from nonvegetarian diets because animal proteins are the richest source of bioavailable zinc.[1] In addition, vegetarians typically eat high levels of legumes and whole grains, which contain phytates that bind zinc and inhibit its absorption.[8] Because animal protein is also a premier source of bioavailable iron, low zinc and low iron often occur simultaneously. Low iron in the bloodstream leads to iron-deficiency anemia, characterized by listlessness in adults and physical and neurological abnormalities in young children.[9] Alcoholics commonly present with zinc efficiency, because alcohol consumption decreases zinc absorption and increases urinary zinc excretion.[10]

FOOD SOURCES

Zinc is found in a wide range of plant and animal sources, but animal protein foods provide the highest and most bioavailable form of zinc.[1] Oysters contain more zinc per serving than any other food (with six oysters providing as much as 76.7 mg of zinc). Beef contains 8.9 mg of zinc per 3-ounce serving, and other animal protein foods, including poultry, fish, and beans contain anywhere between 1 and 3 mg zinc per 3-ounce serving.[1]

MECHANISMS OF ACTION AND PRIMARY USES

The most common primary uses for zinc supplements are related to the following mechanisms of action of zinc:

Zinc Boosts Antioxidant Function

Zinc is an essential component of the antioxidant Cu/Zn SOD,[11,12] whose main task in the body is to disarm superoxide free radicals (by breaking them down in hydrogen peroxide, which quickly converts to water and oxygen).[13] High levels of superoxide free radicals would otherwise damage lipids, proteins, and DNA, leading to cellular damage.[14] Oxidative damage to the enzyme itself has recently been implicated in a variety of pathologies, including Alzheimer's and Parkinson's diseases.[15] However, studies linking zinc to brain function and Alzheimer's disease in particular seem to be paradoxical, with some studies showing a neuroprotective effect and some showing neurodegenerative effects, according to a review study.[16]

Zinc, together with other antioxidants (like beta-carotene and vitamin C), has been found to delay the progression of age-related macular degeneration (AMD) and vision loss, possibly by preventing cellular damage in the retina.[17,18]

It has been hypothesized that oxidative damage can lead to poor sperm quality and male infertility. Low zinc levels and poor zinc nutrition may be an important risk factor for low quality of sperm and idiopathic male infertility.[19]

Zinc Improves the Immune System

Zinc helps the body to develop and activate T-lymphocyte immune cells,[1,20] and mild to moderate zinc deficiency can impair macrophage and neutrophil functions, natural killer cell activity, and complement activity.[21] Zinc has been shown to help with the healing of wounds[21,22] and in the prevention and treatment of childhood diarrhea.[21]

It is hypothesized that zinc prevents the influenza virus from attaching to the respiratory tract cells, thus preventing its replication.[23] The role that zinc plays in the treatment of the common cold, however, is controversial. In September 2007, Caruso and colleagues published a structured review of the effects of zinc lozenges, nasal sprays, and nasal gels on the common cold.[24] Of the 14 randomized, placebo-controlled studies included, 7 (5 using zinc lozenges, 2 using a nasal gel) showed that the zinc treatment had a beneficial effect, and 7 (5 using zinc lozenges, 1 using a nasal spray, and 1 using lozenges and a nasal spray) showed no effect. A Cochrane review of the effects of zinc lozenges on cold symptoms also reported inconclusive findings.[25]

Because of zinc's role in increasing the number of circulation T-lymphocytes, zinc status may be especially important to help boost immunity in patients with conditions that affect T-lymphocyte function, such as HIV.[26]

Zinc Aids Growth and Development

Zinc is vital for normal growth and development in infants, children, and adults. Zinc deficiency has been shown to cause cognitive deficits as well as growth delays in humans, including delays in sexual maturation, as well as deficits in bone mineralization and maturation.[27,28] The mechanism of action may be linked to zinc's ability to stimulate insulin-like growth factor 1 (IGF-1) and other proteins and polypeptides involved in bone and overall growth as well as in DNA synthesis.[29] Zinc supplementation in children at risk for deficiency can help boost poor growth in terms of both weight and height increments.[30]

COMMON DOSAGES

According to the Dietary Reference Intakes (DRIs) developed by the Food and Nutrition Board (FNB) at the Institute of Medicine of the National Academies (formerly National Academy of Sciences),[1] the Recommended Daily Allowance (RDA) for zinc is 8 mg per day for adult females and 11 mg per day for adult males. Studies showing a protective effect for zinc on cold severity symptoms used a dosage of 13.3 mg per day.[31]

Supplements contain several forms of zinc, including zinc gluconate, zinc sulfate, and zinc acetate, with the percentage of elemental zinc varying by form. Research has not determined whether differences exist among forms of zinc in absorption, bioavailability, or tolerability.

TOXICITY

The Tolerable Upper Limit for zinc as set out by the FNB for adults is 40 mg per day.[1] Intakes of 150–450 mg of zinc per day have been associated with chronic effects, including low copper status, altered iron function, lowered high-density lipoproteins, and reduced immune function.[1,32]

FACT VERSUS FICTION

Whether or not most people actually need zinc supplements is controversial, since severe zinc deficiency is rare in developed nations.

Zinc supplementation does appear to boost antioxidant function through the action of Cu/Zn SOD, which may play a role in the prevention of certain neurodegenerative conditions; however, zinc has not consistently shown a neuroprotective effect in this regard. Zinc supplements have, through antioxidant effects, shown to be effective in preventing macular degeneration and improving sperm quality. These conditions, however, have multifactorial causative factors, which may indicate other causative angles besides zinc deficiency. Although zinc supplements may boost immune function, their role in reducing the duration and severity of the common cold remains controversial. Zinc supplementation can help improve growth and development variables in children, but these effects are more relevant in developing countries, where zinc deficiency is common.

REFERENCES

1. Institute of Medicine. Food and Nutrition Board. *Dietary reference intakes for vitamin A, vitamin K, arsenic, boron, chromium, copper, iodine, iron, manganese, molybdenum, nickel, silicon, vanadium, and zinc.* Washington, DC: National Academies Press, 2001.
2. Alaimo, K, McDowell, MA, Briefel, RR, et al. Dietary intake of vitamins, minerals, and fiber of persons ages 2 months and over in the United States: Third National Health and Nutrition Examination Survey, Phase 1, 1988–91. *Adv Data.* 1994 Nov 14;(258):1–28.
3. Maret, W, Sandstead, HH. Zinc requirements and the risks and benefits of zinc supplementation. *J Trace Elem Med Biol.* 2006;20:3–18. [PubMed abstract]
4. Prasad, AS. Zinc deficiency: Its characterization and treatment. *Met Ions Biol Syst.* 2004;41:103–137.
5. Heyneman, CA. Zinc deficiency and taste disorders. *Ann Pharmacother.* 1996;30:186–187.
6. Hambidge, KM. Mild zinc deficiency in human subjects. In: Mills, CF. (Ed). *Zinc in human biology.* New York: Springer-Verlag, 1989;281–296.
7. Ploysangam, A, Falciglia, GA, Brehm, BJ. Effect of marginal zinc deficiency on human growth and development. *J Trop Pediatr.* 1997;43:192–198.
8. Hunt, JR. Bioavailability of iron, zinc, and other trace minerals from vegetarian diets. *Am J Clin Nutr.* 2003;78(3 Suppl):633S–639S.
9. Castejon, HV, Ortega, P, Amaya, D, et al. Co-existence of anemia, vitamin A deficiency and growth retardation among children 24–84 months old in Maracaibo, Venezuela. *Nutr Neurosci.* 2004 Apr;7(2):113–119.
10. Kang, YJ, Zhou, Z. Zinc prevention and treatment of alcoholic liver disease. *Mol Aspects Med.* 2005;26:391–404.
11. Kasperczyk, S, Birkner, E, Kasperczyk, A, Zalejska-Fiolka, J. Activity of superoxide dismutase and catalase in people protractedly exposed to lead compounds. *Ann Agric Environ Med.* 2004;11(2):291–296.

12. Kocaturk, PA, Kavas, GO, Erdeve, O, Siklar, Z. Superoxide dismutase activity and zinc and copper concentrations in growth retardation. *Biol Trace Elem Res*. 2004;102(1–3):51–59.

13. Kato, S, Saeki, Y, Aoki, M, et al. Histological evidence of redox system breakdown caused by superoxide dismutase 1 (SOD1) aggregation is common to SOD1-mutated motor neurons in humans and animal models. *Acta Neuropathol (Berl)*. 2004 Feb;107(2):149–158.

14. Landis, GN, Tower, J. Superoxide dismutase evolution and life span regulation. *Mech Ageing Dev*. 2005 Mar;126(3):365–379.

15. Olin, KL, Golub, MS, Gershwin, ME, et al. Extracellular superoxide dismutase activity is affected by dietary zinc intake in nonhuman primate and rodent models. *Am J Clin Nutr*. 1995 Jun;61(6):1263–1267.

16. Cuajungco, MP, Faget, KY. Zinc takes the center stage: Its paradoxical role in Alzheimer's disease. *Brain Res Brain Res Rev*. 2003 Jan;41(1):44–56.

17. Evans, JR. Antioxidant vitamin and mineral supplements for slowing the progression of age-related macular degeneration. *Cochrane Database of Systematic Reviews*. 2006;2. Art. No.: CD000254. doi: 10.1002/14651858.CD000254.pub2.

18. Age-Related Eye Disease Study Research Group. A randomized, placebo-controlled, clinical trial of high-dose supplementation with vitamins C and E, beta carotene, and zinc for age-related macular degeneration and vision loss: AREDS Report No. 8. *Arch Ophthalmol*. 2001;119:1417–1436.

19. Colagar, AH, Marzony, ET, Chaichi, MJ. Zinc levels in seminal plasma are associated with sperm quality in fertile and infertile men. *Nutr Res*. 2009 Feb;29(2):82–88.

20. Beck, FW, Prasad, AS, Kaplan, J, Fitzgerald, JT, Brewer, GJ. Changes in cytokine production and T cell subpopulations in experimentally induced zinc-deficient humans. *Am J Physiol*. 1997;272:E1002–E1007.

21. Wintergerst, ES, Maggini, S, Hornig, DH. Contribution of selected vitamins and trace elements to immune function. *Ann Nutr Metab*. 2007;51:301–323.

22. Lansdown, AB, Mirastschijski, U, Stubbs, N, Scanlon, E, Agren, MS. Zinc in wound healing: Theoretical, experimental, and clinical aspects. *Wound Repair Regen*. 2007;15:2–16.

23. Hulisz, D. Efficacy of zinc against common cold viruses: An overview. *J Am Pharm Assoc*. (2003);44:594–603.

24. Caruso, TJ, Prober, CG, Gwaltney, JM, Jr. Treatment of naturally acquired common colds with zinc: A structured review. *Clin Infect Dis*. 2007;45:569–574.

25. Marshall, I. Zinc for the common cold. *Cochrane Database of Systematic Reviews*. 2000;2. Art. No.: CD001364. doi: 10.1002/14651858.CD001364.pub2.

26. Patrick, L. Nutrients and HIV: Part two—vitamins A and E, zinc, B-vitamins, and magnesium. *Altern Med Rev*. 2000 Feb;5(1):39–51.

27. Salgueiro, MJ, Weill, R, Zubillaga, M, et al. Zinc deficiency and growth: Current concepts in relationship to two important points: Intellectual and sexual development. *Biol Trace Elem Res*. 2004;99(1–3):49–69.

28. Wagner, PA, Bailey, LB, Christakis, GJ, Dinning, JS. Serum zinc concentrations in adolescents as related to sexual maturation. *Hum Nutr Clin Nutr*. 1985 Nov;39(6):459–462.

29. Imamoglu, S, Bereket, A, Turan, S, Taga, Y, Haklar, G. Effect of zinc supplementation on growth hormone secretion, IGF-I, IGFBP-3, somatomedin generation, alkaline phosphatase, osteocalcin and growth in prepubertal children with idiopathic short stature. *J Pediatr Endocrinol Metab*. 2005 Jan;18(1):69–74.

30. Brown, KH, Peerson, JM, Rivera, J, Allen, LH. Effect of supplemental zinc on the growth and serum zinc concentrations of prepubertal children: A meta-analysis of randomized controlled trials. *Am J Clin Nutr*. 2002 Jun;75(6):1062–1071.

31. Turner, RB, Cetnarowski, WE. Effect of treatment with zinc gluconate or zinc acetate on experimental and natural colds. *Clin Infect Dis*. 2000;31:1202–1208.

32. Hooper, PL, Visconti, L, Garry, PJ, Johnson, GE. Zinc lowers high-density lipoprotein-cholesterol levels. *JAMA*. 1980;244:1960–1961.

36

Magnesium

BRIEF OVERVIEW

Magnesium is a naturally occurring mineral. It is the fourth most common mineral found in the human body. Half of the magnesium in the body can be found in the bones. Almost all of the rest is in the body's organs and tissues, with only 1 percent of the total in the blood.

There are mechanisms to keep the blood level of magnesium constant. This is important because magnesium is involved in at least 300 biochemical reactions.[1]

In general terms, magnesium is involved in muscle contraction and relaxation, the production as well as transport of energy, the production of protein, and the function of hundreds of enzymes. Even though a significant percent of people, perhaps as high as 20 percent, do not ingest enough magnesium, it is not measured during routine blood tests.

THE HYPE

Magnesium maintains normal nerve and muscle function. It helps perpetuate

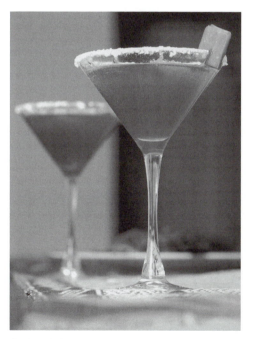

Cactus juice cocktails. Low in fat, the nopal is high in energy-boosting complex carbohydrates as well as calcium, magnesium, potassium, iron, and water-soluble fiber and pectin, which captures fats and disease-causing free radicals, making tasty nopales a natural preventive against cancer and other diseases. (AP Photo/LM Otero)

a normal heart rhythm. It is involved in keeping the bones and the immune system strong.

Magnesium is thought to help regulate blood sugar and is involved in keeping blood pressure normal. It is involved in the synthesis of protein and energy metabolism.

Magnesium may be useful in preventing or treating high blood pressure, diabetes, and cardiovascular disease as well as many other conditions.[1]

Oral supplements may be useful for people who do not get enough magnesium in their diet. However, many of the potential uses for magnesium are in medical/hospital settings.

Asthma

Magnesium has been used both by vein and by inhalation for acute asthma attacks in emergency room settings. Results have shown benefits to using intravenous magnesium for children.[2] There is less evidence for the effectiveness of magnesium in adults.[3]

There does seem to be some benefit to magnesium given by inhalation.[4] The improvements are reflected as lower hospital admission rates and/or improved lung function for those treated. In these cases, magnesium is used in addition to all the standard hospital emergency room care of severe asthma.

There is some evidence that giving children magnesium supplements on a daily basis can lessen the frequency of asthma attacks.[2]

Blood Pressure

There have been many epidemiologic studies that correlate high intake of magnesium with lower blood pressure, including the DASH (Dietary Approaches to Stop Hypertension) Study in the late 1990s. However, the ARIC (Atherosclerosis Risk in Communities) Study found that decreased magnesium intake raised the risk of developing hypertension in women only.[1]

The Joint National Committee on Prevention, Detection, Evaluation, and Treatment of High Blood Pressure has indicated that magnesium-rich diets are good for people with hypertension or those at risk for it. The DASH diet has been recommended to prevent hypertension. The NIH (National Institutes of Health) says that the plan "is clinically proven to significantly reduce blood pressure." It includes fruits, vegetables, low-fat or nonfat milk and milk products, whole grains, nuts, beans and seeds, fish, and poultry. The diet is low in salt, added sugars, fats (especially saturated fat, transfat, and cholesterol), and red meats, as compared with what most Americans usually eat. The DASH diet includes lots of nutrients thought to help lower blood pressure, including magnesium, calcium, and fiber, among others.[5]

While this may be true, it is impossible to separate magnesium from the other elements in the diet when looking at the observational studies. Prospective trials are needed to determine whether or not people given supplemental magnesium will be less likely to develop high blood pressure.

Diabetes

There is a relationship between magnesium and blood sugar. Low levels of the mineral are associated with type 2 diabetes. Type 2 diabetes, which is also known as adult-onset diabetes, occurs when the body cannot use insulin properly, usually in obese people. It is not known if the low magnesium levels make the diabetes worse, or if the diabetes causes the lower magnesium levels.

Low magnesium definitely can make insulin resistance worse, which can make blood sugar harder to control. Elevated blood sugar can cause more magnesium to be lost in the urine, leading to low magnesium levels. There is some evidence that supplemental magnesium can improve control of diabetes in older people.

Two long-term studies, the Nurses' Health Study and the Health Professionals Follow-up Study, which lasted 12 to 18 years, showed a greater risk for type 2 diabetes associated with lower magnesium intake.[1]

The Iowa Women's Health Study and the Women's Health Study came to similar conclusions. However, the ARIC Study (mentioned above) found no relationship between magnesium intake and diabetes. There have been some small prospective studies giving diabetics supplemental magnesium. There was improvement in diabetic control in one such study, and no effect in another study. There is no definitive proof that giving supplemental magnesium to diabetic patients who are not actually low on magnesium will be of benefit.[1]

There is some limited evidence that magnesium supplementation might improve the pain of peripheral neuropathy in diabetics.[6]

Cardiovascular Disease

There is evidence from animal studies that lowered magnesium levels can contribute to heart damage and heart failure. There is also a cardiomyopathy associated with the genetic condition of low magnesium called hereditary hypomagnesemia.[7]

Magnesium given by vein is one way to prevent a heart arrhythmia called atrial fibrillation from occurring during heart surgery.[8]

In the ARIC Study, low magnesium levels were associated with higher rates of coronary artery disease.[9] There have been other observational studies, and a few small studies using supplements that show a potential benefit to taking magnesium as far as heart health is concerned. There is nothing conclusive as yet to indicate that people should take magnesium unless they are deficient.

The American College of Cardiology and the American Heart Association have published guidelines listing measured low magnesium levels and/or a specific arrhythmia of the heart ventricles called "torsade de pointes-type ventricular tachycardia" as reasons to give magnesium to patients having acute heart attacks.[10]

Stroke

There is some evidence that higher levels of dietary magnesium can decrease the risk of stroke.[1]

Magnesium can also be used in a specific way to help manage a stroke. When a person has a stroke from lack of blood flow, protecting the brain tissue until the blood flow can be improved can limit the extent of the damage. This is called neuroprotection. The earlier it can be started, the better. There has been enough success with early studies using magnesium as a neuroprotectant to warrant a large trial, called FAST-MAG.[11,12]

FAST-MAG is a Phase III trial testing in-the-field administration of magnesium to stroke victims. It is the first trial using magnesium quickly, within the first two hours after onset of symptoms. Some 1,300 patients will be involved in the trial, which is currently underway.[13]

Magnesium may work best along with hypothermia in stroke neuroprotection. Some believe slightly cooling the person as well as giving the magnesium will protect the brain better.[14]

Pregnancy

Deficiency of magnesium in pregnancy is fairly common, with some 20 percent of pregnant women deficient. Some investigators believe that this can cause the uterus to be more excitable and make preterm labor more common. In these cases, giving magnesium can stop premature labor.

Higher doses of magnesium sulfate may be able to stop uterine contractions even in women who are not deficient.[15] This is an area of controversy. At least one analysis of available data indicated that magnesium sulfate was not useful for this purpose and might cause more fetal death.[16] A more recent review concluded that magnesium sulfate given to women at risk of preterm birth can protect the baby's brain.[17]

There is also speculation that low levels of maternal magnesium can contribute to congenital birth defects as well as sudden infant death syndrome (SIDS).[15]

Preeclampsia is a condition of the last trimester of pregnancy that includes high blood pressure, protein in the urine, and swelling of the feet and hands. Untreated preeclampsia can progress to eclampsia, with seizures and coma. Magnesium sulfate is used to prevent and treat seizures in pregnant women with preeclampsia/eclampsia.

Miscellaneous

Magnesium has been used with some success to prevent migraine headaches.[18]

Magnesium levels may play a role in the development of depression. In animals, low magnesium levels affect behavior. NMDA is a brain receptor that may be involved in both seizure activity as well as mood. Magnesium is an antagonist of this receptor complex. Blocking NMDA may be an important part of the way antidepressants work. This may eventually help develop other treatments for depression.[19]

Low magnesium can cause seizures. It may be useful to treat seizures in patients who might be magnesium deficient and in pregnant patients with preeclampsia. There is no evidence at the current time that it is a good treatment for people without low magnesium levels.[20]

Magnesium metabolism is related to calcium metabolism, and increased magnesium intake may help improve bone density.[1]

DEFICIENCY

Although studies have shown that many people do not get the recommended amount of magnesium in their diets, frank deficiency is unusual in otherwise healthy individuals. The kidneys are able to retain magnesium when it is needed, and the healthy intestine can absorb the necessary amount.[1]

Low magnesium levels can occur because of impaired absorption as the result of any illness that damages the intestinal tract. Examples include Crohn's disease, gluten-sensitive enteropathy (celiac disease), and regional inflammation in the intestine. Intestinal surgery may remove regions needed for magnesium absorption. Magnesium can also be lost during prolonged vomiting and diarrhea.

Magnesium can be lost in the urine because of diabetes, alcohol abuse, and also the use of certain medications. Medications that can cause magnesium loss in the urine are in the general categories of diuretics, antibiotics, and drugs used to treat cancer.

The cancer-treating medicine cisplatin causes magnesium loss, as do the antibiotics gentamicin and amphotericin. These two antibiotics are not in common use. However, diuretics like Lasix, hydrochlorthiazide, Bumex, and Edecrin are taken by many people to treat high blood pressure or congestive heart failure.[1] A relatively new drug used to treat cancer, cetuximab, also causes significant loss of magnesium.[21]

Low magnesium can occur after severe burns or surgery.

Symptoms of magnesium deficiency include loss of appetite, nausea, and vomiting. Other symptoms are weakness and fatigue. Lower levels can lead to personality changes, seizures, muscle cramps, twitching, hyperexciteability, tingling, and numbness. With lower levels, abnormal rhythms of the heart and spasm of the coronary arteries can occur. With severe deficiency, muscle spasms can be unrelenting, heart rhythms may be abnormal, and a person can have hallucinations or delirium.[22]

Unfortunately, blood tests to measure magnesium do not always reflect the amount of magnesium in the body and miss many cases of low magnesium. The best test may be a magnesium challenge test, in which magnesium is administered and urinary and blood levels then measured. Magnesium levels in red blood cells may better reflect magnesium status.

Low levels of magnesium are often associated with low levels of calcium as well as potassium in the blood.[1]

FOOD SOURCES

Magnesium is absorbed by the small intestine. It leaves the body through the kidneys.

Magnesium is in chlorophyll, found in all plants. Therefore, green vegetables are good sources of magnesium. Magnesium can also be found in some nuts, seeds, legumes, fruits, and unrefined grains.

The content of magnesium in water depends on the source. Hard water, which contains minerals, usually has magnesium in it.

Other sources of magnesium include certain fish, like halibut, dairy products, raisins, and bananas.

Some examples:[1]

- One serving of frozen, cooked spinach has 75 mg of magnesium.
- Three ounces of cooked halibut has 90 mg.
- One ounce of dry roasted almonds has 80 mg.
- One baked potato with skin has 50 mg.
- Two tablespoons of wheat bran have 45 mg.
- One serving of brown, long-grain rice has 40 mg.
- One banana has 30 mg.
- One cup of reduced or fat-free milk has 27 mg.

MECHANISM OF ACTION: HOW DOES IT WORK?

Magnesium is involved in hundreds of the human body's biochemical and metabolic reactions. Magnesium is distributed throughout the body. Half of the magnesium is in bones; 27 percent is in muscles; 19 percent is in the heart and liver.

Most of the magnesium found inside cells is bound to other chemical compounds, including nucleic acids (parts of the genetic code), ATP and ADP (energy sources), and proteins. Ninety percent is bound to compounds or structures made from these building blocks. Magnesium helps stabilize proteins, nucleic acids, and cell membranes. The small amount of free magnesium inside cells ensures that there will be enough magnesium when needed.

Magnesium is involved in the flux of molecules through membranes. It has an effect on various brain receptors that are involved with mood.

Adequate levels of magnesium are necessary for the normal regulation of many hormonal systems, for example, the complex relationships of hormones and minerals that manage bone structure and density. Parathyroid hormone stimulates the absorption of magnesium from the intestine and kidney, as well as the release of magnesium from bone. Magnesium affects the parathyroid glands and the action of vitamin D. There is an important, complex relationship between calcium and magnesium levels.[19]

Magnesium is also found in the blood—in the serum portion and in red blood cells. Some of it is bound, and some is free. There is a balance between magnesium in the blood and the central nervous system that is maintained by an active transport mechanism. The mechanism at the blood-brain barrier serves to keep the amount of magnesium in the brain up even if there is a generally low level in the blood.[19]

When extra magnesium is given by vein, it gets rapidly into the fluid around the brain at higher levels than the blood. It has many actions in the brain, including blocking the NMDA receptor, blocking certain chemical channels, and relaxing the blood vessels to allow more blood flow, among other things. All together, its actions can be neuroprotective (see "The Hype") in the case of stroke.[13]

The amount of magnesium getting through the blood-brain barrier may change as the result of seizure activity. After a seizure occurs, more magnesium may be able to enter the brain, where it acts to prevent more seizures. Magnesium sulfate is used to prevent seizures in women with preeclampsia and to treat seizures in pregnant women with eclampsia.

Magnesium sulfate is a vasodilator: it can cause the relaxation of blood vessel walls. Magnesium does this by acting as a calcium antagonist, acting on calcium channels in smooth muscle. It is believed that magnesium sulfate may lower blood pressure and the resistance of the blood vessels. This is the reason that it is thought to reduce seizures in eclampsia, not because it causes vasodilation in the brain.[23]

However, it is not completely clear how magnesium reduces seizures in eclampsia. Magnesium has effects on various factors in pregnancy. It can stimulate the production of prostacyclin, which also causes vasodilation. It can inhibit the clumping of platelets. In pregnant women with high blood pressure, magnesium sulfate lowers angiotensin-converting enzyme, one cause of high blood pressure.

Magnesium is an NMDA receptor antagonist, which may explain some of its anticonvulsant activity. NMDA is a brain receptor that may be involved in both seizure activity as well as mood.[23]

PRIMARY USES

Magnesium sulfate is used intravenously to prevent and control seizures in pregnant women with preeclampsia. This is accepted practice, although the way in which magnesium sulfate works is not completely understood.[23]

Supplements may be useful for people with asthma.[2]

Magnesium supplements should be given to anyone with a known or suspected deficiency. Supplementation may be especially needed for the following groups of people:[1]

- People with intestinal diseases causing poor absorption of calcium
- Pregnant women
- Alcoholics
- Poorly controlled diabetics
- Patients on the medications listed in "Deficiency" above
- People who have low levels of calcium and potassium
- People with high blood pressure
- Older adults

Since many people do not get enough magnesium, it is reasonable for people to take magnesium as a daily supplement.

COMMON DOSAGES

Dietary Requirements

These were set in 1999 by the Institute of Medicine. There were Recommended Dietary Allowances (RDAs) set for all groups except infants. The RDA is an amount sufficient for most healthy people.[1]

- For 1- to 3-year-olds, the RDA is 80 mg/day. For 4- to 8-year-olds, the RDA is 130 mg/day. For those ages 9 to 13, it is 240 mg/day.
- For men ages 14 to 18, the RDA is 410 mg/day. This drops down to 400 mg for men ages 19 to 30, and goes up to 420 mg/day for men ages 31 years and above.
- For women ages 14 to 18, the RDA is 360 mg/day. This drops down to 310 mg for women ages 19 to 30, and goes up to 320 mg/day for women ages 31 years and above.
- Women ages 14 to 18 who are pregnant need 400 mg/day; they need 360 mg/day while breast-feeding. Women ages 19 to 30 who are pregnant need 350 mg/day; they need 310 mg/day while breast-feeding. Women over 31 years of age who are pregnant need 360 mg/day, and 320 mg/day while breast-feeding. There is no difference in magnesium RDAs for breast-feeding women as opposed to nonpregnant women of the same age.
- For infants, the AI (Average Intake) is 30 mg/day for ages 0 to 6 months, and 75 mg/day for ages 7 to 12 months.

When people are slightly low on magnesium, oral supplements can help. The amount of elemental magnesium varies depending on what it is combined with. Magnesium carbonate is 45 percent magnesium; magnesium citrate is 16 percent magnesium. The amount of magnesium absorbed by the body also has to do with the preparation of the supplement.

For migraine prevention, 600 mg of trimagnesium dicitrate a day has been used.[18]

Symptomatic, severely low levels of magnesium must be treated with intravenous magnesium.

POTENTIAL SIDE EFFECTS

Both low and high magnesium levels can be dangerous. Normal amounts of magnesium in supplements and food are very safe. Magnesium excess can cause diarrhea and cramping. There is more risk of toxicity in people with kidney failure who cannot eliminate enough magnesium.

High magnesium levels can cause other symptoms somewhat similar to low magnesium levels, such as weakness, nausea, loss of appetite, and a change in personality/awareness (mental state). Trouble breathing, low blood pressure, and irregular heartbeat occur with low magnesium levels and not high levels.

Very high magnesium levels can cause death. This may happen to elderly people taking cathartics (for constipation) or antacids that contain magnesium. If their kidney function is deteriorating, magnesium levels can rise. Routine blood tests are not usually done to check magnesium and are not accurate.[24]

Magnesium is present in many laxatives and antacids. It is important to be aware of how much magnesium is in any of these over-the-counter preparations.[1]

FACT VERSUS FICTION

Magnesium is an essential mineral. Many people do not ingest enough of it in their diet. Taking magnesium supplements is reasonable, especially for people more likely than others to have low levels of magnesium.

It is possible that taking magnesium may lower the risk of high blood pressure, diabetes, and/or heart disease, but this has not been proven.

Magnesium is used in the medical treatment of pregnant women with eclampsia/preeclampsia. It can be used to prevent atrial fibrillation during heart surgery. It may become part of the standard emergency treatment of asthma, but this is not certain. It may also become standard as a neuroprotective agent for people suffering a stroke. There are probably many other medical uses that will eventually be better understood.

REFERENCES

1. National Institutes of Health. Office of Dietary Supplements. *Magnesium.* Updated July 13, 2009. http://ods.od.nih.gov/factsheets/magnesium.asp. Accessed June 14, 2010.
2. Bichera, MD, Goldman, RD. Magnesium for treatment of asthma in children. *Canadian Family Physician.* 2009;55:887–889.
3. Mohammed, S, Goodacre, S. Intravenous and nebulised magnesium sulphate for acute asthma: Systematic review and meta-analysis. *Emerg Med J.* 2007;24:823–830.
4. Blitz, M, Blitz, S, Beasely, R, Diner, B, Hughes, R, Knopp, JA, Rowe, BH. Inhaled magnesium sulfate in the treatment of acute asthma. *Cochrane Database of Systematic Reviews.* 2005;4. Art. No.: CD003898 (updated 2009). doi:10.1002/14651858.
5. National Institutes of Health. Your guide to lowering your blood pressure with DASH. http://www.nhlbi.nih.gov/health/public/heart/hbp/dash/dash_brief.pdf. Accessed June 17, 2010.
6. Head, KA. Peripheral neuropathy: Pathogenic mechanisms and alternative therapies. *Altern Med Rev.* 2006;11(4):294–329.
7. Weber, KT, Weglicki, WB, Simpson, RU. Macro- and micronutrient dyshomeostasis in the adverse structural remodelling of myocardium. *Cardiovascular Research.* 2009;81:500–508.
8. Dunning, J, Treasure, T, Versteegh, M, Nashef, SAM. Guidelines on the prevention and management of de novo atrial fibrillation after cardiac and thoracic surgery. *Eur J Cardiothorac Surg.* 2006;30:852–872.

9. Liao, F, Folsom, A, Brancati, F. Is low magnesium concentration a risk factor for coronary heart disease? The Atherosclerosis Risk in Communities (ARIC) Study. *Am Heart J* 1998;136:480–490.

10. Anbe, DT, Armstrong, PW, Bates, ER, et al. ACC/AHA Guidelines for the Management of Patients with ST-Elevation Myocardial Infarction. *Circulation.* 2004;110;588–636.

11. Kidd, PM. Integrated brain restoration after ischemic stroke—medical management, risk factors, nutrients, and other interventions for managing inflammation and enhancing brain plasticity. *Altern Med Rev.* 2009;14(1):14–35.

12. Guidelines for the Early Management of Adults with Ischemic Stroke: A Guideline from the American Heart Association/American Stroke Association Stroke Council, Clinical Cardiology Council, Cardiovascular Radiology and Intervention Council, and the Atherosclerotic Peripheral Vascular Disease and Quality of Care Outcomes in Research Interdisciplinary Working Groups. The American Academy of Neurology affirms the value of this guideline as an educational tool for neurologists. *Circulation.* 2007;115:e478–e534.

13. The Field Administration of Stroke Therapy-Magnesium Phase 3 Clinical Trial. FAST-MAG. http://www.fastmag.info/index.htm. Accessed June 21, 2010.

14. Meloni, BP, Campbell, K, Zhu, H, Knuckey, NW. In search of clinical neuroprotection after brain ischemia: The case for mild hypothermia (35°C) and magnesium. *Stroke.* 2009;40:2236–2240.

15. Durlach, J. New data on the importance of gestational Mg deficiency. *Journal of the American College of Nutrition.* 2004;23(6):694S–700S.

16. Crowther, CA, Hiller, JE, Doyle, LW. Magnesium sulphate for preventing preterm birth in threatened preterm labour. *Cochrane Database of Systematic Reviews.* 2002;4. Art. No.: CD001060. doi:10.1002/14651858.

17. Doyle, LW, Crowther, CA, Middleton, P, Marret, S, Rouse, D. Magnesium sulphate for women at risk of preterm birth for neuroprotection of the fetus. *Cochrane Database of Systematic Reviews.* 2009;1. Art. No.: CD004661. doi:10.1002/14651858.

18. Modi, S, Lowder, DM. Medications for migraine prophylaxis. *Am Fam Physician.* 2006;73:72–78.

19. Szewczyk, B, Poleszak, E, Sowa-Kucma, M, et al. Antidepressant activity of zinc and magnesium in view of the current hypotheses of antidepressant action. *Pharmacological Reports.* 2008;60:588–599.

20. Gaby, AR. Natural approaches to epilepsy. *Altern Med Rev.* 2007;12(1):9–24.

21. Schrag, D, Chung, KY, Flombaum, C, Saltz, L. Cetuximab therapy and symptomatic hypomagnesemia. *Journal of the National Cancer Institute.* 2005;97(16):1221–1224.

22. Medline Plus. Magnesium in diet. Updated March 9, 2009. http://www.nlm.nih.gov/medlineplus/ency/article/002423.htm. Accessed June 21, 2010.

23. Euser, AG, Cipolla, MJ. Magnesium sulfate treatment for the prevention of eclampsia: A brief review. *Stroke.* 2009;40(4):1169–1175.

24. Onishi, S, Yoshino, S. Cathartic-induced fatal hypermagnesemia in the elderly. *Internal Medicine.* 2006;45(4):207–210.

37

Vanadyl Sulfate

BRIEF OVERVIEW

Vanadium is a naturally occurring metal that was discovered more than 200 years ago. While it is an essential nutrient in some animal species, it has not been proven to be essential for humans.

Most people have very low levels of vanadium in their body tissues. It has been estimated that adults in the United States consume approximately 9 µg a day. If vanadium is essential, it would have to be considered a micronutrient that is needed only in very small amounts.

Vanadium can mimic some of the properties of insulin. In the body, it seems to increase insulin sensitivity and may lower blood sugar. It has be given, usually as vanadyl sulfate, to diabetics to help control their diabetes. Vanadium was discovered before insulin and was used by French physicians in the early 20th century to treat diabetes mellitus. However, it is not clear how useful it is compared to the medications available now.

THE HYPE

Vanadyl Sulfate can Help Treat Diabetes

As noted above, vanadyl sulfate was used 100 years ago to treat diabetics. It is now known that vanadium mimics or enhances insulin to some degree. However, the overwhelming majority of the research on vanadium has been biochemical analysis in a laboratory or animal studies on mice, rats, gerbils, and goats.

There are two types of diabetes. In type 1 diabetes, also called insulin-dependent diabetes, the body does not make enough insulin. This type of diabetes frequently comes on early in life. In type 2, the body is resistant to the effects of insulin, along with some decreasing amounts of insulin produced. This often comes on later in life and is usually associated with obesity. Glucose intolerance, or prediabetes, means that the body is not handling sugar as well as it should, and fasting glucose levels may be slightly elevated.

In 2008, reviewers searched the medical literature for high-quality trials of vanadium supplements used to treat type 2 diabetes. It is established in research that high-quality clinical trials include comparing the medicine to placebo, "blinding," which means that the patients and preferably also the doctors don't know who is getting active medication. Trials need to have enough participants so that any differences will be statistically significant, and they need to last long enough to get an idea of long-term safety and efficacy.

In the case of vanadium, that would mean that the researchers compared vanadium to placebo, with participants randomized as to what they received, that the study lasted at least two months, and that there were a minimum of 10 subjects in each part of the trial. Of 151 studies found, none met these criteria. This means that there was no available high-quality research to support the use of vanadium in treating diabetes in 2008.[1]

The reviewers looked at the same clinical trials a second time with less-strict criteria. They looked for studies in which vanadium supplementation was given to diabetics, and at least 30 to 150 mg of vanadium a day was used. They found only five studies. There was some evidence of improved control of fasting blood sugars with use of vanadium. However, the total number of diabetics given vanadium adding all five studies together was only 48. The trials were not conducted in the manner necessary to accurately judge the results. The investigators did not test vanadium against placebo in every case. These studies were too short to measure an important indicator of long-term blood sugar control, HbA1c, or glycosylated hemoglobin. In no case had long-term safety of what were high doses of vanadium been examined. The authors of this study suggested that high-quality research should be performed, but in the absence of such research at this point, vanadyl sulfate should not be recommended to help control type 2 diabetes.[1]

Reviewers writing in the *Canadian Family Physician* in 2009, looking at the same information, also concluded that there is not enough evidence to recommend the use of vanadium for treatment of diabetes.[2]

However, the *Alternative Medicine Review* in 2009 described the results of four of the five of these studies, noting that they showed vanadyl sulfate could be effective in type 2 diabetes.[3] This same review made note of a study of patients with impaired glucose tolerance given vanadyl sulfate with no effect on blood sugar. In the study, 14 overweight or obese patients with evidence of impaired glucose tolerance were given vanadyl sulfate (50 mg twice a day) for four weeks. This trial was double-blind and placebo-controlled. There were no significant effects on blood glucose levels. However, it is important to note that the patients who got vanadyl sulfate experienced a rise in triglyceride levels.[4] Triglycerides are a type of fat in the blood.

It is considered possible that type 1 diabetics could lower their insulin dose by adding vanadyl sulfate. In rats, large amounts of vanadium improve glucose tolerance. However, the amount of vanadium needed to achieve insulin dose reductions may be high, and the research relative to doing this is very sparse and out of date.[5]

One study that included five insulin-dependent diabetics given 125 mg of vanadyl sulfate a day for two weeks found that it caused a "significant decrease" in insulin requirements for those studied.[6] Another study showed no effect on glucose levels or insulin requirements in five type 1 diabetics given 100 mg of vanadyl sulfate a day. It has been suggested that vanadyl sulfate may only work in type 2 diabetics because it increases insulin action and reduces insulin resistance.[7] Type 1 diabetics do not make enough insulin, so there is nothing to enhance.

While there are no long-term studies of high-dose oral vanadium or vanadyl sulfate, there is evidence that occupational exposure to vanadium can cause DNA damage, which puts people at risk of cancer.[8]

Researchers today are trying to put vanadium into a chemical compound that can deliver large amounts of vanadium without toxicity, studying a variety of vanadium-containing compounds and their effects on blood sugar. They are trying to keep all the positive effects of vanadyl sulfate and vanadium but in a more tolerable and safe drug. Bis(maltolato)oxovanadium (IV) (BMOV) and the ethylmaltol analog, bis(ethylmaltolato)oxovanadium (IV) (BEOV), are being tested. As of 2009, BEOV was in Phase IIa clinical trials, being tested successfully on a small group of type 2 diabetics.[9] There are other vanadium-containing drugs being studied.

Weight Training

Vanadyl sulfate is used by athletes during weight training to increase performance and muscle mass. Because vanadium mimics insulin, it is thought it might help promote protein growth. Vanadyl sulfate is marketed as a muscle builder. A dose of 60 mg a day is usually taken. However, there is no evidence as yet that vanadium increases lean body mass, builds muscle, or helps decrease fat mass.[10]

In one study involving 31 weight-training volunteers, there were no differences in body parameters or body composition after 12 weeks of treatment with vanadyl sulfate. There was only a slight suggestion of performance enhancement in number of leg extension repetitions. This was not considered definitive.[11]

Cancer

As a trace mineral/metal, vanadium shares properties with other chemicals that are used to treat cancer, the best-known of which is the group related to platinum, including cisplatin. Vanadium has been shown in countless animal studies to have an effect on both primary cancers and metastatic cancers. In animals, vanadium has many complicated and varied effects on cancer cells. This has not yet been translated into any actual treatment.[12]

Bone Structure and Strength

In rats, there have been studies showing that vanadium being tested as a treatment for diabetes accumulates in bone and may strengthen bones that have been weakened by the diabetic state.

One study demonstrating vanadium's effect on bones used BEOV, one of the new vanadium-containing compounds.[13]

DEFICIENCY

There is no known function of vanadium in humans. Without a biological role, the Institute of Medicine has not made an Average Daily Requirement, Recommended Dietary Allowance, or Adequate Intake.[5]

No deficiency state has been found or described in humans.[3]

As one author put it in 1994, "Is vanadium of human nutritional importance yet?" At that time, no definitive role had been found.[14] The same is true today. While most people consume trace amounts of vanadium, a specific and necessary function for vanadium has not been discovered.

FOOD SOURCES

There is a variety of foods that contain vanadium. Some research suggests that processed foods have more vanadium than unprocessed foods. Mushrooms and shellfish contain vanadium, as do dill seed, parsley, and black pepper. Beer and wine are sources of vanadium, as are grains and grain products, as well as other beverages. The average intake of people in the United States may be approximately 9 μg a day.[5] The average diet contains between 6 to 18 μg a day.[3]

Most vanadium in the diet is not absorbed. The 1 to 10 percent that is absorbed is excreted quickly via the kidneys.[3,15]

Humans also can absorb some vanadium from the environment, through the skin and mucous membranes. It is in the air as a byproduct of various types of combustion and refining processes.[8,12]

MECHANISM OF ACTION: HOW DOES IT WORK?

All the actions of vanadium in the human body are still not fully understood.[2] Vanadium stimulates cell growth and differentiation. How it mimics the effects of insulin is not entirely clear. Vanadium inhibits a number of enzymes. The effects of inhibiting these enzymes have only been ascertained in animals such as rats and goats.[5]

It is believed that inhibition of phosphotryosine phosphatase enzymes affects the insulin receptors of cells.[2] This may up-regulate the insulin receptors, which would make them more sensitive to insulin. In animal studies, vanadium enhances insulin sensitivity and makes the uptake of glucose into cells easier. In humans, it may increase the synthesis of glycogen (a way to store glucose) and moderate the amount of glucose that leaves the liver.[16]

While the vanadate form is active in a laboratory setting, in the body, most vanadium is in the vanadyl form.[5]

There are dozens of ways that vanadium interacts with cancer cells in vitro. Key may be its modification of enzymes in the malignant cells. These modifications may cause cell death or inhibit cell growth.[12]

PRIMARY USES

- At the current time there are very few definite uses for vanadyl sulfate. Vanadium may be a necessary micronutrient, in which case a very small amount can be taken as a dietary supplement.

- Athletes trying to stimulate muscle growth while weight training may take much higher doses of vanadyl sulfate.

- Diabetics trying to control their blood sugar may take vanadyl sulfate, again, in much higher doses.

COMMON DOSAGES

Vanadium occurs in a number of forms. Vanadyl sulfate is 31 percent vanadium. Sodium metavanadate is 42 percent vanadium. Sodium orthovanadate is 23 percent vanadium.[3] Vanadyl sulfate is the most commonly used form of vanadium.

Considering vanadium as a necessary micronutrient, 20 µg a day has been recommended.[3]

As a treatment for diabetes, usually 100 mg/day of vanadyl sulfate is used, often 50 mg twice a day. Sometimes 125 mg of sodium metavanadate can be used instead.[3,5]

Athletes may take up to 60 mg a day of vanadyl sulfate during weight training.[15]

POTENTIAL SIDE EFFECTS

There is a Tolerable Upper Limit (UL) of vanadium set by the Institute of Medicine. The IOM recommends that doses above the UL only be taken during clinical trials and/or under medical supervision.

There are no adverse events reported to have occurred from vanadium in the diet. However, there have been adverse effects from vanadium in supplements.

There have been no reports of acute vanadium toxicity in humans due to ingested vanadium. There have also been no reports of kidney damage. In animal studies, kidney and liver damage can be caused by excessive vanadium intake, as can diarrhea and death.

Humans taking large amounts of vanadium for diabetes have had loose stools and mild cramps. Studies of these effects have been very small, including anywhere from 6 to 10 adults, many reporting gastrointestinal side effects when being treated.[5] People have also experienced more severe stomach upset, bloating, and nausea.[2] Patients given vanadium for up to six months in one study lost weight, possibly because of the gastrointestinal symptoms, including anorexia and abdominal pain.[12]

One small trial giving vanadium sulfate to patients who had impaired glucose tolerance reported it raised their triglyceride levels.[4]

Other observed effects, inconsistently noted and not dose-related include:

- Green tongue
- Fatigue
- Lethargy

The EPA used a study in rats to set an oral reference dose at 0.009 mg/kg/day for humans and animals. The IOM did not use this study to set an UL, but rather used data from kidney toxicity in rats and extended it to humans. The Lowest Observed

Adverse Effects Level (LOAEL) was 7.7 mg/kg body weight/day, based on rat data. Since this is clearly just an estimate, it has a high level of uncertainty. Using a specific formula including the LOAEL and the uncertainty, the IOM set an UL of 1.8 mg/day. The 1.8 refers to elemental vanadium. Since 60 mg of vanadyl sulfate contains 18.6 mg of vanadium, the UL would be about 5.8 mg of vanadyl sulfate, which is much less than what has been given to diabetics and athletes.

The IOM does not want setting the UL to prevent studies of the higher doses. However, since the damage in animals has been to the kidneys, and since the vanadyl sulfate is being given to diabetics who are already at risk for kidney problems, it is an area of concern.

Others have suggested a supplement dose of 10 to 100 µg a day should be safe.[3]

Airborne vanadium pentoxide in high concentrations from industrial exposure is the source of most vanadium toxicity. This toxicity is most obvious as irritation to the eyes, nose, mouth, and respiratory tract.[15] However, there has been DNA damage and other changes in blood that indicate that inhalation exposure to certain forms of vanadium can cause more serious damage.[8]

FACT VERSUS FICTION

It is clear that vanadium does have an effect on glucose metabolism. It is not clear if vanadyl sulfate can benefit both type 1 and type 2 diabetics. It is not clear if vanadyl sulfate can be effective and safe in treating diabetes over long periods of time. The reasons are not clear as to why no one has done large and well-designed clinical trials to answer these questions.

Many people working with vanadium believe that vanadyl sulfate and other commonly used forms of vanadium cannot deliver enough of the vanadium to be effective without causing toxicity and side effects. Many vanadium-containing compounds have been made to try and overcome these problems, and some of them are now in early clinical trials.

Hopefully, there will be more answers about the efficacy and safety of vanadyl sulfate and other vanadium-containing chemicals in the near future.

It is also unclear if vanadyl sulfate can help weight lifters. More research is necessary.

In the meantime, anyone who is taking vanadyl sulfate in high doses should be monitored carefully. Diabetics especially should be followed closely. Athletes taking vanadium should have periodic blood tests.

For many people, the amount of vanadyl sulfate needed for any significant effect on blood sugar or muscle mass will cause them gastrointestinal distress, and they will discontinue the supplement.

REFERENCES

1. Smith, DM, Pickering, RM, Lewith, GT. A systematic review of vanadium oral supplements for glycaemic control in type 2 diabetes mellitus. *Q J Med.* 2008;101:351–358.

2. Nahas, R, Moher, M. Complementary and alternative medicine for the treatment of type 2 diabetes. *Can Fam Physician.* 2009;55:591–596.
3. Thorne Research. Vanadium/vanadyl sulfate. *Altern Med Rev.* 2009;14(2): 177–180.
4. Jacques-Camarena, O, González-Ortiz, M, Martínez-Abundis, E, et al. Effect of vanadium on insulin sensitivity in patients with impaired glucose tolerance. *Ann Nutr Metab.* 2008;53:195–198.
5. Institute of Medicine. Food and Nutrition Board. *Dietary reference intakes for vitamin A, vitamin K, arsenic, boron, chromium, copper, iodine, iron, manganese, molybdenum, nickel, silicon, vanadium, and zinc.* Washington, DC: National Academies Press, 2001.
6. Goldfine, AB, Simonson, DC, Folli, F, Patti, ME, Kahn, CR. Metabolic effects of sodium metavanadate in humans with insulin-dependent and noninsulin-dependent diabetes mellitus in vivo and in vitro studies. *J Clin Endocrinol Metab.* 1995;80:3311–3320.
7. Aharon, Y, Mevorach, M, Shamoon, H. Vanadyl sulfate does not enhance insulin action in patients with type 1 diabetes. [letter]. *Diabetes Care.* 1998;21(12): 2194–2195.
8. Ehrlich, VA, Nersesyan, AK, Hoelzl, C, et al. Inhalative exposure to vanadium pentoxide causes DNA damage in workers: Results of a multiple end point study. *Environ Health Perspect.* 2008;116:1689–1693.
9. Thompson, KH, Lichter, J, LeBel, C, et al. Vanadium treatment of type 2 diabetes: A view to the future. *Journal of Inorganic Biochemistry.* 2009;103(4): 554–558.
10. Patel, DR, Greydanus, DE. Nutritional supplement use by young athletes: An update. *Int Pediatr.* 2005;20(1):15–24.
11. Fawcett, JP, Farquhar, SJ, Walker, RJ, et al. The effect of oral vanadyl sulfate on body composition and performance in weight-training athletes. *Int J Sport Nutr.* 1996;6(4):382–390.
12. Evangelou, AM. Vanadium in cancer treatment. *Critical Reviews in Oncology/ Hematology.* 2002;42:249–265.
13. Facchini, DM, Yuen, VG, Battell, ML, et al. The effects of vanadium treatment on bone in diabetic and non-diabetic rats. *Bone.* 2006;38(3):368–377.
14. Harland, BF, Harden-Williams, BA. Is vanadium of human nutritional importance yet? *Journal of the American Dietetic Association.* 1994;94(8):891–894.
15. Barceloux, DG. Vanadium. *J Toxicol Clin Toxicol.* 1999;37:265–278.
16. Yeh, GY, Eisenberg, DM, Kaptchuk, TJ, Phillips, RS. Systematic review of herbs and dietary supplements for glycemic control in diabetes. *Diabetes Care.* 2003;26:1277–1294.

38

Probiotics

BRIEF OVERVIEW

Probiotics are living microbes that are beneficial to human health. As noted in Chapter 27, "Saccharomyces Boulardii," there is a great deal of advertising for probiotics at the current time, especially those in yogurt and other milk products. This makes probiotics seem like a new idea, but that is not the case. In 1935, Dr. Minoru Shirota discovered a bacterium that could improve health, which was named after him, Lactobacillus casei Shirota. It has been used in Japan for decades. The acceptance of yogurt-containing bacteria as a health supplement goes back centuries in many cultures.

The first official definition of a probiotic was written in 1989 by Robert Fuller. A probiotics is, he said, "A live microbial feed supplement which beneficially affects the host animal by improving its intestinal microbial balance."[1] According to the World Health Organization, it now includes "live micro-organisms that, when administered in adequate amounts, confer a health benefit to the host."[2]

More people than ever are taking probiotics. One reason is that more brands are being produced, advertised, and sold in the grocery store. Another is that the medical community is discovering which conditions probiotics can improve and which probiotics work best. Probiotics are being used as medical treatment in some cases.

The bacterial probiotics found in milk products are being sold to promote good gastrointestinal health, for example, regular bowel movements. There are more specific reasons to take them and some reasons not to take them.

This chapter will cover probiotic bacteria. S. boulardii, a probiotic yeast, is covered in Chapter 27.

THE HYPE

The claim has been made that all probiotics are good for everyone, to improve gastrointestinal health as well as general health. Since this is probably an overstatement, there has been much research to try and define the best uses for these organisms.

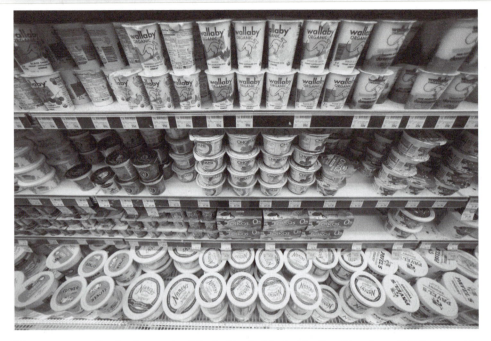

The yogurt section is shown at a Whole Foods Market in San Francisco, 2010. Yogurt is often a source of probiotics. (AP Photo/Eric Risberg)

Prevention of Traveler's Diarrhea

Diarrhea is a common problem for people visiting areas where there is a lot of bacterial contamination of food and water. This is more likely in some areas than others. For example, 50 percent of visitors to Latin America may contract traveler's diarrhea. It can even happen just because there are different bacteria in other parts of the world than those a person is exposed to at home, even if none of the bacteria are normally considered to cause disease. However, traveler's diarrhea is more likely to occur where there are pathogenic (disease-causing) bacteria found in food sources.

In these cases, the diarrhea can be accompanied by cramps and nausea. More severely affected individuals may have fever, vomiting, bloody diarrhea, and prolonged symptoms.

There has been much research into the use of probiotics for traveler's diarrhea. An analysis of good-quality studies included those using a variety of bacteria. There is some evidence that Lactobacillus rhamnosus can lower the risk of developing traveler's diarrhea, without significant side effects. Mixtures of bacteria also show some benefit. Tested mixtures included Lactobacillus acidophilus, Lactobacillus bulgaris, Bifidobacter bifidum, and Streptococcus thermophilus. While there have been positive results in some tests with these bacteria, this particular analysis indicated that yeast S. boulardii was the most effective probiotic to prevent traveler's diarrhea.[3]

Treatment of Acute Diarrhea

In Children

Acute diarrhea in children is usually viral. Probiotics can help shorten the course of viral diarrheal illnesses in children. In one large, placebo-controlled study, for example, L. casei was effective, as was a mix of L. delbrueckii var bulgaricus, L. acidophilus, S. thermophilus, and B. bifidum. Each of these shortened the course of the diarrheal illness by about a day and a half as well as lessening the severity.[4]

A number of studies and analyses of multiple trials have found many probiotics useful in shortening the duration and symptoms of acute diarrhea in children.[5]

A number of studies have found probiotics useful for reducing the length and severity of diarrhea specifically associated with rotavirus infection.[6]

In Adults

Other analysis of multiple studies has indicated that probiotics can shorten the course of acute infectious diarrhea in adults.[5]

Prevention of Antibiotic-Associated Diarrhea

General

Antibiotic-associated diarrhea is a common problem. Antibiotics do not just kill the infectious agent being treated. They also kill a number of safe bacteria that normally live in the intestine. Upsetting the bacterial balance in the intestine allows those that are more likely to cause diarrhea to grow. Probiotics formulas can offset this effect because they are good bacteria that do not cause diarrhea; they can prevent the overgrowth of pathogenic bacteria.

A review of 31 good-quality studies involving probiotic use to prevent antibiotic-associated diarrhea in both children and adults found that probiotics are effective in preventing antibiotic-associated diarrhea. Three types of probiotics seem to be most effective—S. boulardii, Lactobacillus rhamnosus GG, and mixtures of probiotic organisms.[7]

Another review found a 52 percent reduction of antibiotic-associated diarrhea with the use of probiotics, and that most of the probiotics in general use are effective.[8]

Children

Analysis of a number of studies of antibiotic-associated diarrhea specifically in children found that probiotics help prevent it. The analyzed studies used Lactobacilli species, Bifidobacterium species, Streptococcus species, and Saccharomyces boulardii alone or in combination. These bacteria (as well as the yeast) were said to "show promise" with larger, good-quality research suggested.[9]

Adults

In one study, half of a group of 135 elderly, hospitalized patients on antibiotics were randomized to take a commercially prepared yogurt drink containing

Lactobacillus casei imunitass, S. thermophilus, and L. bulgaricus. They took it twice a day, continued a week past the end of antibiotic use. This definitely decreased the incidence of diarrhea, from 34 to 12 percent.[10] Additionally, the group taking probiotics did not have evidence of C. difficile (see next section). There were no adverse results reported.

Prevention and/or Treatment of C. Difficile Diarrhea

The bacterium Clostridium difficile can cause diarrhea during and after antibiotic treatment. C. difficile can grow while a person takes antibiotics and cause diarrheal disease through toxins it secretes. Hospitalized elderly, or those in nursing homes, are more at risk for C. difficile illness.[11] The range of this disease is from a simple, diarrheal illness to something much more serious called pseudomembranous colitis, which can lead to intestinal perforation and even death. C. difficile is difficult to treat because it is resistant to many antibiotics.

In the study mentioned above, 17 percent of the patients not given probiotics, all of whom had diarrhea, were positive for C. difficile toxin, whereas none of the patients taking the probiotic were positive for toxin, including those with diarrhea. This particular group of patients did not include anyone taking the antibiotics known to be most closely associated with C. difficile, but some of them manifested it anyway.[10] This provides some evidence that probiotic administration may be helpful in preventing C. difficile illness.

This is an area of ongoing research. Bacterial probiotics are not yet recommended for this purpose.[6]

Treatment of Inflammatory Bowel Diseases

There are a number of pathogenic bacteria that may contribute to the development of inflammatory bowel diseases or may cause flare-ups of the diseases. It is thought that a combination of genetics, bacteria, and a person's immune status can lead to one of these diseases. It therefore seems reasonable that probiotic bacteria might be able to help treat inflammatory bowel diseases.

Probiotics may help treat inflammatory bowel diseases, including Crohn's disease and ulcerative colitis. These bacteria may make some anti-inflammatory chemical substances. They also may be able to stabilize the intestinal lining, as well as send signals to host cells to lower inflammation.

A number of clinical trials have demonstrated that probiotics can maintain remission in ulcerative colitis. In one study, a nonpathogenic strain of E. coli maintained remission as long as the standard treatment of mesalamine. Other probiotics, such as a mixture of Lactobacilli, Bifidobacteria strains, and S. salivariius thermophilus (VSL #3), have also been able to maintain remission in ulcerative colitis, Crohn's disease, and pouchitis, which is an inflammation of remaining bowel after the rest has been surgically removed.[12] However, large placebo-controlled studies are needed.

Treatment of Irritable Bowel Syndrome

The causes of irritable bowel syndrome are not completely understood. They may include a change in the movements of the intestinal walls, overgrowth of bacteria in the small intestine, tiny areas of inflammation, and oversensitivity to pain from the intestine. Probiotics could be helpful in treating a number of these factors. However, there have only been a small number of trials. Many have used similar bacteria to those used in inflammatory bowel disease testing, including Lactobacillus, Bifidobacterium, and mixtures of bacteria. In one small study using VSL#3, there was a slight decrease in bloating, but it was not statistically significant. In another, there was a delay in the time it takes food residue to go through the large intestine and a reduction of flatulence.[13]

Other studies using different probiotics have shown decreases in symptoms. These studies have been small, often lack control groups, and have not been randomized. However, some have shown improvement in symptoms, such as pain and bloating, and quality-of-life scores. Bifidobacterium seem to be more effective than Lactobacillus species.

One meta-analysis of multiple trials has shown a tendency toward improvement of patients with irritable bowel syndrome. Another concluded that only one of the Bifidobacterium species showed any promise.[13]

One study of 86 patients randomized to receive a multispecies probiotic or placebo for five months showed a significant improvement in symptoms for the treated patients.[14]

Large, placebo-controlled, randomized trials need to be done.

Allergy

The use of probiotics to prevent allergic diseases from developing in children is extremely controversial.

The incidence of allergic diseases, including eczema and asthma, seems to be rising, and no one is sure why. One theory called the "hygiene hypothesis" states that there are less normal bacteria around to help babies' immune systems develop. The immune system is thought to develop by learning to tolerate intestinal bacteria. Compared to the past, the food is more sterile, hygiene is improved, vaccination reduces the spread of some of the communicable diseases, and antibiotics kill some of the bacteria. Infants might have fewer bacteria in their intestines, so the immune system does not develop normally. Infants with skin allergy—eczema and atopic dermatitis—have been found to have different intestinal bacteria than nonallergic babies, which lends some support to this theory.

Allergic tendencies run in families. Infants with allergic parents or siblings are more likely to become allergic than those without allergic family members. Proponents of the hygiene hypothesis believe that giving infants at risk probiotics may help their immune systems develop properly. There has been some success giving probiotics to infants, including Bifidobacterium lactis, Lactobacillus rhamnosus, and combinations of bacteria. These have been used in some trials with an improvement in eczema among children who are positive to skin prick tests, meaning that when a tiny amount of an allergic substance is put into the skin with a pinprick, they have a red, raised area showing a reaction.

There have also been attempts at preventing eczema by giving probiotics to pregnant mothers with allergies and subsequently to their infants. In one study, allergic mothers were given L. rhamnosus GG or placebo for two to four weeks before they were expected to have their babies. Afterward, the infants received the same for six months; 46 percent of the children in the placebo group developed eczema, as opposed to 26 percent of those given probiotics.[15]

Another trial used two strains of Lactobacillus rhamnosus, Bifidobacterium breve, and Propionibacterium freudenreichii given in capsules to mothers two to four weeks before delivery, and the same mixed in sugar drops to their babies for six months. There was a matched placebo group. The children were followed until two years of age. The risk of eczema was 26 percent less in the children who took probiotics, and they had a 34 percent less risk of what was called atopic eczema. This is eczema in children with high blood levels of IgE, an immunoglobulin that is higher in people with allergy. They concluded that probiotics lowered the risk of eczema, atopic eczema, and any IgE-associated disease. These authors believe that probiotics should be given to mothers and babies at high risk of developing allergies.[16]

However, not all trials using probiotics this way have had the same results. Another group of researchers working at about the same time took a group of newborns whose mothers were allergic and gave half placebo and half probiotics, in this case Lactobacillus acidophilus. The probiotic preparation had no detectable milk protein in it. The babies who took the probiotic did show the bacteria in their intestines at six months of age. However, at six months they did not have any less skin allergy than the babies who took placebo. At a year of age, the babies who took probiotics had a higher incidence of skin allergy together with skin prick positivity than the babies who got placebo. Also, at six months, the babies who got the Lactobacillus had an increased incidence of sensitivity to cow's milk.[17]

Another double-blind, placebo-controlled trial in which the treated mothers took probiotic Lactobacillus GG four to six weeks before delivery and then the infants were given the same for six months did not show a benefit from the probiotics. The children were followed until two years of age. They did not have less atopic dermatitis (eczema), less severe dermatitis, or diseases with wheezing (asthma) than the children given placebo.[18]

The American Academy of Pediatrics does not believe there is enough information to make guidelines establishing the use of probiotics to prevent allergy.

Miscellaneous Uses

Urinary tract infections in women are often caused by E. coli, thought to come from the intestine or vaginal tract. If probiotics can change the bacterial colonization, they might be able to prevent urinary tract infections. There have only been limited studies with oral probiotics for this purpose, including a trial using

L. rhamnosus GG to prevent urinary tract infections in premature infants. There was a trend toward a decreased infection rate, but it was not statistically significant. L. acidophilus was reported to be useful in a case report of one six-year-old girl with recurrent urinary tract infections.[19] More research needs to be done in this area.

Probiotics, usually Lactobacilli, have been used to treat H. pylori infections associated with gastritis or gastric ulcer. While they do not eradicate the infection when used alone, they can improve gastritis and reduce the numbers of H. pylori. In conjunction with standard treatment, probiotics improve the eradication rate and significantly reduce side effects.[20]

DEFICIENCY

Probiotics are not a vitamin or essential nutrient. There is no deficiency state.

FOOD SOURCES

Bacterial probiotics are cultures of bacteria that can be introduced into milk products such as yogurt. They can also be put into a powdered form.

Many probiotics can be found in the dairy and cheese section of the supermarket or grocery store. The difference between different products has to do with which bacteria are in them, how many bacteria are in them, and if the bacteria are all alive.

The FDA does not certify probiotics unless they are marketed to treat a specific disease.

Often when probiotics are independently tested, they are found not to have as many live bacteria as stated.

MECHANISM OF ACTION: HOW DOES IT WORK?

Bacteria that are useful as probiotics have many things in common. They must be of human origin. They must be regarded as safe and not pathogenic bacteria. They must be able to reach the intestine. To do that, they have to be able to resist stomach acid as well as bile. They have to survive for some time in the intestine. The bacteria have to be able to attach to the intestinal wall. They have to be able to make substances that will damage other pathogenic bacteria, as well as substances that can activate local immunity. They can also make the lining of the intestine more difficult to penetrate.[12]

It is not known with any certainty how the bacteria improve allergy. In allergic children, probiotic bacteria may improve the tightness of the intestinal lining to prevent possibly allergic substances from getting through. The bacteria also make chemicals that can affect the amount of immunoglobulins in the intestine, possibly also helping to keep allergic substances from getting into the bloodstream.[15]

They have been said to act as immunomodulators. In one study involving healthy middle-aged and elderly volunteers, administration of Lactobacillus casei strain Shirota had an effect on the activity of natural killer cells. Killer cells are white blood cells that are part of the immune system. The placebo-controlled, crossover trial involved giving the probiotic daily for three weeks. Natural killer cell activity increased in the middle-aged participants (ages 30 to 45 years). In the older patients (55 to 75 years of age), the killer cell activity did not increase in the group given probiotics but stayed the same. However, those given placebo showed a decrease in natural killer cell activity.

The researchers noted that natural killer cells are very important to the immune system, helping prevent tumor development as well as stopping viral infections.[21]

Probiotics stimulate a nonspecific immune response. This includes secretion of a number of chemical mediators as well as activating white blood cells. One type of white blood cell, the T cell, secretes substances called cytokines. Probiotics stimulate T cells to secrete cytokines that help confer protective immunity. There have been suggestions that probiotics help maintain the correct balance between active immunity and overreaction such as occurs with allergy.[22] Perhaps they should be called "immunobiotics."

PRIMARY USES

Probiotics are marketed and taken to improve intestinal health.
Probiotics can also be used for:

- Prevention of antibiotic-associated diarrhea
- Treatment of acute diarrhea in children and adults
- Prevention and treatment of traveler's diarrhea in children and adults
- Prevention of C. difficile diarrhea (not proven with bacteria)
- Treatment of irritable bowel syndrome
- Help in maintaining remission in patients with inflammatory bowel disease

The use of probiotics for allergies in infants and young children is not established at this time.

Many other medical uses are under investigation as indicated.

COMMON DOSAGES

One of the difficulties in evaluating information about probiotics is the different strains of bacteria used, as well as the varying numbers of live bacteria. The majority of trials use 1 to 20 billion CFUs per day, a CFU being a colony-forming unit. Each colony-forming unit is a bacterium that could be removed and a colony of bacteria could be grown from it.

Generally speaking, the studies that have had the most positive outcomes have used higher amounts of probiotics, more than 5 billion CFUs a day in children and 20 billion CFUs a day in adults. There is no evidence that higher doses are less safe. There is a question as to whether higher doses are necessary and worth the expense.

Most people are aware that probiotics in milk products can be purchased from any grocery store. Examples include Activia, which contains 5 to 10 billion CFUs of B. animalis, and Danactive, which contains 10 billion CFUs of L. casei. Yo-Plus and Stonyfield contain B. lactis and L. reuteri, but the amounts are not made available. There are other products on the market. It is never clear if the CFU amounts in these yogurts and drinks are accurate.

Probiotics can also be obtained as capsules, tablets, and powders. Many contain a combination of various Lactobacilli and Bifidobacteriae.

There have been studies demonstrating that many of the preparations do not contain the amount of live bacteria stated.[5]

It is reasonable to try a well-known brand, or purchase from a trusted source. Depending on a person's age and what condition they are trying to manage, aiming for the higher dose may mean two servings of one of the milk-containing products a day or more.

When treating illness, discussing the specific product and amount with a physician is reasonable.

POTENTIAL SIDE EFFECTS

Probiotics are generally well tolerated. Those marketed to the general public are advertised as improving gastrointestinal health and making people feel better.

There have been reports of mild bloating and gas associated with L. rhamnosus GG.[7]

Infants have demonstrated vomiting, excessive crying, and apparent abdominal discomfort from probiotics.[16]

Since these are live bacteria, there is the potential for serious illness if they should get into the circulation. There have been cases of bacteria in the bloodstream (bacteremia and sepsis), bacteria on heart valves, and other systemic infections related to the use of probiotics. This occurs rarely with the probiotics discussed in this chapter, and usually to people with abnormal immune systems who are critically ill. Great care must be taken when using probiotics in a hospital setting.[7]

A 2006 review noted that there had been no cases reported of sepsis in healthy individuals.[23]

A review of the available information in 2008 found no cases of sepsis specifically from Lactobacillus rhamnosus GG and Bifidobacterium sp. during the published trials.[5] However, people with serious medical illnesses that lower the effectiveness of their immune system should discuss the use of probiotics with their physicians.

FACT VERSUS FICTION

Probiotics are marketed to be taken for good intestinal health. Whether that is generally true is not proven. However, since they are safe, otherwise healthy individuals can try them to see how they feel.

Bacterial probiotics are definitely useful in the prevention and treatment of many kinds of diarrheal illnesses in children and adults, including viral diarrheal illnesses, antibiotic-associated diarrhea, and traveler's diarrhea. They may prove useful in preventing C. difficile–caused diarrhea.

Probiotics may play a role in managing other intestinal problems, both inflammatory bowel disease and irritable bowel disease. Probiotics may also be useful in treating H. pylori infections associated with gastritis or gastric ulcer.

The use of probiotics to prevent allergy in infants is still controversial and unproven. Since some studies have found increased incidence of some allergic problems in infants treated with probiotics, it seems prudent to wait until there is more evidence before giving them to newborns.

For other conditions, like urinary tract infections, the usefulness of probiotics has not been proven. However, there is no reason that people without serious medical illnesses should not try them. They should probably not be taken by those who are very ill, especially hospitalized patients, until it is better understood how to prevent them from causing systemic infections.

REFERENCES

1. Fuller, R. A review: Probiotics in man and animals. *Journal of Applied Bacteriology*. 1989;66:365–378.
2. Food and Agriculture Organization of the United Nations and World Health Organization. *Evaluation of health and nutritional properties of probiotics in food including powder milk with live lactic acid bacteria*. Cordoba, Argentina: FAO/WHO, 2001.
3. McFarland, LV. Meta-analysis of probiotics for the prevention of traveler's diarrhea. *Travel Medicine and Infectious Disease*. 2007;5:97–105.
4. Canani, RB, Cirillo, P, Terrrin, G, et al. Probiotics for treatment of acute diarrhoea in children: Randomised clinical trial of five different preparations. *BMJ.com online first*. 2007. doi:10.1136/bmj.39272.581736.55.
5. Kligler, B, Cohrssen, A. Probiotics. *American Family Physician*. 2008; 78(9):1073–1078.
6. Culligan, EP, Hill, C, Sleator, RD. Probiotics and gastrointestinal disease: Successes, problems and future prospects. *Gut Pathogens*. 2009;1:19. doi:10.1186/1757–4749–1–19.
7. McFarland, LV. Meta-analysis of probiotics for the prevention of antibiotic associated diarrhea and the treatment of Clostridium difficile disease. *Am J Gastroenterol*. 2006;101:812–822.
8. Sazawal, S, Hiremath, G, Dhingra, U, et al. Efficacy of probiotics in prevention of acute diarrhoea: A meta-analysis of masked, randomised, placebo-controlled trials. *The Lancet Infectious Diseases*. 2006;6(6):374–382.
9. Johnston, BC, Supina, AL, Ospina, M, Vohra, S. Probiotics for the prevention of pediatric antibiotic-associated diarrhea. *Cochrane Database of Systematic Reviews*. 2007;18;2. Art. No.: CD004827. doi: 10.1002/14651858.CD004827.pub2.
10. Hickson, M, D'Souza, AL, Muthu, N, et al. Use of probiotic Lactobacillus preparation to prevent diarrhoea associated with antibiotics: Randomised double blind placebo controlled trial. *BMJ.com online first*. 2007. doi:10.1136/bmj.39231.599815.55.

11. Miller, K, Fraser, T. What is the role of probiotics in the treatment of acute Clostridium difficile-associated diarrhea? *Cleveland Clinic Journal of Medicine*. 2009;76(7):391–392.

12. Sheil, B, Shanahan, F, O'Mahoney, L. Probiotic effects on inflammatory bowel disease. *J Nutr*. 2007;137:819S–824S.

13. Aragon, G, Graham, DB, Borum, M, Doman, DB. Probiotic therapy for irritable bowel syndrome. *Gastroenterology & Hepatology*. 2010;6(1):39–44.

14. Kajander, K, Myllyluoma, E, Rajilić-Stojanović, M, et al. Clinical trial: Multispecies probiotic supplementation alleviates the symptoms of irritable bowel syndrome and stabilizes intestinal microbiota. *Aliment Pharmacol Ther*. 2008;27(1):48–57.

15. Ouwehand, AC. Antiallergic effects of probiotics. *J Nutr*. 2007;137: 794S–797S.

16. Kukkonen, K, Savilahti, E, Haahtela, T, et al. Probiotics and probiotic galacto-oligosaccharides in the prevention of allergic diseases: A randomized, double-blind, placebo-controlled trial. *J Allergy Clin Immunol*. 2007;119:192–198.

17. Taylor, AL, Dunstan, JA, Prescott, SL. Probiotic supplementation for the first 6 months of life fails to reduce the risk of atopic dermatitis and increases the risk of allergen sensitization in high-risk children: A randomized controlled trial. *J Allergy Clin Immunol*. 2007;119:184–191.

18. Kopp, MV, Hennemuth, I, Heinzmann, A, Urbanek, R. Randomized, double-blind, placebo-controlled trial of probiotics for primary prevention: No clinical effects of Lactobacillus GG supplementation. *Pediatrics*. 2008;121;e850–e856.

19. Head, KA. Natural approaches to prevention and treatment of infections of the lower urinary tract. *Altern Med Rev*. 2008;13(3):227–244.

20. Lesbros-Pantoflickova, D, Corthesy-Theulaz, I, Blum, AL. Helicobacter pylori and probiotics. *J Nutr*. 2007;137:812S–818S.

21. Takeda, K, Okumura, K. Effects of a fermented milk drink containing Lactobacillus casei strain Shirota on the human NK-cell activity. *J Nutr*. 2007;137:791S–793S.

22. Clancy, RL, Pang, G. Probiotics—industry myth or a practical reality? *Journal of the American College of Nutrition*. 2007;26(6):691S–694S.

23. Boyle, RJ, Robins-Browne, RM, Tang, MLK. Probiotic use in clinical practice: What are the risks? *Am J Clin Nutr*. 2006;83:1256–1264.

39

Strontium Ranelate

BRIEF OVERVIEW

Strontium is an element chemically very similar to calcium. Calcium plays a very important role in the formation of bone in human body. When the formation of bone is reduced, combined with increased resorption of bone, it results in structural damage and fragility of bones causing osteoporosis.[1] Osteoporosis is a disease of bone where the bone mineral density (BMD) is reduced, leading to an increased risk of fracture. This disease is most common in women after menopause, when it is called postmenopausal osteoporosis, although it may develop in men and pre-menopausal women due to hormonal disorders or other factors.

Various studies have shown that strontium effectively reduces the risk of vertebral,[1] peripheral (nonvertebral),[2,3] and hip[2] fractures and increases bone mineral density (BMD) in postmenopausal women with osteoporosis.

Strontium ranelate (strontium salt of ranelic acid) is registered as a prescription medicine (POM) in the European Union for the treatment of osteoporosis in postmenopausal women. Strontium ranelate is not approved by the FDA in the United States and Canada for the treatment of osteoporosis in postmenopausal women. However, other salts of strontium like strontium citrate, strontium gluconate, strontium lactate, and strontium carbonate are presented as natural therapies and sold at much higher doses than is required, which can disturb calcium metabolism in the body.[12]

THE HYPE

Positive

Strontium has the following positive effects in postmenopausal women with osteoporosis:

1. It effectively reduces the risk of vertebral,[1] peripheral (nonvertebral),[2,3] and hip[2] fractures in postmenopausal women with osteoporosis.

2. Increases the lumbar and femoral bone mineral density (BMD), thus reducing the risk of new vertebral and hip fractures.[4]

3. Oral strontium reduces the incidence of bone fractures in individuals with metastatic bone cancer.[13]

4. Prevents or reduces the risk of dental cavities in individuals who consumed water naturally rich in strontium.[14]

5. Strontium might also improve cartilage metabolism in osteoarthritis (OA).

Negative

Supplemental strontium is often mistaken for radioactive strontium (Sr-90), produced as a result of above-ground nuclear testing that contaminated the environment and foods, which when consumed accumulates in the bones, bone marrow, teeth, and other tissues surrounding the bones of affected individuals causing bone cancer, leukemia, and cancer of surrounding tissues.

DEFICIENCY

Strontium is used to treat osteoporosis in postmenopausal women. There is no requirement for strontium in other age groups. Hence, there are no deficiency symptoms for strontium.

FOOD SOURCES

Strontium is not naturally present in any of the food sources.

MECHANISM OF ACTION: HOW DOES IT WORK?

Strontium ranelate reduces the risk of fractures in postmenopausal women with osteoporosis by the following functions:

- Reduces the resorption of bone
- Stimulates the mineralization of bone
- Increases the bone mineral density (BMD)
- Increasing the deposition of calcium in the bone

Resorption of Bone

This is a process by which the bone tissue is broken down by osteoclasts. The minerals from the bone are transferred to the blood making the bone soft and fragile.

This process is mainly stimulated or inhibited by the calcium levels in the blood. Lower levels of calcium in the blood stimulate the secretion of parathyroid hormone (PTH), which in turn stimulates the differentiation and activity of osteoclasts resulting in the resorption of the bone. On the other hand, high levels of calcium decrease the secretion of parathyroid hormone (PTH), which reduces the production and activity of osteoclasts resulting in the reduction of bone resorption.

Strontium ranelate appears to reduce the resorption of bone by decreasing the differentiation and activity of osteoclasts.[9]

Mineralization of Bone

Mineralization of bone is also called ossification. It is a highly regulated process where calcium phosphate crystals are incorporated into the matrix of the bone by the bone-forming cells called osteoblasts.

Strontium ranelate stimulates this process by increasing the replication of pre-osteoblast cells, in turn leading to increased synthesis of the bone matrix.[9]

Bone Mineral Density

Strontium has a higher atomic weight (84–88) than calcium (40). As the atomic radius of strontium is similar to that of calcium, it easily substitutes calcium in the body. Strontium ranelate aids the growth of bone and increases the bone density.

The increase in bone mineral density (BMD) in women on strontium ranelate is attributed to two factors:

1. Higher atomic weight of strontium compared with calcium
2. True increase in bone mass

Along with an increase in bone mineral density (BMD), administration of strontium ranelate in ovariectomized rats (similar to postmenopausal women) also improved the bone mechanical properties of vertebrae and midshaft femur leading to a decrease in the incidence of vertebral and hip fractures.[9]

The Spinal Osteoporosis Therapeutic Intervention Study and the Treatment of Peripheral Osteoporosis Study showed that administration of strontium ranelate also increased the BMD of femoral neck associated with a proportional reduction in vertebral fracture incidence.[10]

The strontium ranelate for treatment of osteoporosis (STRATOS) trial also showed an increase in the vertebral BMD that reduced the incidence of vertebral fractures.[4]

Increases the Deposition of Calcium in the Bone

Administration of strontium ranelate in optimal doses also results in a significant increase in the calcium contents in the bone, indicating an increase in the absorption of intestinal calcium without significantly altering any other metabolic parameters of calcium.[5]

Strontium ranelate is able to increase pre-osteoblast replication, osteoblast differentiation, collagen type I synthesis, and bone matrix mineralization probably through a calcium-sensing receptor (CaR)-dependent mechanism. Along with this effect, there is inhibition of osteoclast differentiation and activity mediated by an increase in osteoprotegerin (OPG) and a decrease in RANK ligand (RANKL), resulting in a rebalanced bone turnover that enhances the bone strength.[5]

PRIMARY USES

Treatment of osteoporosis in postmenopausal women with strontium ranelate has the following uses:

- Reduced risk of vertebral,[1] peripheral,[2,3] and hip[2] fractures in postmenopausal women with osteoporosis
- Increased bone mineral density (BMD) of the lumbar and femoral bones, resulting in early and sustained reduction in the incidence of osteoporotic nonvertebral fractures, including hip fractures and vertebral fractures[1,3,4]
- Reduced incidence of bone fractures in individuals with metastatic bone cancer[13]
- Reduced risk of new dental cavities in individuals who consumed water naturally rich in strontium[14]
- Improved cartilage metabolism in osteoarthritis (OA)
- Reduce the resorption of bone by decreasing the differentiation and activity of osteoclasts[9]
- Stimulation of mineralization of bone by increasing the replication of pre-osteoblast cells, leading to increased synthesis of the bone matrix[9]
- Stimulation of absorption of intestinal calcium[5]
- Increased bone formation and reduces bone resorption simultaneously, thus re-balancing bone turnover in favor of bone formation

COMMON DOSAGES

Recommended dose of strontium is 2 g orally, once daily, preferably at bedtime.

The 2 g/day dose was considered to offer the best combination of efficacy and safety evidenced by a significant increase in serum levels of bone alkaline phosphatise (ALP), and a decrease in urinary excretion of cross-linked N-telopeptide, a marker of bone resorption, compared with placebo.[4]

This dose of 2 g/day is recommended for all age groups and no dosage adjustments are required in relation to age.[17]

Strontium ranelate (2 g/day) was shown to prevent bone loss, increase bone strength, and reduce vertebral and peripheral fractures.[7]

Strontium ranelate must be consumed mixed with at least 30 mL of water.[16,17]

TOXICITY AND INTERACTIONS

There is not enough literature on the long-term effects of consuming high doses of strontium and its toxicity profile. However, excessive doses can lead to strontium toxicity as well as disturb calcium metabolism in the body.[12]

Strontium should be taken at least two hours after food, milk, or other dairy products, calcium-containing medicines or tetracyclines, as the bioavailability of strontium is reduced by calcium, oral tetracyclines, and food.[16,17,18] Co-administration of strontium with calcium appears to impair strontium absorption.[15]

Strontium should not be taken along with antacids containing aluminum or magnesium. The two should be separated by at least two hours.[16,17,18]

Women at increased risk of thromboembolism should use caution before considering strontium.

POTENTIAL SIDE EFFECTS

Though no major side effects are documented, a small percent of individuals exhibited some common side effects like nausea, diarrhea, headache, and eczema, which are later tolerated.

Strontium ranelate as an orally prescription drug for the treatment of postmenopausal osteoporosis has been extensively studied. Evidence for the safety and efficacy of strontium ranelate comes from two large multinational trials, the SOTI (Spinal Osteoporosis Therapeutic Intervention) and TROPOS (Treatment of Postmenopausal Osteoporosis) studies and is as follows.

1. Treatment of postmenopausal osteoporosis with strontium ranelate results in a sustained reduction in the incidence of osteoporotic nonvertebral fractures, including hip fractures, and vertebral fractures over five years.[3]

2. Strontium ranelate is a bone-seeking element that has been assessed in postmenopausal osteoporosis in various studies. Treatment with strontium ranelate is able to decrease the risk of vertebral fractures, by 41 percent over three years, and by 49 percent within the first year of treatment. This risk of nonvertebral fractures is decreased by 16 percent and, in patients at high risk for such a fracture, the risk of hip fracture is decreased by 36 percent over three years. Recent five-year data from these double-blind, placebo-controlled studies show that the antifracture efficacy is maintained over time.[6]

3. Treatment efficacy with strontium ranelate has been documented across a wide range of patient profiles: age, number of prevalent vertebral fractures, BMI, as well as family history of osteoporosis and addiction to smoking are not determinants of antifracture efficacy. During these clinical trials, safety was good. Its large spectrum of efficacy allows the use of strontium ranelate in the different subgroups of patients with postmenopausal osteoporosis.[6]

4. Strontium ranelate is an effective and safe treatment for long-term treatment of osteoporosis in postmenopausal women.[7]

5. Strontium ranelate is a useful addition to the range of antifracture treatments available for treating postmenopausal women with osteoporosis and is the only treatment proven to be effective at preventing both vertebral and hip fractures in women aged 80 years and over.[8]

FACT VERSUS FICTION

Efficacy: Strontium ranelate is very effective in reducing the risk of vertebral, nonvertebral, and peripheral fractures in postmenopausal women with osteoporosis.

But this has been indicated only in postmenopausal women, who had been post-menopausal for more than 20 years.[2,1]

Toxicity: Strontium at low doses has been effectively used to treat osteoporosis. However, excessive doses can lead to strontium toxicity as well as disturb calcium metabolism in the body.[12]

Cost-effectiveness: Though strontium ranelate is effective, it appears to be less cost-effective than the bisphosphonate alendronate.[11]

Advice: Fractures in osteoporotic women can be prevented with lifestyle advice and medication, as well as preventing falls in people with known or suspected osteoporosis.

Strontium ranelate is recommended for women:

- Who cannot tolerate bisphosphonates (e.g., because of gastrointestinal adverse effects, including oesophageal ulceration)
- Who are unable to administer bisphosphonates correctly (e.g., needing to sit upright after administration)
- For whom bisphosphonates are contraindicated (e.g., oesophageal abnormalities that delay oesophageal emptying, such as stricture or achalasia)

REFERENCES

1. Meunier, PJ, Roux, C, Seeman, E, et al. The effects of strontium ranelate on the risk of vertebral fracture in women with postmenopausal osteoporosis. *N Engl J Med.* 2004 Jan 29;350(5):459–468.
2. Reginster, JY, Seeman, E, De Vernejoul, MC, Adami, S, Compston, J, Phenekos, C, Devogelaer, JP, Curiel, MD, Sawicki, A, Goemaere, S, Sorensen, OH, Felsenberg, D, Meunier, PJ. Strontium ranelate reduces the risk of non-vertebral fractures in postmenopausal women with osteoporosis: Treatment of Peripheral Osteoporosis (TROPOS) Study. *J Clin Endocrinol Metab.* 2005 May;90(5):2816–2822.
3. Reginster, JY, Felsenberg, D, Boonen, S, Diez-Perez, A, Rizzoli, R, Brandi, ML, Spector, TD, Brixen, K, Goemaere, S, Cormier, C, Balogh, A, Delmas, PD, Meunier, PJ. Effects of long-term strontium ranelate treatment on the risk of nonvertebral and vertebral fractures in postmenopausal osteoporosis: Results of a five-year, randomized, placebo-controlled trial. *Arthritis Rheum.* 2008 Jun;58(6):1687–1695.
4. Meunier, PJ, Slosman, DO, Delmas, PD, Sebert, JL, Brandi, ML, Albanese, C, Lorenc, R, Pors-Nielsen, S, De Vernejoul, MC, Roces, A, Reginster, JY. Strontium ranelate: Dose-dependent effects in established postmenopausal vertebral osteoporosis—a 2-year randomized placebo controlled trial. *J Clin Endocrinol Metab.* 2002 May;87(5):2060–2066.
5. Fonseca, JE. Rebalancing bone turnover in favour of formation with stron-tium ranelate: Implications for bone strength. *Rheumatology (Oxford).* 2008 Jul;47(Suppl 4):iv17–19.

6. Roux, C. Strontium ranelate: Short- and long-term benefits for post-menopausal women with osteoporosis. *Rheumatology (Oxford)*. 2008 Jul;47(Suppl 4):iv20–22.

7. Meunier, PJ, Roux, C, Ortolani, S, Diaz-Curiel, M, Compston, J, Marquis, P, Cormier, C, Isaia, G, Badurski, J, Wark, JD, Collette, J, Reginster, JY. Effects of long-term strontium ranelate treatment on vertebral fracture risk in postmenopausal women with osteoporosis. *Osteoporos Int*. 2009 Oct;20(10):1663–1673.

8. Blake, GM, Fogelman, I. Strontium ranelate: A novel treatment for post-menopausal osteoporosis: A review of safety and efficacy. *Clin Interv Aging*. 2006;1(4):367–375.

9. Tournis, S. Improvement in bone strength parameters: The role of strontium ranelate. *J Musculoskelet Neuronal Interact*. 2007 Jul–Sep;7(3):266–267.

10. Bruyere, O, Roux, C, Detilleux, J, Slosman, DO, Spector, TD, Fardellone, P, Brixen, K, Devogelaer, JP, Diaz-Curiel, M, Albanese, C, Kaufman, JM, Pors-Nielsen, S, Reginster, JY. Relationship between bone mineral density changes and fracture risk reduction in patients treated with strontium ranelate. *J Clin Endocrinol Metab*. 2007 Aug;92(8):3076–3081.

11. Stevenson, M, Davis, S, Lloyd-Jones, M, Beverley, C. The clinical effectiveness and cost-effectiveness of strontium ranelate for the prevention of osteoporotic fragility fractures in postmenopausal women. *Health Technol Assess*. 2007 Feb;11(4):1–134.

12. Morohashi, T, Sano, T, Yamada, S. Effects of strontium on calcium metabolism in rats. I. A distinction between the pharmacological and toxic doses. *Jpn J Pharmacol*. 1994 Mar;64(3):155–162.

13. Skoryna, SC. Effects of oral supplementation with stable strontium. *Can Med Assoc J*. 1981;125:703–712.

14. Gaby, AR. *Preventing and reversing osteoporosis*. Rocklin, CA: Prima Publishing, 1994.

15. Reginster, JY, Deroisy, R, Dougados, M, Jupsin, I, Colette, J, Roux, C. Prevention of early postmenopausal bone loss by strontium ranelate: The randomized, two-year, double-masked, dose-ranging, placebo-controlled PREVOS Trial. *Osteoporos Int*. 2002 Dec;13(12): 925–931.

16. Rossi, S. (Ed). *Australian medicines handbook*. Adelaide: Australian Medicines Handbook Pty Ltd, 2007.

17. Servier Laboratories (Australia) Pty Ltd. Protos product information. May 28, 2007.

18. Sweetman, S. (Ed). *Martindale: The complete drug reference updated periodically (Thomson Micromedex)*. London: Pharmaceutical Press, 2006.

Index

sources, 195–96; hype, 191–95; hypertension and, 193; interactions, 199; mania and, 193; mechanism of action, 196–97; memory and, 194; migraine headaches and, 194; overview, 191; Parkinson's disease and, 194; phenylalanine and, 198; protein, recommended amounts of, 197–98; side effects, potential, 199; stress and, 193–94; uses, primary, 197
Lung cancer, 46
Lung diseases, 46, 219–20
Lysine. *See* L-lysine

Macular degeneration, 293, 316
Magnesium, 339–47; asthma and, 340; blood pressure and, 340; cardiovascular disease and, 341; deficiency, 343; diabetes and, 341; dosages, 346; fact *versus* fiction, 347; food sources, 343–44; hype, 339–42; mechanism of action, 344–45; overview, 339; pregnancy and, 342; side effects, potential, 346–47; stroke and, 341–42; uses, primary, 345
Mania, 193
Melatonin, 203–8; cancer and, 205; deficiency, 206; depression and, 204; dosages, 207; fact *versus* fiction, 208; food sources, 206; hype, 203–6; mechanism of action, 206–7; neurodegenerative diseases and, 205–6; side effects, potential, 207–8; sleep and, 203–4; uses, primary, 207
Memory, 194
Metabolism abnormalities, 32–33, 126–27
Methylsulfonylmethane. *See* MSM
Migraine headaches, 194
Mood, 269
Mortality: beta-carotene and, 279; calcium and, 39, 46; vitamin A and, 279; vitamin E and, 316, 320
MSM, 211–16; allergic rhinitis (hay fever) and, 214; cancer and, 214; deficiency, 214; dosages, 215; fact *versus* fiction, 216; food sources, 214–15; hype, 211–14; interstitial cystitis and, 214; mechanism of action, 215; osteoarthritis and, 211–12, 213; overview, 211; for pain relief, 211–14; side effects, potential, 216; uses, primary, 215
Multiple sclerosis: beta-sitosterol and, 20–21; glutathione (GSH) and, 119; vitamin D and, 302
Multistep immune targeting for radioimmunotherapy, 33
Muscle mass/strength, 81, 300

N-acetylcysteine (NAC), 219–25; acetaminophen overdose and, 221; cancer and, 222; chronic obstructive pulmonary disease and, 219–20; deficiency, 223; fact *versus* fiction, 225; food sources, 223; hype, 219–23; intravenous contrast media used in x-ray studies and, 221–22; kidney damage/failure and, 221–22; liver disease and, 221; lung diseases and, 219–20; mechanism of action, 223; overview, 219; polycystic ovary syndrome and, 222; Raynaud's phenomenon and, 223; side effects, potential, 224–25; surgery and, 222; upper respiratory illnesses and, 220; uses, primary, 223–24; viral illnesses and, 220. *See also* Glutathione
Nails, brittle, 30
Neural tube defects, 101–2
Neurodegenerative diseases: coenzyme Q_{10} and, 57–58; copper and, 67; glutathione (GSH) and, 118–21; melatonin and, 205–6
Neurologic development, 160, 239
Niacin (vitamin B3), 227–33; deficiency, 228–29; dosages, 230–31; dyslipidemia and, 231; fact *versus* fiction, 232–33; food sources, 229; hype, 228; mechanism of action, 229–30; overview, 227; pellagra and, 231; side effects, potential, 231–32; uses, primary, 230
Nicotinic acid. *See* Niacin (vitamin B3)
Nitric oxide (NO), 135

Omega-3 fatty acids, 235–44; asthma and, 238–39; cancer and, 240; cardiovascular health and, 236–38; central nervous system disorders and, 239; coronary heart disease and, 238; deficiency, 240; dosages, 242–43; fact *versus* fiction, 243–44; food sources, 241; heart rhythm disorders and, 238; hype, 236–40; mechanism of action, 241–42; neurologic development and, 239; organ transplantation and, 239; overview, 235; side effects, potential, 243; uses, primary, 242
Organ transplantation, 239
Ossification, 371
Osteoarthritis: glucosamine and, 111–13; MSM and, 211–12, 213; S-Adenosylmethionine (SAMe) and, 255–56, 260
Osteoporosis: calcium and, 37–38, 42–43, 44, 45; L-lysine and, 181; vitamin D and, 298–300; vitamin K and, 323–25

About the Author

Dr. Zina Kroner is the founder and medical director of Advanced Medicine of New York, a unique center that caters to patients who want a comprehensive and personal approach to their health concerns and prevention strategies. Dr. Zina Kroner attended New York University College of Arts and Sciences for undergraduate work, after which she graduated from New York College of Osteopathic Medicine. She then became a board-certified internist after completing a three-year residency at North Shore University Hospital, an NYU School of Medicine affiliate, in Manhasset, NY. She also served as the Associate Medical Director of the Hoffman Center in New York for four years. She is actively practicing medicine.

Her initial medical objective is to intelligently find a cause to a set of medical concerns. She uses astute history taking and state-of-the-art integrative and traditional laboratory and radiologic tests. Then, she customizes evidence-based nutritional and medical treatments and integrates them into a patient's treatment regimen. Dr. Kroner engages in proactive (rather that reactive) medical and nutritional management, encouraging discussion of cause and effect, patient education, and application of up-to-date prevention strategies. Thus, living smarter, and therefore, living longer.

Dr. Kroner has an informative blog on her Web site, www.advanced-medicine.com, to which she actively contributes up-to-date medical information. She has published an article in *Alternative Medicine Review* entitled, "The Relationship between Alzheimer's Disease and Diabetes: Diabetes Type 3?" She is the author of a chapter in *The Biography of Diabetes: Alternatives to Conventional Diabetic Care*. She is an active writer for the American Academy for the Advancement of Medicine and a bimonthly contributor to *Manhattan Women's Journal*.